T0344489

The Handbook of DOHaD and Society

Research in the field of the Developmental Origins of Health and Disease (DOHaD) has had a fundamental impact on our understanding of how environmental experiences and contexts influence the development of health and disease over the entire lifecourse. This book provides a comprehensive overview of this research and provides models and tools for the future. Covering a wide range of geographic regions, this volume includes an overview of the field, key concepts, and cutting-edge examples of interdisciplinary collaboration. The first reference text covering the interdisciplinary work of DOHaD, this book has a broad list of contents: it maps the history of DOHaD, showcases examples of biosocial collaboration in action, offers a conceptual toolkit for interdisciplinary research, and maps future directions for the field. This definitive volume on biosocial collaborations in DOHaD will be indispensable for scholars working at the intersections of public health, lifecourse epidemiology, and the social science of DOHaD. This title is also available as Open Access on Cambridge Core.

Michelle Pentecost is a physician-anthropologist based in the Department of Global Health and Social Medicine at King's College London and in the School of Clinical Medicine at the University of the Witwatersrand. She is the author of *The Politics of Potential: Global Health and Gendered Futures in South Africa* (Rutgers University Press, 2024).

Jaya Keaney is a lecturer in Gender Studies at the University of Melbourne. Her work in feminist science studies explores how reproduction is shaped by technoscientific practices and regimes of race, gender, sexuality, and coloniality. She is the author of *Making Gaybies: Queer Reproduction and Multiracial Feeling* (Duke University Press, 2023).

Tessa Moll is a medical anthropologist in South Africa. Her work explores the possibilities of life-making and life-sustaining that arise from new technologies and new knowledges of reproduction. She is currently completing her first solo-authored monograph on reproductive politics, fertility care, and race in the afterlife of apartheid.

Michael Penkler is a medical sociologist and science and technology studies scholar based at the University of Applied Sciences Wiener Neustadt, Austria. His work explores the social, ethical, and political aspects and implications of life science innovations, biomedical technologies, and healthcare.

This magnificent collection crosses disciplines and continents in its synthesis of exciting scholarship around the past, present, and future of DOHaD. It is a singular achievement, and its readers will be multiple.

Martyn Pickersgill, Professor of the Sociology of Science and Medicine, Edinburgh Medical School

The clearest and most comprehensive account of DOHaD in society ever. Framing the field in terms of its history and with a biosocial lens, the many distinguished authors of this Handbook offer, in combination, a very thorough and erudite reading of DOHaD in its strength (and sometimes weakness). Understanding child health from this perspective queries and questions approaches in public health, clinical practice and policy. A book that sets the standard in this field; a book to cherish and keep close to hand by all those interested and involved in child health, from any perspective.

Stanley Ulijaszek, Emeritus Professor of Human Ecology, University of Oxford

In a masterful manner, this Handbook weaves together a rich tapestry of perspectives from across the globe and various disciplines, offering a nuanced yet concise overview of the state of the art of research on DOHaD. Irrespective of your own field—whether you're a medical researcher, a nurse, social scientist, or a policy maker—prepare to see your work in a new light after reading this book.

Barbara Prainsack, Department of Political Science, University of Vienna, Austria

The Handbook of DOHaD and Society

Past, Present, and Future Directions of Biosocial Collaboration

Edited by

Michelle Pentecost
King's College London

Jaya Keaney
University of Melbourne

Tessa Moll
University of the Witwatersrand

Michael Penkler
University of Applied Sciences Wiener Neustadt

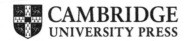

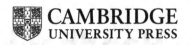

Shaftesbury Road, Cambridge CB2 8EA, United Kingdom

One Liberty Plaza, 20th Floor, New York, NY 10006, USA

477 Williamstown Road, Port Melbourne, VIC 3207, Australia

314–321, 3rd Floor, Plot 3, Splendor Forum, Jasola District Centre, New Delhi – 110025, India

103 Penang Road, #05-06/07, Visioncrest Commercial, Singapore 238467

Cambridge University Press is part of Cambridge University Press & Assessment, a department of the University of Cambridge.

We share the University's mission to contribute to society through the pursuit of education, learning and research at the highest international levels of excellence.

www.cambridge.org
Information on this title: www.cambridge.org/9781009201728

DOI: 10.1017/9781009201704

First published 2024

A catalogue record for this publication is available from the British Library

A Cataloging-in-Publication data record for this book is available from the Library of Congress.

ISBN 978-1-009-20172-8 Hardback

Contents

Contributors

Salma Ayis
School of Life Course and Population Sciences, Faculty of Life Sciences & Medicine, King's College London, UK

Lara Azevedo
School of Medicine, Deakin University, Australia

Celeste Barrett-Watson
Cook Islands Ministry of Education, Cook Islands

Jacquie L. Bay
Liggins Institute; Koi Tū: Centre for Informed Futures, The University of Auckland (Waipapa Taumata Rau), New Zealand

Astrid Berg
Department of Psychiatry, FMHS, Stellenbosch University, South Africa

Neera Bhatia
Deakin University, School of Law School, Australia

Chani Bonventre
Department of Anthropology, Faculty of Social Sciences, Université Laval, Canada

Edna N. Bosire
Brain and Mind Institute, Aga Khan University, Nairobi Kenya
SAMRC/Wits Developmental Pathways for Health Research Unit, Faculty of Health Science, University of the Witwatersrand, South Africa

Sarah Bourke
National Centre for Epidemiology and Population Health, The Australian National University, Australia

Tatjana Buklijas
Koi Tū: Centre for Informed Futures, Europe Institute, University of Auckland (Waipapa Taumata Rau), New Zealand

Henrietta Byrne
School of Social Sciences, University of Adelaide, Australia

Luca Chiapperino
STS Lab, Institute of Social Sciences, Faculty of Social and Political Sciences, University of Lausanne, Switzerland

Jennifer Cohen
Department of Global and Intercultural Studies, Miami University, USA
Ezintsha, Faculty of Health Sciences, University of the Witwatersrand, South Africa

Jeffrey M. Craig
School of Medicine, Deakin University, Australia

Lillian Dipnall
School of Psychology, Deakin University, Australia

Catherine E. Draper
SAMRC-Wits Developmental Pathways for Health Research Unit, Faculty of Health Sciences, University of the Witwatersrand, South Africa

Emily H. Emmott
UCL Anthropology, University College London, UK

Cindy Gerber
STS Lab, Institute of Social Sciences, Faculty of Social and Political Sciences, University of Lausanne, Switzerland

Sahra Gibbon
UCL Anthropology, University College London, UK

Peter Gluckman
Koi Tū: Centre for Informed Futures, Liggins Institute, University of Auckland (Waipapa Taumata Rau), New Zealand
Singapore Institute for Clinical Sciences, Singapore

Jaclyn M. Goodrich
Environmental Health Sciences Department, University of Michigan, USA

Mark Hanson
Institute of Developmental Sciences, University of Southampton, UK

Ayuba Issaka
Non-communicable Disease and Implementation Science Lab, Baker Heart and Diabetes Institute, Australia

Chandni Maria Jacob
Institute of Developmental Sciences, University of Southampton, UK

Erica C. Jansen
Nutritional Health Sciences Department, University of Michigan, USA

Drollet Joseph
Araura College, Cook Islands Ministry of Education, Cook Islands

Isabel Karpin
Faculty of Law and Centre for Law Health Justice, University of Technology Sydney, Australia

Shivani Kaul
Faculty of Social and Behavioural Sciences, University of Amsterdam, the Netherlands

Jaya Keaney
School of Social and Political Sciences, University of Melbourne, Australia

Evie Kendal
Department of Health Sciences and Biostatistics, Swinburne University of Technology, Australia

Martha Kenney
Women and Gender Studies, San Francisco State University, USA

Emma Kowal
Alfred Deakin Institute, Deakin University, Australia

Christopher Kuzawa
Department of Anthropology, Northwestern University, USA

Anusha Lachman
Department of Psychiatry, FMHS, Stellenbosch University, South Africa

Martine Lappé
Social Sciences Department, California Polytechnic State University, USA

Stephanie Lloyd
Department of Anthropology, Faculty of Social Sciences, Université Laval Canada

Raymond Lovett
National Centre for Epidemiology and Population Health, The Australian National University, Australia

Felicia Low
Koi Tū: The Centre for Informed Futures, University of Auckland, (Waipapa Taumata Rau) New Zealand

Pierre-Eric Lutz
National Centre for Scientific Research (CNRS), Institute of Cellular and Integrative Neurosciences (UPR 3212), University of Strasbourg, France

Khuthala Mabetha
SAMRC-Wits Developmental Pathways for Health Research Unit, Faculty

of Health Sciences, University
of the Witwatersrand, South Africa

Ziyanda Majombozi
Department of Sociology and Social
Anthropology, Stellenbosch University,
South Africa

Marguerite Marlow
Institute for Life Course Health
Research, Department of Global Health,
Stellenbosch University, South Africa

Maurizio Meloni
School of Humanities and Social Sciences,
Deakin University, Australia

Emily Mendenhall
SAMRC/Wits Developmental Pathways for
Health Research Unit, Faculty of Health
Science, University of the Witwatersrand,
South Africa
Edmund A. Walsh School of Foreign
Service, Georgetown University, USA

Amelia van der Merwe
Institute for Life Course Health
Research, Department of Global Health,
Stellenbosch University, South Africa

Tessa Moll
Postdoctoral Research Fellow, School of
Public Health, University of
Witwatersrand, South Africa

Vivienne Moore
School of Public Health and Robinson
Research Institute and Fay Gale Centre for
Research on Gender, University of
Adelaide, Australia

Ruth Müller
School of Social Sciences and Technology,
Technical University of Munich, Germany

Mutsawashe Mutendi
Department of Anthropology, University of
the Witwatersrand, South Africa

Belinda L. Needham
Epidemiology Department, University of
Michigan, USA

Jörg Niewöhner
Department of Science, Technology and
Society, Technical University of Munich,
Germany

Shane A. Norris
SAMRC-Wits Developmental Pathways
for Health Research Unit, Faculty
of Health Sciences, University of
the Witwatersrand, South Africa
School of Human Development
and Health, University of
Southampton, UK

Francesco Panese
STS Lab, Institute of Social Sciences,
Faculty of Social and Political
Sciences, University of Lausanne,
Switzerland

Michael Penkler
Institute of Market Research and
Methodology, University of Applied
Sciences Wiener Neustadt, Austria

Michelle Pentecost
Department of Global Health and
Social Medicine, King's College
London, UK
SAMRC-Wits Developmental Pathways
for Health Research Unit, Faculty of
Health Sciences, University of the
Witwatersrand, South Africa

Simone M. Peters
Department of Anthropology, University of
Cape Town, South Africa

Teaukura Puna
Ministry of Education, Cook Islands

Sarah S. Richardson
Department of the History of Science,
Committee on Degrees in Studies of

Women, Gender, and Sexuality, Harvard
University, USA

Elizabeth F.S. Roberts
Anthropology Department, University of
Michigan, USA

Martha M. Téllez Rojo
Instituto Nacional de Salud Publica,
Nutrition and Health Research,
Mexico

Natasha Rooney
Alfred Deakin Institute for Citizenship
and Globalisation, Deakin University,
Australia

Fiona C. Ross
Department of Anthropology, University of
Cape Town, South Africa

Sophia Rossmann
Department of Science, Technology and
Society, TUM School of Social Sciences and
Technology, Technical University of
Munich, Germany

Georgia Samaras
Department of Science, Technology
and Society, TUM School of Social
Sciences and Technology, Technical
University of Munich,
Germany

Kura Samuel-Ioane
Te Marae Ora Cook Islands Ministry of
Health, Cook Islands

Brisa N. Sánchez
Epidemiology and Biostatistics
Department, Drexel University, USA

Kaleb Saulnier
Social Sciences and Humanities Research
Council, Tri-Agency Institutional
Programs Secretariat, Canada

Julie Nihouarn Sigurdardottir
Department of Forensic and
Neurodevelopmental Sciences, Institute
of Psychiatry, Psychology &
Neuroscience, King's College
London, UK

Umberto Simeoni
DOHaD Laboratory & Clinics of
Pediatrics, Woman-Mother-Child
Department, Centre Hospitalier
Universitaire Vaudois and University of
Lausanne, Switzerland

Sarah Skeen
Institute for Life Course Health
Research, Department of Global Health,
Stellenbosch University, South Africa

Larske M. Soepnel
SAMRC-Wits Developmental Pathways
for Health Research Unit, Faculty of
Health Sciences, University of the
Witwatersrand, South Africa

Garth Stephenson
School of Medicine, Deakin University,
Australia

Mark Tomlinson
Institute for Life Course Health
Research, Department of Global
Health, Stellenbosch University, Cape
Town, South Africa; and School of
Nursing and Midwifery, Queens
University, Belfast, UK

Siobhan Tu'akoi
Pacific Health section, School of
Population Health, The University of
Auckland, (Waipapa Taumata Rau)
New Zealand

Natali Valdez
Department of Anthropology, Purdue
University, USA

Mark H. Vickers
Liggins Institute, The University of
Auckland, (Waipapa Taumata Rau)
New Zealand

Megan Warin
School of Social Sciences and Robinson
Research Institute and Fay Gale Centre for
Research on Gender, University of
Adelaide, Australia

Emily Yates-Doerr
School of Language, Culture & Society,
Oregon State University, USA

Foreword

Mark Hanson, Peter Gluckman, and Lucilla Poston

The title of this book – *The Handbook of DOHaD and Society* – suggests the need for a greater integration between two broad fields: one an area of biomedicine and the other in social studies. But linking them also indicates a synthesis of these areas. The nature of a handbook is to provide a go-to source of information on a particular subject or, in this case, on convergent fields. It should give a guide to underlying concepts and current methodologies and offer insights into new ideas and research possibilities. It is therefore far more ambitious than a multi-author book comprising disparate chapters, perhaps resulting from a symposium where diverse topics were presented but not synthesised. As past and current presidents of the International DOHaD Society and researchers and advocates for Developmental Origins of Health and Disease (DOHaD) who have worked with colleagues in the social sciences for some time, we believe that this volume does indeed meet the expectations raised by its title. The chapters have been carefully considered and commissioned by thought leaders in their subject areas, and they have been written to avoid unnecessary overlap whilst demonstrating linkages. The authors have shared drafts and engaged in discussions, and all chapters have been reviewed by the editors and others and modified appropriately. It has been a huge task, and we congratulate the editors on their achievement.

Why is this handbook so timely? When the term DOHaD was developed to supersede Fetal Origins of Adult Disease (FOAD) two decades ago, it was seen as a burgeoning field that would need to encompass the social as well as the biomedical sciences. This was because 'development' was clearly a broad term that described life from conception to maturity and the environments in which it takes place, as opposed to the phase of mammalian life in utero. It recognised the importance of a range of comparative studies and insights from developmental biology and evolutionary biology. Moreover, by extending consideration to include health as well as disease and considering health and disease across the lifecourse rather than just in adulthood, DOHaD recognised the importance of much broader contexts. This included integrating growing understandings of developmental plasticity as well as what are now termed the social determinants of health. Of course, this broader conceptualisation of development in itself was far from new; Hippocrates, for instance, expounded on the connection between public health and the environment and indeed the importance of the early environment for the development of the individual. Nonetheless, as social science studies of DOHaD have shown, the concept of environment tends to be overly simplified in DOHaD research, a tension grappled with across many of this handbook's chapters.

DOHaD had to confront a growing imbalance in biomedical sciences that privileged the reductionism of genetics, which dominated the last decades of the twentieth century and led to the claims that the Human Genome Project would reveal the primary causes of common traits and diseases. Against this background, the drivers of global health issues were becoming clear, with particular emphasis on inequalities and social justice between high- and low-income countries, and the formulation of the Millennium Development Goals led to a renewed focus on maternal and child health. It was during this period that the global importance of non-communicable diseases (NCDs) was, belatedly, recognised, alongside the realisation that NCD risk at the population level was not substantially attributable to fixed genetic factors. By late 2011, global bodies such as the United Nations and the World Health Organization (WHO) had recognised the importance of wider environmental influences acting on human development to increase NCD risk. Laboratory sciences had moved on from genetics to epigenetics to account for such processes. By 2015, when the Sustainable Development Goals (SDGs) were announced, DOHaD researchers were actively engaged with colleagues in many other disciplines, especially in the social sciences. At around the halfway mark for the SDGs, it is appropriate to take stock of these collaborations and stress the need to expand them. This handbook is the resource essential to this endeavour.

The handbook illustrates the benefits and new insights gained from interdisciplinarity, but also its challenges. As with other truly interdisciplinary explorations, what might be seen as 'biosocial DOHaD' does more than cross disciplines to benefit from different perspectives whilst leaving the field of exploration the same. Rather, it integrates the disciplines, recognising the value and understanding of the concepts, methodologies, and working practices of each discipline. This is easily said but hard to undertake. It requires a deep understanding of the epistemology of the contributing disciplines, going beyond just the language used (although misunderstandings here often create barriers to interdisciplinarity in themselves), and a respect for the insights that very different academic traditions might bring. As with all sciences, the evidence base for both biomedical and social sciences changes, being at best only provisional: studies once seen as the 'gold standard' are no longer as pivotal or relevant today. Thus, an understanding of disciplinary histories is also critical to interdisciplinary conversations. The handbook demonstrates the value of such informed interdisciplinary interactions, and it gestures towards future opportunities for collaboratively exploring human development and the impact of early life factors on later life and indeed across generations.

Acknowledgements

This is a book about developmental origins and, as such, a book about how people and things grow in networks that provide nourishment and care. Similarly, this book is the product of the care, support, and commitment that many have provided. We are especially grateful for the generous support of our mentors, who offered encouragement and guidance on this mammoth undertaking. We offer special thanks to Mark Hanson, Lucilla Poston, Shane Norris, Maurizio Meloni, Megan Warin, Emma Kowal, Ruth Müller, and Fiona Ross. We also gratefully acknowledge the time and commitment of all of the handbook contributors, a diverse group of scholars who span six continents and who have all thoroughly engaged in the generous intellectual exchanges that have brought this handbook to fruition. Holding the space together have been four early-career scholars who have navigated the challenges of the contemporary academy alongside the challenges wrought by the COVID-19 pandemic and their own reproductive and kinship commitments. (Two babies were born in the intervening three years since the inauguration of this project, alongside other kin who were cared for and nurtured as we created this book.) From formative meetings in 2021 to writing this in 2023, this handbook is a product of imagination and planning, some good luck, and a deliberate collaborative and critical stocktaking of the DOHaD landscape.

We thank Nicholas Eppel for permission to use his artwork from the Thermal Optimum series as our cover image, and Stanley Ulijaszek for his role as workshop rapporteur – his reflections have been invaluable in corralling this interdisciplinary conversation. Many thanks also to Anna Whiting from Cambridge University Press, whose always helpful assistance as an editor was crucial in bringing this project to completion.

We acknowledge our funders. Michelle Pentecost is funded by a UKRI Future Leaders Fellowship (MR/T040181/1) and this book is open access courtesy of UKRI funding. Tessa Moll acknowledges funding through the Australian Research Council via a Future Fellowship Award (FT180100240, PI M. Meloni) and Discovery Research Award (DP200101270, PI A. Whittaker). Jaya Keaney was funded by an Australian Research Council Discovery Project Award (DP190102071, PIs E. Kowal, M. Warin, and M. Meloni). Michael Penkler was supported by the DFG German Research Foundation through the project 'Situating Environmental Epigenetics' (403161875, PI R. Müller).

Finally, we are grateful to our families for their support during the completion of this volume. Michelle Pentecost dedicates this work to Thomas and Julian Cousins. Jaya Keaney gratefully acknowledges Mariana Podesta-Diverio. Tessa Moll dedicates this work to Rasmus Bitsch and Aya Ukhanye Bitsch Moll. And Michael Penkler dedicates this book to Nevena and Malina Born-Penkler.

DOHaD Pasts, Presents, and Futures
An Introduction

Michael Penkler, Jaya Keaney, Tessa Moll, and
Michelle Pentecost

In the photograph on the cover of this book, we peer into the lives of three figures: two children and an adult caregiver. They are balanced at play on a seesaw in an urban park. Modernist hierarchies of distinction are rendered opaque here; it is not easy to discern any markers of gender, ethnicity, and class through which we might read the relationships between these figures and place them in a broader social order. Yet this absence perhaps amplifies the intimacy between the figures, sensed in the throbbing colours that weave them together. The image glows with intensity, and the figures seem to blur at their edges, spilling into one another and the environment of the playground.

This striking photograph was created with thermography, where a thermal camera captures an image using infrared waves rather than the light of traditional photography. Originally developed for military purposes, the technology was adapted here as part of a collaboration between photographer Nicholas Eppel and anthropologist Fiona Ross about the 'First 1000 Days', a health paradigm emphasising the developmental significance of the period from conception to age two. In the broader suite of photographs from which this cover image is drawn, Eppel and Ross sought new ways of depicting the social and biological relations that comprise development, autonomy, and caregiving. They sought, as they write, 'a way to open questions about how the "hard facts" of biology are given force and presence through "soft" actions of care' [1, p. 66].

The image resonates with a central concern of our book, which traces how the folded relations of sociality, interdependence, and biological life play out at one particular site: the field of the *Developmental Origins of Health and Disease* or DOHaD. DOHaD is one crucial body of research informing the First 1000 Days paradigm on which Eppel and Ross fix their gaze. The DOHaD field argues that environmental factors such as nutrition, stress, and toxic exposure shape health and well-being over extended periods of time [2]. DOHaD has had a far-reaching impact on understandings of how life experiences — and the social contexts in which they occur — become embodied, and how the effects of these embodiments are potentially passed on between generations. In this handbook, we consider the broad-ranging implications of the DOHaD hypothesis, the ways of seeing and thinking that have historically structured its uptake by diverse audiences and publics, and new conceptual apertures through which we might more effectively and equitably harness the insights of this field.

While focusing on health across the lifecourse, DOHaD has a strong focus on early life, where experiences during critical developmental windows – such as pregnancy, preconception, and from birth until age two – are seen as particularly impactful for future health across generations. Scientific research in this field has revolutionised

1

understandings of pregnancy and health, highlighting the inseparability of fetal development from broader social contexts and material inequities, and the entanglement of a
child and their caregivers. Yet in honing attention on pregnancy and early life, research
has at times over-emphasised the maternal–fetal relation to a concerning degree, strip-
ping it of context and obscuring the distributed relations through which pregnancy,
birth, and child-rearing proceed.

A key reason we are drawn to Eppel's covering image is that it offers a perceptual
reorientation of sorts in relation to the keystone figures of DOHaD analysis and the
undue historical focus on the pregnant body. It offers us a compelling route for conceptualising intergenerational inheritance, in all its intimacy and vulnerability, without
falling into the trap of reproductive sentimentality and highly gendered, heteronormative
images of the mother–child dyad. While the figures depicted on the cover may well be a
mother and children, it is not definitively apparent, and indeed, it is beside the point.
What matters here is the evident intimacy between the three, regardless of biological or
gestational ties; the pulses of heat depict an elemental kinship that is one crucial
developmental environment, among others. When untethered from dominant gendered
and racialising modes of perception in such a way, we might better account for the
embodied intensities of care, the material environments through which we move, and the
imprints we leave on the earthly surfaces that also imprint us.

This handbook grapples with these questions from the diverse perspectives of the
authors assembled here, working in a wide range of fields in the life sciences, the social
sciences, and the humanities. DOHaD is often described as an interdisciplinary scientific
paradigm that incorporates multiple subdivisions within the life sciences and which social
scientists and feminist scholars have subjected to critique. In this handbook, we define the
field in more capacious terms, including scientists working with the DOHaD paradigm
alongside social scientists and feminist scholars who have theorised DOHaD as an increasingly powerful discourse of health and inheritance. This editorial framing reflects our
conviction that DOHaD as it is constituted today is not thinkable without the preceding
decades of engagement from social theorists and feminists, who have indissolubly shaped
the development of scientific research and its translation into policy and clinical care.
Simultaneously, the history of scientific research in DOHaD has fundamentally reshaped
critical social theories of embodiment, inheritance, and kinship, playing a fundamental role
in the turn to the 'biosocial' in social theory, by providing insight into how social relations
and inequalities literally shape biology at molecular scales [3, 4]. This handbook is a
testament to the increasing collaboration between life and social scientists under the
DOHaD banner, with DOHaD an exemplar of interdisciplinary collaboration.

In this introductory chapter, we set the scene for the rich contributions that follow by
providing an overview of the field of DOHaD in a distinctly interdisciplinary tenor.
We first trace the evolution of DOHaD over the past two decades, charting the historical
conditions that have informed the emergence of this handbook. We then discuss the
biosocial perspective that DOHaD offers as its central premise and promise, allowing for
questions of socio-environmental justice and equity to be centred in science and biomedicine. Yet, as we explore, a range of obstacles complicate this biosocial agenda,
requiring attention to questions of research translation, interdisciplinary lexicons, and
genealogies of inequality.

Responding to the fundamental tension between a biosocial approach and its challenges, the handbook as a whole offers a comprehensive overview of contemporary

biosocial collaborations in DOHaD. The handbook foregrounds a critical moment when the field is at a threshold of interdisciplinary innovation and maps future directions for research and collaboration. It serves as both an account of the field to date and a conceptual toolkit for future research, collecting histories, key concepts, and case studies of biosocial collaboration in action.

1.1 DOHaD: The Last 20 Years

Theories of DOHaD were developed in the late 1980s and 1990s through the convergence of epidemiological work investigating links between deprivation and later life disease, and experimental work in animals conducted by developmental physiologists (see Buklijas and Hanson in this volume). The DOHaD field was based on the hypothesis that environmental experiences can condition a developing organism in ways that heighten or lower the risk of disease in later life, a hypothesis with profound implications for health interventions and policy [5]. The field was formally established through the founding of the International DOHaD Society at the Second World Congress on Fetal Origins of Adult Disease in Brighton in 2003. In the subsequent two decades, the field has grown considerably, both in terms of research output and wider scientific and social recognition [5, 6]. During this time, DOHaD has developed institutionally, conceptually, and methodologically and is now a significant research agenda in health and well-being.

The change of the field's name from 'fetal origins of adult disease' to 'developmental origins of health and disease' in the early 2000s signalled a broadening of the research agenda. Early work in the field by David Barker and others had a strong focus on the prenatal period, linking nutritional restrictions in utero to later-life cardiovascular disease [7]. This focus has since expanded to consider how developmental factors influence health and disease over the entire lifespan, beginning in the so-called 'pre-conception' period before a child is conceived and continuing into advanced age [2, 6]. The field has also expanded in terms of the factors, conditions, and end points considered. While originally focussed on nutrition and metabolic disease, the fields of toxicology and psychiatry have widened the scope to include the study of teratogens and stress [8, 9]. In recent years, DOHaD research has also investigated the developmental origins of human well-being more broadly, including in topics such as adolescent cognitive function and educational attainment [10, 11].

Over the past two decades, the conceptual aperture for understanding 'development' in DOHaD has also shifted from a focus on pathological processes to a wider enquiry into normal development. Hanson and Gluckman [12] have argued that developmental effects are the result of physiological processes of developmental plasticity that have adaptive purposes insofar as they help the developing organism adapt to prospective environments, thereby linking DOHaD to current thinking in evolutionary biology. Similarly, the reversibility of developmental effects is increasingly discussed in DOHaD. Whereas early DOHaD thinking tended to view developmental effects as deterministic and permanent, as reflected in the language of 'developmental programming' (for a critique of the term, see 12), current DOHaD thinking increasingly eschews environmental determinism by attending to how the effects of early life adversity might be reversed in later life (Lloyd et al. in this volume).

The move towards a non-deterministic and non-pathological vision of development in DOHaD is inseparable from the interdisciplinary expansion of the field. Having emerged from the confluence of fetal physiology and epidemiology, DOHaD has been interdisciplinary from the outset (Buklijas and Hanson in this volume). Over time, it has coalesced diverse disciplinary approaches, including molecular biology, public health, data studies, different clinical specialties, and evolutionary biology, as well as economics, the social sciences, and humanities. At this stage, these interdisciplinary modes of knowledge-making typically occur across departments rather than in dedicated research centres, with only a few dedicated DOHaD research departments around the world [6].

A major site for the interdisciplinary expansion of DOHaD is recent advances in environmental epigenetics, a field that offers an explanatory model for the underlying mechanism of DOHaD observations [3, 13]. Environmental epigenetics studies how environmental factors influence the way genetic information – encoded in DNA – is transcribed and translated into biological processes, potentially influencing development, health, and disease. The first foundational studies in environmental epigenetics [14–16] in the early 2000s were quickly taken up in DOHaD. Buklijas and Hanson (in this volume) argue that the DOHaD field was, for a variety of reasons, originally uninterested in genomics; however, broader trends in science funding, such as the move towards funding genomic science and away from other areas like experimental physiology, are likely one key reason for the field's embrace of epigenomics in the mid-2000s. Both environmental epigenetics and DOHaD have profited from the links between the two fields [17]. In its early days, the fetal origins hypothesis was critiqued due to the absence of a clear mechanism; the entry of epigenetics has offered a 'molecular proof' of sorts. Concurrently, environmental epigenetics researchers have framed the medical and policy relevance of their work with reference to the DOHaD hypothesis [17].

The credibility tied to having a plausible mechanism in epigenetics may have contributed, among other factors, to the growing policy traction of the field since the mid-2000s. In 2010, the then-named DOHaD council launched the *Journal of DOHaD* to congregate the 'integrative, interdisciplinary, and translational' [18, p. 1] work of the field. Mark Hanson, then President of the DOHaD Society, wrote that the field had garnered sufficient acceptance in biomedical research, policy, and development agendas as to legitimate the journal's launch. Indeed, DOHaD has enjoyed significant traction in the last decades, especially in a global health context, which is increasingly concerned with the growing burden of non-communicable diseases (NCDs) in low- and middle-income countries [19]. There are regional DOHaD Societies that span six continents, including DOHaD Africa, DOHaD Society of Australia and New Zealand, DOHaD Latin America, US DOHaD, DOHaD Canada, DOHaD Japan, DOHaD China, the Pakistan DOHaD Society, and the French-Speaking DOHaD Society. International organisations such as the World Health Organization (WHO) and the World Bank have also integrated DOHaD frameworks into their agendas, as seen in the WHO's Childhood Obesity Report and the Bank's increasing investment in early childhood and maternal care [20].

At the same time, there is also a widespread feeling among DOHaD scientists that the field has not yet realised its full policy potential. In a recent editorial, former and current DOHaD society presidents Peter Gluckman, Mark Hanson, and Lucilla Poston have argued that the field has not yet found its footing in national and international health policy arenas [21]. They attribute this to DOHaD's emphasis on long-term effects in contrast to policy interest in short-term gains; a lack of coherent framing that presents a simple moral or ethical message; and the complexity of pathways within DOHaD that make it less amenable to identifying discrete points of effective intervention.

Another possible reason for the limited uptake of DOHaD in health and social policy is that the field is open to contestation both for its central hypothesis and for its policy relevance [22]. Part of this is the experimental complexity of investigating how diverse factors influence health and disease over time [23]. While evidence for long-term developmental effects has been demonstrated in animal models [24], such evidence is much more difficult to obtain in human populations. Epidemiological cohort studies, the go-to method in DOHaD research, are prone to confounding effects and are ill-equipped to prove causal effects, limiting the translatability of the evidence base (though recent methodological advances in regard to Mendelian randomisation are promising in this regard) [25].

To expand the evidence base for DOHaD, scientists have turned to intervention studies or clinical trials. However, the results of interventions during pregnancy thus far have been disappointing [26]. In pregnancy trials drawing on DOHaD that focus on obesity, for example, to date no cohort studies have established conclusively that lifestyle interventions have a positive impact on obesity across the lifecourse [27]. Meanwhile, social and feminist theorists have cautioned that intervention studies can reinforce gendered and racialised assumptions about normative development, health, and parenting that maintain unjust racial hierarchies and centre the mother–child dyad to the detriment of broader socio-environments [27].

An additional methodological critique is that existing intervention studies have been limited (only targeting a limited set of factors) and constrained (only for a set time period). Currently, there is hope within the field that complex intervention studies like the HeLTI trial, which are interdisciplinary in nature and incorporate a critical, feminist understanding of social factors, will provide a sought-after evidence base that may better inform health policy and improved healthcare (see Pentecost et al. in this volume). These complex intervention studies try to account for the complexities of the biosocial processes in which they seek to intervene. Against the background of the COVID-19 pandemic, which exacerbated global inequalities in health, DOHaD researchers have also argued for the importance of considering developmental origins to promote social resilience and health equity [28].

In 2024, then, DOHaD is on a threshold. The field has expanded disciplinarily and conceptually. It has formulated an ambitious research programme in its quest to account for the complexity of how socio-environmental factors influence health and disease across the lifecourse, and studies have moved from observation to intervention to generate evidence with policy traction. Interdisciplinary DOHaD research promises to improve our understanding of how we can contribute to social and health equity. And it promises a deeper understanding of how social environments and biological processes intertwine to produce health and disease on both individual and population scales. It is this promise to which we now turn.

1.2 Promises of the Biosocial

The promise of DOHaD lies in large part in its biosocial understanding of health and well-being. That is, it offers tools to articulate — in both biological and social terms — the intergenerational mechanisms of health inequality. Through a DOHaD prism, social contexts and unequal living conditions are understood as directly impacting biological outcomes across generations, thus construing social contexts as having biological effects, and vice versa. As a result, DOHaD has opened new avenues for conceptualising the biological and the social as entangled and inextricable.

The biosocial is a conceptual frame and heuristic that seeks to bridge the divide between biology, typically seen as the remit of the life sciences, and the social and the cultural, traditionally the remit of the social sciences and humanities. In their 2018 introduction to the *Handbook of Biology and Society*, Maurizio Meloni and co-authors characterise the biosocial as an emerging research horizon defined by interdisciplinary convergences and a shift in proper objects of research and modes of knowledge production [4]. As they write, 'the life sciences, broadly conceived, are currently moving toward a more social view of biological processes, just as the social sciences are beginning to reincorporate notions of the biological body into their investigations' [4, p. 2]. Biology is revealed as thoroughly social, while social theory turns to biological data and methods as a lively site for understanding social relations. This is not simply attention to the socially constructed nature of scientific knowledge, although literature in this vein is a vital precursor to biosocial thinking [29–31]. Rather, a biosocial approach, as we understand it here, construes the biological and the social as inseparable domains that are always already co-constituted.

As a framework for thinking about biological development, the biosocial gathered momentum in social science literature in the early and mid-2000s. The idea of the 'biosocial' has been expressed in a range of ways by social theorists, who have introduced concepts like 'biocultural' [32], 'biosocial becomings' [33], 'embedded bodies' [34], 'impressionable biologies' [35], 'situated biologies' [36], and 'exposed biologies' [37], to highlight how biology is always processual and culturally embedded. These concepts build on vital scholarly antecedents that sought to bridge the divide between nature and culture. Most notable in this respect is Donna Haraway's feminist theorisation of 'naturecultures' [38]; Bruno Latour's elaboration of nature–culture hybrids [39]; and Paul Rabinow's work on 'biosociality', which challenged the silo-ing of biology and society implicit in the then emergent paradigm of 'sociobiology' [40].

This biosocial momentum emerged concurrently with a postgenomic turn in the sciences, characterised by greater attention to the relationships between genes and environments and an increasing awareness that the development of an organism cannot be separated from its milieu [35]. The past two decades have seen a shift in attention in the life sciences, from a focus on the 'blueprint' of DNA as exemplified by the Human Genome Project completed in 2003 to a greater examination of the role of context in biological processes in fields like epigenetics, microbiomics, and immunology [4]. These varied approaches conceptualise the body as open-ended and embedded in various environments that shape and reshape collective embodiment across generations [3, 35].

While findings in epigenetics boosted the public profile of DOHaD in recent decades, it may have come at the cost of DOHaD's earlier attention to the relationship between health outcomes and social contexts via pathways unrelated to genomics. In their foundational work from the late-1980s developing the fetal origins hypothesis, for example, David Barker and colleagues foregrounded structural factors, emphasising 'geographical and socio-economic constraints on the health of women and children' [41, p. 455] as paramount in shaping disparate susceptibility to chronic disease and mortality rates. As feminist scholars have cautioned, this early attention to social contexts and structural inequalities has since given way to a narrowed view of pregnant bodies and individualised lifestyle choices, with health and disease 'telescoped into a bodily environment of the womb' ([41, p. 458]; see also [6, 27, 42]).

Many researchers have nonetheless welcomed DOHaD as an important field for critiquing the silo-ing of biology and society and reconceptualising health and disease in biosocial terms. Feminist accounts have drawn on DOHaD and allied postgenomic sciences to challenge the cultural iconicity of the mother–fetus dyad as the primary locus of reproduction and inheritance [43], pointing to how DOHaD enables an understanding of the 'reproductive environment' as situated in broader socio-environmental contexts [27, 44]. The liveliness of gestational and developmental biology is one capacious place from which to critique discourses that emphasise maternal responsibility and fetal personhood and to instead elaborate more complex models of human development [27, 43, 45]. As van Wichelen and Keaney write in their introduction to a recent special issue on *The Reproductive Bodies of Postgenomics,* 'postgenomics offers new models and conceptual horizons for understanding how we are materially related to one another beyond the fictive confines of the nuclear biogenetic family' [43, p. 1113]. This feminist mode of biosocial theorising is central to this handbook (see, for instance, chapters by Moore and Warin and by Karpin), as is the interdisciplinary concern with DOHaD's potential for securing health justice.

Another related site of biosocial thinking in DOHaD is changing understandings of categories of difference, such as race, class, and geographic location, and the material inequalities that accompany them. DOHaD analyses have generated new understandings of racialisation as a biosocial process (as explored in the chapters by Meloni et al. and Valdez and Lappé in particular). Social categories of race shape differential access to things like nutritious food, housing stability, protection from environmental toxins, and access to education and healthcare; as DOHaD research has illustrated, these factors directly shape unequal susceptibility to chronic disease, chronic stress, and mortality across generations, with disadvantaged and historically marginalised communities particularly affected [28, 46, 47]. A DOHaD approach confirms that racist social environments are exposures that become biological outcomes over time – or, as Clarence Gravlee put it, race *'becomes* biology' [48, p. 47]. As Shannon Sullivan argues, the racial health disparities often studied in health research are better conceptualised as *'racist* disparities' due to the way that social categories of race are not predetermined, but are rather biosocially materialised over time [49, p. 193].

Biosocial frameworks in DOHaD also offer new articulations of health justice. As Penkler and colleagues write, 'based on its key assumptions – that life circumstances, health, and disease are closely linked on a molecular scale – DOHaD is an inherently political research field' [6, p. 268]. DOHaD research is increasingly mobilised as a useful evidence base for attesting to the embodied intergenerational impacts of what are typically considered social or historical harms, including the processes and policies of dispossession associated with colonisation and slavery (see Keaney et al. in this volume and [50]). For example, Black and Indigenous communities are increasingly deploying epigenetic research to advocate for state reparations [51]. DOHaD and epigenetic insights hold the potential for creating more effective health and social policy responses to inequality by shifting the focus away from individuals and towards social contexts, which are in turn understood as impacting developmental outcomes. A biosocial frame may also resonate with Indigenous understandings of health and well-being and non-Western worldviews that regard personhood as inextricable from surrounding environments ([51]; see also Meloni and Rooney, and Bourke and Lovett in this volume).

In a range of ways, the enthusiasm surrounding DOHaD hinges on its biosocial model of bodies and inheritance. And yet, despite the great promise of such a way of thinking, many challenges remain. Chief among them is the disentangling and re-siloing of the biological and the social when it comes to how scientific research is conducted in practice and translated into policy.

1.3 Challenges of the Biosocial

Radically interdisciplinary research in DOHaD is necessary to fulfil the potential of biosocial thinking. While the field is uniquely placed to produce innovative modes of collaboration, in part because of its deeply interdisciplinary history, it is vital to account for the challenges of a biosocial approach in practice.

Several scholars have highlighted the difficulties of representing biosocial complexity within traditional research models and methods, despite good faith efforts and clear frustrations [23, 52, 53]. For instance, DOHaD research often reduces 'the environment' to single, fixed variables – such as food (measured as calories), pollution exposures (often singular toxicants), and stress (measured by cortisol levels). From the pressures to present research in a more linear fashion, to producing publications quickly, to using cost-effective research methods, DOHaD research is embedded within institutional structures that compel scientists to make pragmatic choices around variables and proxies. Penkler [23] points in this respect to Knorr-Cetina's description of the 'decision-ladenness' [31] of research: decisions regarding variables and measures must be made among multiple, competing interests (costs, feasibility, and reliability) but also considerations such as the burden on participants and retention rates, and all this often across multiple contexts. Together, these factors can steer scientific research in reductionist directions.

While the use of single and fixed variables as environmental proxies is often a pragmatic necessity in scientific research, it has the effect of neglecting the complex histories and social relations that shape developmental environments (see Rossmann and Samaras in this volume). For instance, pinpointing a deficient diet among pregnant women may offer an experimentally feasible research question; however, it comes at the risk of backgrounding the more complex question of *why* certain populations face nutritional challenges. By defining the problem as one of individual behaviours, such research justifies interventions that also target individual choices. This renders interventions potentially futile, as these 'choices' remain deeply shaped by access and acceptability. It also potentially reproduces injustice by reinforcing gendered, classed, and racist patterns of responsibilisation and blame, siphoning the structural forces of racism, sexism, and poverty into a problem of individual behaviours [3, 6, 27]. While all research involves decisions that delineate a research object by focusing on certain aspects of the world at the expense of others [29, 31], it is crucial to be self-reflexive about and accountable for the kinds of decision we make as researchers, the histories of thought from which they emerge as sensible or even automatic, and the relations and futures that they preclude.

Working across disciplines may provide an opportunity to reflect on the decisions that delineate a research problem. Interdisciplinary teams could provide 'ethical safeguards' [54] against some of the critiques levelled at DOHaD research, such as its continuing focus on individual factors and behaviours. This individual focus dovetails with existing and historical assumptions about who and what is in need of intervention – what Pentecost terms DOHaD geographies [55]. The challenges here are multiple. Scientific research needs to reframe studies away from individual behaviours and mother-blaming [56, 57]. It also needs to remain attentive to the ways that research messaging overlaps with local histories and can reproduce stigmatising narratives (see Kenney and Müller in this volume). When brought into policy or public health messaging, DOHaD research needs to be adapted and reworked to fit within the needs of local communities (see Tu'akoi and colleagues in this volume).

The methodological and translational challenges facing biosocial research are heightened by the structural features of the contemporary university, often characterised by silo-ed disciplinary boundaries and employment structures. As with all academic knowledge creation, DOHaD research unfolds within the confines of institutional practices, knowledge and funding economies, and epistemic environments that can hinder fruitful biosocial collaboration. In the current context, quantitative data and the 'hard sciences' garner greater legitimacy and credibility than the social sciences and humanities [52]. This is particularly true in health research where implicit epistemic hierarchies result in the accommodation of social science approaches in biomedicine, rather than their full integration [58]. This problem is reflected in research funding culture [59], peer review [60], pedagogy [61], and academic recognition [58]. As a result, projects may only accommodate the 'addition' of social components and social scientists to biological and biomedical research teams, when the research problem has already been defined by scientists. Barry and Born [62] describe this kind of interdisciplinarity as the 'subordination-service model'. Such an arrangement perpetuates the bracketing of the 'social' from the 'biological' and offers little space for iterative learning from 'the social' in crafting and orienting future research. In thinking about the efficacy of biosocial collaboration, it is also important to extend the notion of collaboration beyond the academy to foster collaborative knowledge-making practices with the communities that DOHaD researchers recruit and study (see Tu'akoi and colleagues in this volume). Collaborative research may challenge the fundamental assumptions of biomedicine: for example the primacy of the individual versus Indigenous notions of collective personhood. At the same time, iterative, engaged, and interactive work with communities can be time-consuming and expensive and is thus often in tension with the demands of the neoliberal university. Addressing this tension requires commitment to the longer-term reshaping of research infrastructures.

1.4 Overview of Contributions

In this handbook, a global authorship has come together to reflect on the state of DOHaD today and the questions, tools, and ways of working that will foster the promise of a DOHaD research agenda that promotes health justice. The handbook is the product of our authors' patience with conversations not only across time zones but also across the divisions of disciplinary practice, language, and convention. Across 29 chapters, anthropologists, psychologists, physiologists, gender studies scholars, molecular biologists, clinicians, sociologists, epidemiologists, science and technology studies scholars, and legal scholars have worked towards interdisciplinary legibility as a foundation for generous exchange.

Many of the contributions are themselves the outcome of interdisciplinary engagements; some are explicitly framed as such, while others foreground a healthy scepticism for the interdisciplinarity DOHaD scholarship might meaningfully achieve. Defining interdisciplinarity is itself a fraught question: as Callard and Fitzgerald suggest, it is a term that 'everyone invokes and none understands' [63, p. 4]. The formalisation of 'interdisciplinarity' as a policy concern, academic orientation, and epistemic field has come with its own foreclosures, even as it has held the promise of openings [62, 63]. Yet in fields such as DOHaD, the need for collaborative research practices is irrefutable. We perceive a unique willingness in the DOHaD community to embrace an interdisciplinarity that allows for 'the co-existence of difference', to borrow from science and technology studies scholars Annemarie Mol and Anita Hardon, where 'solutions are sought that aim to do justice to each interlocutor's particular intellectual and practical stakes' [64, p. 4]. This is perhaps facilitated by the contributors' shared interest in intergenerational health, the folding of social inequality into bodies, what it means to live well, and how health interventions can aid this pursuit.

In six sections, the 29 chapters comprising this handbook represent the key debates, concepts, and case studies of interdisciplinary work in DOHaD. Section 1 traces the history of the field and its intellectual precursors. Maurizio Meloni and Natasha Rooney show in their contribution how thinking about 'maternal impressions', that is the idea that maternal experiences and emotions can leave long-lasting effects on the developing organism, has been a recurrent theme in different historical and cultural contexts since antiquity. Tatjana Buklijas traces how this idea has developed in the twentieth century, showing that conceptualisations of the maternal–fetal relationship have undergone marked change during this period. These changes, which are more complex than often assumed in standard historical accounts, are central to the story of DOHaD's emergence as a distinct field in the 'long decade' from 1989 to 2003. Mark Hanson and Tatjana Buklijas' chapter covers these 'first 5000 days' in which DOHaD was established as a distinct biomedical research field, beginning with an influential interdisciplinary meeting in 1989 between epidemiologists, led by David Barker, and fetal physiologists, and ending with the formation of the International DOHaD Society in 2003.

Section 2 is concerned with the social life of DOHaD research, and its interface with questions of injustice. Maurizio Meloni, Christopher Kuzawa, Ayuba Issaka, and Tessa Moll warn that deterministic notions of environment and development mobilised in DOHaD can reproduce an essentialist understanding of racial categories. Moore and Warin show how an overt focus on women's nutrition obscures the broad scope and implications of DOHaD for understanding health inequalities. Natali Valdez and Martine Lappé contend that gender and race are inseparably intertwined as social categories, arguing that a gendered and racialised health discourse disproportionally places the burden of intergenerational health on women of colour. Jennifer Cohen reviews economic research in DOHaD, arguing that it has often been limited by a narrow focus on molecular aspects and a decontextualised use of demographic variables, with the effect of obscuring social structures. Luca Chiapperino, Cindy Gerber, Francesco Panese, and Umberto Simeoni continue the critique of DOHaD's focus on the individual, describing this tendency as a 'moral paradox' characterising how health interventions are generated in the field. Finally, Isabel Karpin highlights the significant implications of DOHaD for intergenerational justice and legal conceptualisations of personhood and harm.

Section 3 is a toolkit that showcases a series of critical concepts for biosocial DOHaD research. The first, profiled by Mark Tomlinson, Amelia van der Merwe, Marguerite

Marlow, and Sarah Skeen, is *lifecourse*, a concept developed in the past 50 years to highlight the role of social and behavioural influences on illness. Edna Bosire, Michelle Pentecost, and Emily Mendenhall's chapter on *syndemics* foregrounds the synergistic characteristics of diseases, calling attention to the importance of studying how diseases cluster and interact across the lifecourse. *Embodiment,* as discussed by Ziyanda Majombozi and Mutsawashe Mutendi, is a social science concept that has been similarly developed to connect the body, subjective experiences, and broader social contexts and is useful to deepen awareness of how social and political factors and contexts influence the development of health and disease over extended periods of time. Sarah Richardson, contends that the ensuing complexity poses a challenge for the field, as DOHaD research investigates causes and effects that are difficult to observe experimentally. She argues that the field is thus characterised by a tolerance to what she calls *causal crypticity* – a characteristic common to many data-rich, postgenomic life sciences. According to Jaya Keaney, Henrietta Byrne, Megan Warin, and Emma Kowal, these difficulties are also evident in research on *intergenerational trauma*, a concept developed to study the long-term physiological consequences of violence and discriminatory social contexts. In the final chapter in Section 3, Elizabeth Roberts and colleagues offer *bioethnography* as a useful interdisciplinary tool for DOHaD research, describing it as a key method and concept to integrate ethnographic research into epidemiological cohort studies.

Section 4 considers how DOHaD research has travelled beyond the lab or academy and into policy and practice. Felicia Low, Peter Gluckman, and Mark Hanson outline the key issues for the field's traction within health policy, while Chandni Maria Jacob, Michael Penkler, Ruth Müller, and Mark Hanson challenge DOHaD researchers to take up insights from communication theory to frame their work in responsible ways for science and society. Involving communities and publics in DOHaD research is an important avenue for creating responsible frameworks, as Siobhan Tu'akoi and colleagues argue in their contribution to community-based participatory methods for translating key DOHaD insights into public health practice in the Cooke Islands. Finally, Anusha Lachman, Astrid Berg, Fiona Ross, and Simone Peters consider how DOHaD ideas are translated into clinical practice, offering the example of the integration of first 1000 days frameworks into a new academic curriculum for infant mental health in Southern Africa.

In Section 5, contributions discuss how biosocial research approaches play out in practice. Emily Emmott and Sahra Gibbon discuss how 'early life' has often been narrowly framed and argue that a biosocial anthropological perspective can contribute to a more nuanced framework for DOHaD-informed research and intervention. Using the example of the HeLTI–South Africa randomised trial, Michelle Pentecost, Larske Soepnel, Khuthala Mabetha, Catherine Draper, and Shane Norris discuss the recent trend towards complex intervention studies within DOHaD. Sophia Rossmann and Georgia Samaras also discuss the challenges of how to adequately capture complex environments in biosocial research, demonstrating that while DOHaD research acknowledges in principle the complexity of lived environments, results often replicate reductionist accounts. Martha Kenney and Ruth Müller's chapter also highlights the importance of framings, by turning their attention to researchers' storytelling practices and how researchers, clinicians, and other actors embed DOHaD knowledge claims as part of larger scientific and societal narratives that have consequences for how DOHaD knowledge circulates in society. Lastly, Shivani Kaul and

Emily Yates-Doerr discuss DOHaD work in Bhutan and Guatemala that advances relational, interdependent models of development.

Section 6 looks at current trends and possible future directions for DOHaD research. Julie Nihouarn Sigurdardottir and Salma Ayis review moves in DOHaD towards Big Data, artificial intelligence, and machine learning, and the ethical and methodological issues that these innovations represent for the field. Stephanie Lloyd, Pierre-Eric Lutz, and Chani Bonventre offer a case study for how to conceptualise and investigate reversibility as an important concept for DOHaD, using the example of neuroepigenetic research on traumatic memories. Kaleb Saulnier and colleagues discuss the lessons that can be learned from engaging with the interdisciplinary field of disability studies for being inclusive in DOHaD knowledge-making and interventions. They argue that research has often occurred without engaging affected disability communities and point to the importance of the slogan, 'nothing about us without us', for conducting socially responsible research into disability. In a similar vein, Sarah Bourke and Raymond Lovett discuss epidemiological research with, for, and by Indigenous people and how applying an Indigenous lens provides valuable lessons for developing health research and interventions that address the determinants of intergenerational health and well-being in a holistic way. Lastly, Jorg Niewöhner argues that recent scientific developments challenge notions of origin and development that are foundational for DOHaD research and considers new ways of conceptualising DOHaD for the Anthropocene. Drawing on themes that connect the entire handbook, he argues for the vital necessity of interdisciplinary research across the nature–culture divide: only by embracing ideas of anthropogenic biology can DOHaD grapple with the pressing current challenges that face human and non-human life on a planet whose habitability is challenged by multiple crises like climate change and novel planetary health threats.

Together, the chapters highlight the manifold contributions that biosocial research in DOHaD can make to not only rethinking development and health but also to furthering health equity on a planet still marked by persistent and shocking health disparities. The contributions gathered here are a testament to the depth and wealth of biosocial thinking within DOHaD and to the value of interdisciplinary collaborations. The interdisciplinary approach in this volume aims for transformational research, where the outcome 'is a paradigm shift that causes the scientific community to see problems in an entirely different way' [65, p. S21]. The DOHaD research paradigm is inherently transformational, having produced key shifts in biomedical thinking from older chronic disease models to the lifecourse frameworks that are now commonly used for understanding health disparities [2]. The relative youth of the DOHaD field affords further opportunities to radically reshape research practices, and this handbook is both a record of the successes and challenges of this project so far and a toolkit for forging a robust interdisciplinary agenda for transformational research going forward.

References

1. Ross FC, Eppel N. Thermal optimum: Time, intimacy and the elemental in the first thousand days of life. *Anthropology Southern Africa*. 2016; 39(1): 64–73.

2. Poston L, Godfrey KM, Gluckman PD, Hanson MA, eds. *Developmental Origins of Health and Disease*. 2nd ed. Cambridge, Cambridge University Press, 2022.

3. Müller R, Hanson C, Hanson M, et al. The biosocial genome? Interdisciplinary perspectives on environmental epigenetics, health and society. *EMBO Reports*. 2017; 18(10): 1677–82.

4.   Meloni M, Cromby J, Fitzgerald D, Lloyd S. Introducing the new biosocial landscape. In: Meloni M, Cromby J, Fitzgerald D, Lloyd S, eds. *The Palgrave Handbook of Biology and Society*. London, Palgrave Macmillan UK. 2018; 1–22.

5.   Gluckman PD, Buklijas T, Hanson M. The developmental origins of health and disease (DOHaD) concept: Past, present, and future. In: Rosenfeld CS, ed. *The Epigenome and Developmental Origins of Health and Disease*. Boston, MA, Academic Press. 2016; 1–15.

6.   Penkler M, Hanson M, Biesma RG, Müller R. DOHaD in science and society: Eemergent opportunities and novel responsibilities. *Journal of Developmental Origins of Health and Disease*. 2019; **10** (3): 268–73.

7.   Barker DJ, Osmond C. Infant mortality, childhood nutrition, and ischaemic heart disease in England and Wales. *Lancet*. 1986; **1**(8489): 1077–81.

8.   Haugen AC, Schug TT, Collman G, Heindel JJ. Evolution of DOHaD: The impact of environmental health sciences. *Journal of Developmental Origins of Health and Disease*. 2015; **6**(2): 55–64.

9.   O'Donnell KJ, Meaney MJ. Fetal origins of mental health: The developmental origins of health and disease hypothesis. *American Journal of Psychiatry*. 2016; **174** (4): 319–28.

10. Chandrashekarappa SM, Krishna M, Krupp K, et al. Size at birth and cognitive function among rural adolescents: A life course epidemiology study protocol of the Kisalaya cohort in Mysuru, South India. *BMJ Paediatric Open*. 2020; **4**(1): e000789.

11. Almond D, Currie J. Killing me softly: The fetal origins hypothesis. *Journal of Economic Perspectives*. 2011; **25**(3): 153–72.

12. Hanson M, Gluckman PD. Early developmental conditioning of later health and disease: Physiology or pathophysiology? *Physiological Reviews*. 2014; **94**(4): 1027–76.

13. Safi-Stibler S, Gabory A. Epigenetics and the developmental origins of health and disease: Parental environment signalling to the epigenome, critical time windows and sculpting the adult phenotype. *Seminars in Cell & Developmental Biology*. 2020; **97**: 172–80.

14. Weaver ICG, Cervoni N, Champagne FA, et al. Epigenetic programming by maternal behavior. *Nature Neuroscience*. 2004; **7**(8): 847–54.

15. Waterland RA, Jirtle RL. Transposable elements: Targets for early nutritional effects on epigenetic gene regulation. *Molecular Cell Biology*. 2003; **23**(15): 5293–300.

16. Lillycrop KA, Phillips ES, Jackson AA, et al. Dietary protein restriction of pregnant rats induces and folic acid supplementation prevents epigenetic modification of hepatic gene expression in the offspring. *The Journal of Nutrition*. 2005; **135**(6): 1382–86.

17. Kenney M, Müller R. Of rats and women: Narratives of motherhood in environmental epigenetics. *BioSocieties*. 2017; **12**(1): 23–46.

18. Hanson MA. Development and after. *Journal of Developmental Origins of Health and Disease*. 2010; **1**(1): 1.

19. Pentecost M. *The Politics of Potential: Global Health and Gendered Futures in South Africa*. New Jersey, Rutgers University Press, 2024.

20. Moll T, Meloni M, Issaka A. Foetal programming meets human capital: Biological plasticity, development, and the limits to 'the economization of life'. *BioSocieties*. 2023; online first. https://doi.org/10.1057/s41292-023-00309-8

21. Hanson MA, Poston L, Gluckman PD. DOHaD – the challenge of translating the science to policy. *Journal of Developmental Origins of Health and Disease*. 2019; **10**(3): 263–67.

22. Richardson SS. *The Maternal Imprint: The Contested Science of Maternal-fetal Effects*. Chicago, University of Chicago Press, 2021.

23. Penkler M. Caring for biosocial complexity. Articulations of the environment in research on the

Developmental Origins of Health and Disease. *Studies in History and Philosophy of Science.* 2022; **93**: 1–10.

24. Ramírez V, Bautista RJ, Frausto-González O, et al. Developmental programming in animal models: Critical evidence of current environmental negative changes. *Reproductive Sciences.* 2023; **30**(2): 442–63.

25. Lawlor DA, Richmond R, Warrington N, et al. Using Mendelian randomization to determine causal effects of maternal pregnancy (intrauterine) exposures on offspring outcomes: Sources of bias and methods for assessing them. *Wellcome Open Research.* 2017; **2**(11): 1-23.

26. Gaillard R, Wright J, Jaddoe VWV. Lifestyle intervention strategies in early life to improve pregnancy outcomes and long-term health of offspring: A narrative review. *Journal of Developmental Origins of Health and Disease.* 2019; **10**(3): 314–21.

27. Valdez N. *Weighing the Future: Race, Science, and Pregnancy Trials in the Postgenomic Era.* Oakland, University of California Press, 2022.

28. Penkler M, Jacob CM, Müller R, et al. Developmental Origins of Health and Disease, resilience and social justice in the COVID era. *Journal of Developmental Origins of Health and Disease.* 2022; 13 (4): 413–416.

29. Haraway D. *Simians, Cyborgs and Women. The Reinvention of Nature.* London, Free Association Books, 1991.

30. Latour B. *Reassembling the Social: An Introduction to Actor-Network-Theory.* Oxford, Oxford University Press, 2005.

31. Knorr-Cetina K. *The Manufacture of Knowledge: An Essay on the Constructivist and Contextual Nature of Science.* Oxford, UK, Pergamon Press, 1981.

32. Frost S. *Biocultural Creatures: Toward a New Theory of the Human.* Durham, NC, Duke University Press, 2016.

33. Ingold T, Gísli Pl. *Biosocial Becomings: Integrating Social and Biological Anthropology.* New York, Cambridge University Press, 2013.

34. Niewöhner J. Epigenetics: Embedded bodies and the molecularisation of biography and milieu. *BioSocieties.* 2011; **6**(3): 279–98.

35. Meloni M. *Impressionable Biologies. From the Archaeology of Plasticity to the Sociology of Epigenetics.* London, Routledge, 2019.

36. Niewöhner J, Lock M. Situating local biologies: Anthropological perspectives on environment/human entanglements. *BioSocieties.* 2018; **13**(4): 681–97.

37. Wahlberg A. Exposed biologies and the banking of reproductive vitality in China. *Science, Technology and Society.* 2018; **23**(2): 307–23.

38. Haraway D. *The Companion Species Manifesto: Dogs, People, and Significant Otherness.* Chicago, IL, Prickly Paradigm Press, 2003.

39. Latour B. *We Have Never Been Modern.* Cambridge, MA, Harvard University Press, 1993.

40. Rabinow P. *Essays on the Anthropology of Reason.* Princeton NJ, Princeton University Press, 1996.

41. Warin M, Moore V, Zivkovic T, Davies M. Telescoping the origins of obesity to women's bodies: How gender inequalities are being squeezed out of Barker's hypothesis. *Annals of Human Biology.* 2011; **38**(4): 453–60.

42. Lappé M. The maternal body as environment in autism science. *Social Studies of Science.* 2016; **46**(5): 675–700.

43. van Wichelen S, Keaney J. The reproductive bodies of postgenomics. *Science, Technology, & Human Values.* 2022; **47**(6): 1111–30.

44. Lappé M, Jeffries Hein R, Landecker H. Environmental politics of reproduction. *Annual Review of Anthropology.* 2019; **48**(1): 133–50.

45. Yoshizawa RS. Fetal–maternal intra-action. *Body & Society.* 2016; **22**(4): 79–105.

46. Kuzawa CW, Sweet E. Epigenetics and the embodiment of race: Developmental origins of US racial disparities in cardiovascular health. *American Journal of Human Biology.* 2009; **21**(1): 2–15.

47. Mansfield B, Guthman J. Epigenetic life: Biological plasticity, abnormality, and new configurations of race and reproduction. *Cultural Geographies.* 2015; **22**(1): 3–20.

48. Gravlee CC. How race becomes biology: Embodiment of social inequality. *American Journal of Physical Anthropology.* 2009; **139**(1): 47–57.

49. Shannon S. Epigenetics and the transgenerational effects of white racism inheriting racist disparities in health. *Critical Philosophy of Race.* 2013; **1**(2): 190–218.

50. Singh G, Morrison J, Hoy W. DOHaD in Indigenous populations: DOHaD, epigenetics, equity and race. *Journal of Developmental Origins of Health and Disease.* 2019; **10**(1): 63–64.

51. Warin M, Keaney J, Kowal E, Byrne H. Circuits of time: Enacting postgenomics in Indigenous Australia. *Body & Society.* 2023; **29**(2): 20–48.

52. Ackerman SL, Darling KW, Lee SS-J, et al. Accounting for complexity: Gene–environment interaction research and the moral economy of quantification. *Science, Technology & Human Values.* 2016; **41**(2): 194–218.

53. Pinel C. What counts as the environment in epigenetics? Knowledge and ignorance in the entrepreneurial university. *Science as Culture.* 2022; **31**(3): 311–33.

54. Saulnier KM, Dupras C. Race in the postgenomic era: Social epigenetics calling for interdisciplinary ethical safeguards. *American Journal of Bioethics.* 2017; **17**(9): 58–60.

55. Pentecost M. The first thousand days: Epigenetics in the age of global health. In: Meloni M, Cromby J, Fitzgerald D, Lloyd S, eds. *The Palgrave Handbook of Biology and Society.* London, Palgrave Macmillan UK. 2018; 269–94.

56. Sharp GC, Schellhas L, Richardson SS, Lawlor DA. Time to cut the cord: Recognizing and addressing the imbalance

of DOHaD research towards the study of maternal pregnancy exposures. *Journal of Developmental Origins of Health and Disease.* 2019; **10**(5): 509–12.

57. Pentecost M, Ross FC, Macnab A. Beyond the Dyad: Making Developmental Origins of Health and Disease (DOHaD) interventions more inclusive. *Journal of Developmental Origins of Health and Disease.* 2018; **9**(1): 10–14.

58. Albert M, Paradis E, Kuper A. Interdisciplinary promises versus practices in medicine: The decoupled experiences of social sciences and humanities scholars. *Social Science & Medicine.* 2015; **126**: 17–25.

59. Huutoniemi K. Communicating and compromising on disciplinary expertise in the peer review of research proposals. *Social Studies of Science.* 2012; **42**(6): 897–921.

60. Mallard G, Lamont M, Guetzkow J. Fairness as appropriateness: Negotiating epistemological differences in peer review. *Science, Technology, & Human Values.* 2009; **34**(5): 573–606.

61. Felt U, Igelsböck J, Schikowitz A, Völker T. Growing into what? The (un-) disciplined socialisation of early stage researchers in transdisciplinary research. *Higher Education.* 2013; **65**(4): 511–24.

62. Barry A, Born G. *Interdisciplinarity: Reconfigurations of the Social and Natural Sciences.* London, Routledge, 2013.

63. Callard F, Fitzgerald D. Introduction: Not another book about interdisciplinarity. In: Callard F, Fitzgerald D, eds. *Rethinking Interdisciplinarity across the Social Sciences and Neurosciences.* London, Palgrave Macmillan UK. 2015; 1–14.

64. Moll A, Hardon A. What COVID-19 may teach us about interdisciplinarity. *BMJ Global Health.* 2020; **5**(12): e004375.

65. Dankwa-Mullan I, Rhee KB, Stoff DM, et al. Moving toward paradigm-shifting research in health disparities through translational, transformational, and transdisciplinary approaches. *American Journal of Public Health.* 2010; **100**(Suppl 1): S19–24.

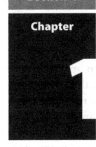

Porous Bodies, Impressible Mothers
A Global and *Longue Durée* Perspective

Maurizio Meloni and Natasha Rooney

1.1 Introduction

To contextualise present biomedical debates on the role of pregnancy in shaping offspring traits, and hence the related notion of maternal responsibility, we review in this chapter the prehistory of the belief in maternal impression. Maternal impression is the enduring notion that the emotions and experiences of a pregnant woman could leave permanent marks on her unborn child. We are not claiming in the following pages that maternal impression, or its historical understanding, is a direct predecessor of the Developmental Origins of Health and Disease (DOHaD). However, with this global historical overview, moving eastward from the Mediterranean to Asian medical systems, we are alerting the reader to the ubiquitous pre-scientific concern with pregnancy, and sometimes pre-pregnancy, as a key time 'requiring self-discipline and work on the part of expectant mothers' [1]. As DOHaD globalises its research and claims about novel forms of soft inheritance [2] to geographical regions that encompass a multiplicity of knowledge systems, this *longue durée* and global view of maternal effects may help understand both its resonance with traditional beliefs in the West and contemporary forms of hybridisation with non-Western systems of medical knowledge, which we will discuss in Section 1.4.

1.2 Maternal Impressions in Europe before Modern Medicine

1.2.1 Greco-Roman and Medieval Medicine

In describing the relevance of maternal impressions in Greco-Roman and Latin medieval medicine, it is important to highlight three major aspects. First is the wider experience of the pre-modern body as a permeable and porous entity, living in a state of *constant apprehension* of the external environment on its physiological balance. Second is the physical power of imagination. Before the modern split between body and mind, a fully materialistic view prevailed in pre-modern medicine where the soul and human temperament were seen as mostly determined by the physical impact of changes in diet, climate, or through the effects of planets' movement. This deep communication between imagination and bodily changes may seem superstitious or only metaphorical in the post-Enlightenment mindset, which neatly separates inwardness and external objects, but it was literal and effective well into early modernity [3]. Scholastic philosophers, for instance, shared the notion that mental images could impress real forms into matter. Al-Kindi (ninth

MM gratefully acknowledges funding from the *Australian Research Council* (Future Fellowship Award FT180100240).

century CE), one of the fathers of Islamic philosophy known in the Latin West for his On Rays (De Radiis) and a translator of Aristotle, held the view that any spiritual substance can induce true forms in the body just through imagination [4, 5]. This widespread understanding of the relationship between matter and mind offers a context to appreciate the impact and ubiquity of the doctrine of maternal impression or the belief that a mother's imagination could imprint both physical and mental characteristics on an unborn child.

Third is the gendering of biological knowledge, at different degrees, in both medical and philosophical views of reproduction. Physiologically, in Greco-Roman and later medieval medicine, it was widely assumed that women were of a softer, more permeable, and less stable nature, more liquid and transparent than men, and hence easily subject to passion [6]. This perceived greater impressionability of the female body finds its validation earlier in Hippocratic texts, where women are considered spongier, 'with a capacity to absorb fluid which makes it directly analogous to wool or sheepskin' [6]. These and other tropes were instrumental in consolidating the image of women as more subject to passions and less shielded 'against corrupting ingestions' [1]. These ingestions included the power of imagination and the susceptibility to several social influences that we would now call shocks or traumas. As we can read in the most influential treatise in female medicine in antiquity, Soranus' *Gynecology* (*c.*125 CE):

> Some women, seeing monkeys during intercourse, have borne children resembling monkeys. The tyrant of the Cyprians who was misshapen, compelled his wife to look at beautiful statues during intercourse and became the father of well-shaped children; and horsebreeders, during covering, place noble horses before the mares. Thus, in order that the offspring may not be rendered misshapen, women must be sober during coitus because in drunkenness the soul becomes the victim of strange fantasies; this furthermore, because the offspring bears some resemblance to the mother as well, not only in body but in soul.

A treatise attributed to Galen [7] enlists the perceived ability of an expectant mother to imprint her child as one of the many 'wonderful works of nature'. The Aristotelian view is even more radically gendered. Whereas the Hippocratic and Galenic tradition sees both men and women as contributing to semen for procreation, for the most influential philosophers of antiquity until early modernity, women contribute only bare matter to the male semen that will inform and shape the female menses. Medieval medicine and natural philosophy would rework these tropes with a few variations. Women being not just less hot but also of a more watery constitution than men, Albert the Great and Thomas Aquinas thought that they would behave as any moist object would: that is, they would receive impressions more 'easily but retain them poorly' [8]. In a moralising rendering of this trope, Albert the Great instead made the claim that the mud-like impressionability of women could explain why 'women are more inconstant and fickle than men' [9]. Their moister constitution made women more easily subject, for instance, to the effects of lunar tides. Throughout the European Middle Ages and into early modern Europe, maternal impression was debated as one of the key environmental influences to explain the specific characteristics of the child, particularly birth defects or the resemblance (or lack of) to the father [10, 11]. The emphasis remained on the negative, and the avoidance of scary sights or stressful emotions was largely advised in the medical literature as a way to counteract the power of a porous womb.

1.2.2 Early Modern European Debates 1500–1700

Maternal impression, and particularly one racialised version of it possibly based on the Hippocratic 'On the Nature of Children' [12], became widespread in the Renaissance and early modern Europe (see [13]). In the medical-teratological work of Ambroise Paré (*Des monstres et prodiges*, 1573), Hippocrates was said to have saved a white princess from the accusation of adultery when she mothered a child 'black as a Moor'. The father of medicine pronounced that a portrait of a Moor in the princess's bedroom was to blame for the case of dissimilarity in generation. (For the racialised aspect of maternal imagination, see [12].) Besides Paré's teratology, a belief in maternal impression was shared by a large number of European intellectuals and doctors of this period from Ficino to Montaigne and Gassendi [14]. Paracelsus claimed that 'the woman is the artist and the child the canvas on which to raise the work' (cited in [15]); Montaigne claimed that 'we know by experience that women transmit marks of their fancies to the bodies of the children they carry in the womb' (cited in [16]).

The seventeenth century saw a progressive collapse of the fluid body of humoralism in favour of an organic understanding of physiology and the fading of teleological explanations replaced by emerging mechanistic science. Maternal impression, however, still found a place in debates on reproduction and heredity. Rather than just being confined to teratological abnormalities, the power of imagination was integrated as another mechanism for explaining resemblance among generations [17]. For this reason, the alleged power of maternal impression was often resisted and criticised by scholars who highlighted instead the stability of natural processes and their relative impermeability to the direct effect of accidents or emotions [18].

Although scientific debates became more cautious in connecting abnormalities to maternal misconceptions, seventeenth- and eighteenth-century medical and midwifery texts, both technical and popular, continued to offer harsh prescriptions to control pregnant women. Unknowingly building on old humoralist tropes of maternal permeability, they taught women that their wombs were sensitive to the external world 'as our senses are' and that 'whatsoever moves the faculties of the mother souls may do like in the child' [19]. John Maubray, in his influential treatise *The Female Physician* (1724), also claimed that when the soul is 'elevated and inflamed with a fervent Imagination, it may not only affect its proper Body, but also that of Another'. Therefore, pregnant women were encouraged to 'suppress all Anger, Passion, and other Perturbations of Mind, and avoid entertaining too serious or melancholic Thoughts; since all such tend to impress a Depravity of Nature upon the Infant's Mind, and Deformity on its Body' (1724 cited in [20]).

1.3 The Middle East: Biblical, Talmudic, and Arabic Commentaries on Maternal Impression

1.3.1 Pre-eugenic Thinking in the Biblical and Talmudic Tradition

Moving to the East Mediterranean and what is today the Middle East, we can see how tropes around maternal impression often took a different form within debates on paternal and maternal power to shape heredity. In the Jewish tradition, for instance, what emerges more vividly is the possibility to control and optimise reproduction through impressions, particularly at the time of conception rather than during the whole pregnancy. The *Torah* offers a clear and oft-cited example. Jacob, the grandson of Abraham, uses something akin to maternal impressions to generate spotted sheep. Genesis (30, 37–39) says:

Jacob, however, took fresh-cut branches from poplar, almond and plane trees and made white stripes on them by peeling the bark and exposing the white inner wood of the branches (38). Then he placed the peeled branches in all the watering troughs, so that they would be directly in front of the flocks when they came to drink. When the flocks were in heat and came to drink, (39) they mated in front of the branches. And they bore young that were streaked or speckled or spotted [21].

While Midrashic disputes or Talmudic commentaries refer to this episode to exonerate white mothers having a black child or vice versa [22–24], in later rabbinic commentaries (14th CE) the passage in Genesis is taken as a platform to suggest a positive possibility of control of heredity among humans:

If animals, who have no intelligence to understand the benefit of a matter or its detriment, and only act out of instinct, have the power to mold their offspring according to their thoughts at the time of copulation, how much more so for human beings, who have great power of intellect to form in their minds perceptions of matters lofty and mundane, and they have the power to direct their thoughts with regard to any given matter, that they need to purify their thoughts for this endeavor [25]

An interesting albeit anecdotal variation to this quasi-eugenic theme (in the sense of better birth) can be found in a story about the famous Rabbi Yohanan (first century) who apparently justified to other rabbis his frequent attendance of Roman public bathhouses by claiming that 'the sight of his physical beauty' would cause women who 'washed before intimacies with their husbands ... to conceive handsome children' [26]. The focus on preventing negative effects, instead, is highlighted by a story in the Talmud of the anxious precaution of a rabbi who only made love to his wife in darkness, so that at the moment of copulation he would not set his eyes on another woman 'begetting sons who are as bastards' (cited in [12]). At least in this case, it is the man and not the woman the possible channel through which impressions or emotions may shape a child's nature.

Finally, Moses Maimonides' work (1135–1204) also emphasises the potential usage of maternal impression to achieve a good or better birth. In his medical aphorisms on Greco-Roman medicine, he writes [7]:

(xxiv.26b) I was informed about an ancient physician that he wished to have a fair son born to him and that he painted a portrait on the wall of a boy as handsome as possible. When he had sexual intercourse with his wife, he ordered her to look at that portrait constantly and not to look away from it even for a short moment. She got a son who was as beautiful as that portrait but did not resemble his father [12, 27].

1.3.2 Muslim Medical Views in the Middle Ages

Medical views in Islam are influenced by four parallel and somehow competing if not conflicting sources and traditions: the Greco (Unani)-Islamic tradition (Avicenna, Al-Razi, etc.); Aristotle's highly influential view of generation and reproduction as determined mostly or only by the power of the male semen to control a recalcitrant maternal matter; Prophetic medicine (medical sayings attributed to Muhammad, which were later turned to a whole discipline); and 'spiritual' saintly healing. References to maternal impression are, however, somehow more contained. Key medical sources from the tenth and eleventh centuries – Al-Qurtubi, al-Rāzī, and Ibn Sina – are more worried about possible miscarriages caused by frightening emotions in women (or undue movement) than maternal impression or influence on the child morphology as such (see, for instance, [28]). Two peculiar aspects of Islamic culture may have deflected the medical view on impressions. One is that the Islamic ban on portraits and statues at home limits the number of eccentric sights (mostly outdoor sights such as animals) (see [29]) that could influence a woman [22]. The diminished impact of images is balanced by a stronger emphasis on smell. According to Ibn Sina, women could abort due to particular smells such as an extinguished candle. And if the smell of some peculiar food generated a craving that was not satisfied immediately, this would lead to a proverbial birthmark (in the shape of the food) or crossed eyes, a punitive sign that not enough attention has been paid to a mother's desire. As commentators noticed, a penalty applied to all tenants of a building if a maternal craving caused by smelling food was not satisfied, illuminating the attention and care that should be reserved for pregnant women under Islamic rules [28].

The second peculiarity of Islamic commentaries is their emphasis on a less *permeable* view of heredity that somehow 'resembles' a contemporary understanding. Indeed, Islamic medieval commentators developed a specific understanding of heredity that sidelined the direct power of impression and instead highlighted how 'traits from distant relatives may skip generations and then suddenly appear in subsequent offspring' [22].

This is important to highlight to avoid a too-deterministic view of direct maternal effects as a ubiquitous monolith in pre-modern traditions. Besides medical advice such as the work of the Persian physician *Ali ibn Sahl Rabban al-Tabari* (d. 870) in his *Firdaws al-Hikma* (*Paradise of Wisdom*), similar notions can be found in the saying of the prophet Muhammad who explicitly advised fathers not to disown sons who look nothing like them because children frequently receive hereditary traits (*naj'a 'irq*) from distant ancestors, just as red camels oftentimes produce ashy-coloured offspring that resemble prior relatives [22]. This is less to attribute to the Prophet a Mendelian view of heredity and more to highlight sociological pressures to avoid a too-easy dismissal of paternal responsibility from men and hence the risk of disintegration of the family [22].

This is not to say that in medieval Islamic medicine there is no emphasis on and hence anxiety about direct environmental influences on the act of procreation and accordingly the quality of birth. Tenth-century embryological debates (Arıb ibn Sad (d. 980), in his *Kita̅b khalq al-janı̅n* (*Creation of the Embryo*)) are ripe with precautions about the presence of certain winds during coitus that may produce lazier or more delicate children, the importance of maternal and paternal mood at the moment of procreation (a happy soul strengthens the body, and a stronger body gives rise to more robust sperm), or avoiding intercourse with women who had refrained from sex for a long time [22]. Both Islamic and Jewish medical traditions present different interpretations of maternal impressions developing out of their specific religious contexts. A shared similarity is the importance placed on the various senses at the time of conception to optimise reproduction, and a framing within legal-theological debates, while references to licit and illicit sexual intercourse and a patriarchal anxiety to control female desire are in continuity with the Greco-Roman experience.

1.4 Eastern Medical Traditions and Fetal Education

Eastern medical traditions, such as Ayurveda in India and traditional Chinese and Japanese medicines, share similar albeit differing perspectives on the mother's ability to influence her child in the womb. Instead of a focus on maternal impressions as seen previously, however, these traditions developed the concept of 'fetal education' or the ability to educate or influence the child from within the womb. The ideas expressed in fetal education have strong roots in ancient texts and beliefs and work to create positive and avoid negative influences on the fetus. Both Ayurveda and Chinese medicine continue as traditional therapeutic medical systems today, unlike European humoralism discussed previously [30], and various forms of fetal education continue to be practiced contemporarily (see [31, 32]). While Ayurveda draws on Hindu moral ideas and a specific medical framework, Chinese and Japanese medicine share very similar resemblances and largely rely on Confucian doctrines.

1.4.1 Garbh Sanskar: Ayurvedic Education in the Womb

The concept of fetal education in Ayurveda is often evoked by the tragic hero Abhimanyu from the Indian classic the *Mahabharata*. In this epic, Abhimanyu learns how to enter an impenetrable city while within his mother's womb [33]. Hindu myths express ideas about maternal impressions during conception or even prior to conception (see [12]). In Ayurvedic medicine, *Garbh Sanskar*, commonly translated as 'education in the womb', prescribes a regime for both men and women to conceive and birth a healthy child. *Garbh Sanskar* interestingly has cited the preconception period as a key component to producing healthy children and advises a variety of purification procedures and timings to ensure good-quality progeny. The focus is not solely on women, and men are included in the procedures and are thought to play an important role in conception.

The classical text, the *Charaka Samhita* explains how at conception the embryo is created by three factors: the mother, the father, and 'the self' or 'life'. All three components are said to influence different organs and dispositions of the child [34]. Here, maternal and paternal health both play an important role before conception, and men are required to undertake actions to produce good-quality semen. Semen, in classical Ayurvedic medicine, is viewed as the 'highest essence' generated by the body [34]. Invoking an agricultural metaphor, the *Caraka Samihita* describes the need to prepare for pregnancy: 'As seed (of a plant) does not sprout if affected by improper time, water, worms, insects and fire, so is the defective semen of man' [35]. For women, menstrual blood plays a similar, but not equivalent, role to semen and is a generative fluid that unites with semen at conception [34]. After the time of conception, the focus shifts to the mother and her actions, behaviours, and nutrition.

1.4.2 Taijiao and Taikyō: Fetal Education in Chinese and Japanese Medicine

Classical Chinese medicine incorporates the cosmology of Yin and Yang. Yin is representative of qualities such as 'darkness, cold, moisture … the moon, the night and the feminine'. Yang is representative of the qualities of 'brightness, the sun, fire, warmth, activity and the masculine principle'. Yin and Yang were seen to regulate the bodily *qi* (fundamental energy) and any changes in the body [30]. In medieval China, the concept of fetal education reflected a particular interconnection between the womb and external stimuli. The sex of the child, for instance, was thought to be malleable during this indeterminate time, and the responsibility for the outcome rested upon the mother's conduct [30]. For instance, in Song Dynasty texts, such as the *Fu Ren Da Quan Liang Fang* (*A Great Complete Collection of Fine Formulas for Women*) (1237 CE), the mother's actions are described as impacting the attractiveness or intelligence of the child:

The child during the first trimester is called the initial fetus. This is the period during which the infant begins to be moulded. If a dignified and elegant stature is desire, the mother should think, speak, and act discretely. If a handsome offspring is wanted, she should wear a piece of jade. If a witty offspring is desired, she should read verses and poems. This is because the exterior reception communicates with the interior plasticity. [36]

Taijiao or 'fetal education' (literally *tai* [fetus] and *jiao* [to instruct]) has roots in the classical text the *Senior Dai's Book of Rites* (*Da Dai Liji*) and was later expanded upon by Liu Xiang (ca. 80–7 BCE), a Han Dynasty Confucian scholar, who claimed that the integrity of kings rested on the morality of their mothers [37]. It has been part of Chinese gynaecology for centuries and returned periodically to prominence at certain historical junctures of Chinese stories, such as the early Republican era from the 1910s. Often, the specific nature of training in the womb reflected the importance of moral transformation within Confucianism and the wider belief that the outside environment could influence the developing fetus. Here, the fetus is responsive to stimuli provided by the mother through her senses, behaviour, emotions, and environment. Taboos, such as not eating or looking at rabbits (which would result in the child developing a harelip), reflect the belief in the ability of the fetus to absorb outside stimuli and incorporate them physically into their own developing body [37].

The influence of the environment on the child is expanded in Japanese fetal education or *Taikyō* to include both parents and the wider society. *Taikyō* was introduced to Japan from China in the tenth century and, like Chinese medicine, was strongly influenced by Confucian ideas [38, 39]. In Japanese, *Taikyō* translates to 'womb teaching' and could be interpreted as teaching the pregnant woman or the fetus within the womb. Originally, the belief was that if a pregnant woman behaved appropriately, she would birth a man of great virtue [38]. Other texts such as the *Onna chōhōki* or *The Record of Women's Great Treasures*, written by Namura Jōhaku in seventeenth-century Japan, show the progression of these beliefs and give an insight into ideas of pregnancy during the Edo period. Namura's recommendations on *Taikyō* included wrapping the belly, prescribing types of food, and producing an ideal environment to bring about an uneventful birth and the health of the child [40].

1.5 Conclusion

Global history has emerged in the last two decades as an attempt to decentre Euro-Atlantic routes of trade, power, and science, as the main site of knowledge production [42]. Through a review of primary and secondary sources about maternal impression from the Mediterranean to China before the rise of modern science, in this chapter we have aimed to contribute to debates on the global history of the permeable body across different cultural and medical contexts. Focusing on a time where there is no techno-logical or scientific gap between East and West is particularly fertile because it avoids the narrative of the diffusion of Western science. It suggests instead circulation, 'connected histories', and networks of exchange across Afro-Eurasia [43, 44]. As the following chapter will show, the trope of maternal impression declined with the rise of modern science, and genetics in particular, but not the emphasis on the maternal body as a site for optimising reproduction and monitoring a mother's behaviour before and during pregnancy. Eighteenth-century embryological debates [41, 45], the rise of 'pre-natal culture' in nineteenth-century European science [46], and more recently, the growing interest in mother–fetal interaction and maternal 'imprint' [51] can undoubtedly be linked with several immediate causes in medical, scientific, and technological changes. In particular, the last half-century changes in Euro-American biomedicine have led to a new visibility and agency of the fetus within a technologically transparent maternal body [47–50]. This chapter has aimed to show that whatever their present iterations and more immediate genealogies, contemporary postgenomic findings – and their related notions of risk, responsibility, gendering of biological knowledge, and blame or optimisation – are not solely a modern invention and have a much wider global and historical resonance. Contemporary scientific labs did not emerge in a historical vacuum but are embedded in sociocultural contexts in which pre-comprehensions of the maternal body as uniquely transparent and impressionable, and hence subject to control and governance, have a long prehistory.

A good example of the persistence and hybridisation of *longue durée* beliefs with contemporary science comes from India. Newspaper articles have reported on specialised ashram-style clinics that have claimed to use the practice of *Garbh Sanskar* not only to help parents conceive and produce healthy children but to also perfect the reproduction process. Some institutions claim that they can help couples produce the 'perfect progeny' or even 'upgrade' or 'repair' dysfunctional genes [31]. It has been suggested that by utilising the knowledge and practices of *Garbh Sanskar*, epigenetic programming can take place and help create healthier offspring [52]. Articles have likened the practice to a modern version of 'genetic engineering' [31]. The practice of *Garbh Sanskar* has also found space in the digital sphere in India with apps, online workshops, webinars, and music advertised to help women increase the likelihood of producing healthy and intelligent children. These trading zones exemplify the globalisation and commercialisation of traditional medical knowledge and ideas about the pre-pregnant and pregnant body. The example of Garbh Sanskar illuminates how the circulation of epigenetic ideas across the world is neither uniform nor bound by bioscience and can be adapted and entangled with pre-existing notions of maternal imprinting and responsibility. As DOHaD develops and expands globally, these entanglements will become important to assess how epigenetic knowledge is being (re)produced in localised contexts. An invitation to look at history not just as a succession of novel discoveries but also as the long-term accretion and sedimentation of mentalities across a long historical time will be helpful for DOHaD scholars and practitioners to situate their work in context.

References

1. Kukla R. Mass Hysteria: Medicine, Culture, and Mothers' Bodies. Lanham: Rowman & Littlefield Publishers; 2005.

2. Hanson MA, Low FM, Gluckman PD. Epigenetic Epidemiology: The Rebirth of Soft Inheritance. Ann Nutr Metab. 2011;58(Suppl. 2):8–15.

3. Kirmayer L. Toward a Medicine of the Imagination. New Lit Hist. 2006 Jun 1;37:583–601.

4. Zambelli P. The Spéculum Astronomiae and Its Enigma: Astrology, Theology and Science in Albertus Magnus and His Contemporaries. Berlin: Springer; 1992. 352 p. (Boston studies in the philosophy of science).

5. al-Kindi Adamson P. In: Zalta EN, editor. The Stanford Encyclopedia of Philosophy [Internet]. Spring 2020. Metaphysics Research Lab, Stanford University; 2020 [cited 2022 Mar 29]. Available from: https://plato.stanford.edu/archives/spr2020/entries/al-kindi/

6. Helen King. Hippocrates' Woman : Reading the Female Body in Ancient Greece [Internet]. London: Routledge;

1998 [cited 2021 Oct 27]. Available from: https://search.ebscohost.com/login.aspx?direct=true&db=e000xww&AN=60796&site=eds-live&scope=site

7. Leigh R. On Theriac to Piso, Attributed to Galen: A Critical Edition with Translation and Commentary [Internet]. Leiden: Brill; 2015 [cited 2022 Apr 4]. Available from: https://brill.com/view/title/32249

8. Aquinas T. The Essential Aquinas: Writings on Philosophy, Religion, and Society [Internet]. Westport: Greenwood Publishing Group; 2002 [cited 2022 Mar 29]. 248 p. Available from: www.abc-clio.com/products/c6853c/

9. Albertus Resnick IM. On the Causes of the Properties of the Elements: Albert the Great [Internet]. Milwaukee: Marquette University Press; 2010 [cited 2022 Mar 29]. Available from: https://public.ebookcentral.proquest.com/choice/publicfullrecord.aspx?p=688676

10. Temkin O, editor. Soranus' Gynecology. Baltimore: Johns Hopkins University; 1991.

11. Tucker HA. Birth Defects before Epigenesis. Clin Genet. 2008 Oct;74(4):338–42.

12. Doniger W, Spinner G. Misconceptions: Female Imaginations and Male Fantasies in Parental Imprinting. Daedalus. 1998;127(1):97–129.

13. Paré A. On Monsters and Marvels [Internet]. Chicago: University of Chicago Press; 1982 [cited 2022 Mar 29]. 256 p. Available from: https://press.uchicago.edu/ucp/books/book/chicago/O/bo37629686.html

14. Hirai H. Imagination, Maternal Desire and Embryology in Thomas Fienus. In: Manning G, Klestinec C, editors. Professors, Physicians and Practices in the History of Medicine: Essays in Honor of Nancy Siraisi [Internet]. Cham: Springer International Publishing; 2017 [cited 2022 Mar 29]. pp. 239–53. Available from: https://doi.org/10.1007/978-3-319-56514-9_11

15. Pagel W. Paracelsus: An Introduction to Philosophical Medicine in the Era of the Renaissance [Internet]. Basel: Karger Medical and Scientific Publishers; 1982 [cited 2022 Apr 4]. Available from: www.karger.com/Book/Home/220262

16. Huet MH. Monstrous Imagination. Cambridge: Harvard University Press; 1993. 334 p.

17. Smith JEH, editor. The Problem of Animal Generation in Early Modern Philosophy [Internet]. Cambridge: Cambridge University Press; 2006 [cited 2022 Apr 4]. (Cambridge Studies in Philosophy and Biology). Available from: www.cambridge.org/core/books/problem-of-animal-generation-in-early-modern-philosophy/36676015DD931A09A6843FF972240E0D

18. De Renzi S. Resemblance, Paternity and Imagination in Early Modern Courts. In: Mueller-Wille S, Rheinberger HJ, editors. Heredity Produced: At the Crossroads of Biology, Politics, and Culture, 1500–1870 [Internet]. Cambridge, MA, USA: The MIT Press; 2007 [cited 2022 Apr 4]. pp. 61–83. Available from: http://mitpress.mit.edu/catalog/item/default.asp?ttype=2&tid=11164

19. Sharp J. The Midwives Book, or, The Whole Art of Midwifery Discovered: Directing Childbearing Women how to Behave Themselves in Their Conception, Breeding, Bearing, and Nursing of Children in Six Books. London: Simon Miller; 1671. 370 p.

20. Shildrick M. Embodying the Monster: Encounters with the Vulnerable Self [Internet]. Thousand Oaks: SAGE Publications; 2001 [cited 2022 Mar 29]. Available from: www.123library.org/book_details/?id=646

21. The Holy Bible. New international version. [Internet]. Hodder and Stoughton; 1979. Available from: https://search.ebscohost.com/login.aspx?direct=true&AuthType=sso&db=cat00097a&AN=deakin.b1069813&authtype=sso&custid=deakin&site=eds-live&scope=site

22. Kueny K. Marking the Body: Resemblance and Medieval Muslim Constructions of Paternity. J Fem Stud Relig. 2014;30(1):65–84.

23. Midrash Rabbah. Numbers IX. Stricker; 1669.

24. Preuss J. Biblical and Talmudic Medicine. J. Aronson. 1993; Lanham, MD.

25. Farber Z. Maternal Impressions: From Sheep to Humans – TheTorah.com [Internet]. TheTorah.com. 2013 [cited 2022 Mar 31]. Available from: www .thetorah.com/article/maternal-impressions-from-sheep-to-humans

26. Barilan YM. Jewish Bioethics: Rabbinic Law and Theology in their Social and Historical Contexts. Cambridge, UK: Cambridge University Press; 2014. 297 p.

27. Bos G. The Medical Works of Moses Maimonides: New English Translations Based on the Critical Editions of the Arabic Manuscripts [Internet]. Boston, MA: Brill; 2021 [cited 2022 Mar 31]. Available from: http://ebookcentral .proquest.com/lib/deakin/detail.action? docID=6811470

28. Kruk R. Pregnancy and Its Social Consequences in Mediaeval and Traditional Arab Society. Quad Studi Arabi. 1987;5(6):418–30.

29. Amster EJ. Harem Medicine and the Sleeping Child: Law, Traditional Pharmacology, and the Gender of Medical Authority. In: Ellen J. Amster, editor Medicine and the Saints: Science, Islam, and the Colonial Encounter in Morocco, 1877–1956 [Internet]. Austin: University of Texas Press; 2021. pp. 142–73. Available from: https://doi.org/10.7560/745445-008

30. Furth C. A Flourishing Yin: Gender in China's Medical History: 960–1665. Berkeley: University of California Press; 1999. 374 p.

31. Garbh Sanskar. Baby by Choice, Not by Chance [Internet]. *Hindustan Times*. 2019 [cited 2020 Apr 1]. Available from: www.hindustantimes.com/cities/garbh-sanskar-baby-by-choice-not-by-chance/story-ZnBSjsaBHAerOTh15kOBUI.html

32. Sleeboom-Faulkner M. Eugenic Birth and Fetal Education: The friction between lineage enhancement and premarital testing among rural households in mainland China. China J. 2010;(64):121–41.

33. Smith John D. The Mahabharata [Internet]. Varanasi, UP, India: Penguin; 2009 [cited 2022 Mar 18]. (Penguin Classics). Available from: www.booktopia .com.au/the-mahabharata-john-d-smith/book/9780140446814.html

34. Wujastyk D. The Roots of Ayurveda. London: Penguin Publishing Group; 2003. 454 p.

35. Samhita Caraka. *Caraka Samhita.* Translated by PV Sharma. 4th ed. Varanasi: Chaukhambha Orientalia, India; 1998.

36. Flaws B. A Handbook of Traditional Chinese Gynecology. Boulder, CO: Blue Poppy Enterprises, Inc.; 1987. 260 p.

37. Richardson N. The Nation in Utero: Translating the Science of Fetal Education in Republican China. Front Hist China. 2012 Mar 1;7(1):4–31.

38. Yoshino A. How Was It in Mummy's Tummy?": Japanese Pregnancy Literature. Womens Stud Int Forum. 2008 Nov;31 (6):483–91.

39. Kamata H. Japanese Childbirth and Childcare [Nihonjin no Koumi Kosodate]. Tokyo: Keiso Shoboh; 1990.

40. Tanimura R, Chart D. The Record of Women's Great Treasures: Pregnancy and Childbirth in the Edo Period: A Translation of Volume Three of Onna chōhōki. Asiat Stud – Études Asiat. 2017 May 1;71(2):545–66.

41. Fischer-Homberger E. On the Medical History of the Doctrine of Imagination. Psychol Med. 1979 Nov;9(4):619–28.

42. Berg M. Writing the History of the Global. Oxford: Oxford University; 2013.

43. Subrahmanyam S. Connected Histories: Notes towards a Reconfiguration of Early Modern Eurasia. Modern Asian Studies. 1997 Jul;31(3):735–62.

44. Raj K. Beyond Postcolonialism . . . and Postpositivism: Circulation and the Global History of Science. Isis. 2013 Jun 1;104(2):337–47.

45. Epstein J. The Pregnant Imagination, Fetal Rights, and Women's Bodies: A Historical Inquiry. Yale J Law Humanit. 2013 May 8;7(1):139–62.

46. Arni C. The Prenatal: Contingencies of Procreation and Transmission in the Nineteenth Century. In: Brandt C, Müller-Wille S, editors. Heredity Explored: Between Public Domain and Experimental Science 1850–1930 [Internet]. Cambridge MA: MIT Press; 2016 [cited 2022 Apr 4]. pp. 285–309. Available from: http://edoc.unibas.ch/43812/

47. Dubow S. Ourselves Unborn: A History of the Fetus in Modern America. 1st edition. Oxford; New York: Oxford University Press; 2010. 320 p.

48. Buklijas T. Histories and Meanings of Epigenetics. In: Meloni M, Cromby J, Fitzgerald D, Lloyd S, editors. The Palgrave Handbook of Biology and Society [Internet]. London: Palgrave Macmillan UK; 2018 [cited 2020 Jul 13]. pp. 167–87. Available from: https://doi.org/10.1057/978-1-137-52879-7_8

49. Löwy I. Imperfect Pregnancies: A History of Birth Defects and Prenatal Diagnosis [Internet]. Baltimore: Johns Hopkins University Press; 2017 [cited 2022 Apr 22]. Available from: https://muse.jhu.edu/book/55867

50. Waggoner MR. The Zero Trimester: Pre-Pregnancy Care and the Politics of Reproductive Risk [Internet]. Oakland: University of California Press; 2017 [cited 2021 Sep 16]. Available from: https://search.ebscohost.com/login.aspx?direct=true&db=e000xww&AN=1571292&site=eds-live&scope=site

51. Richardson SS. The Maternal Imprint: The Contested Science of Maternal–Fetal Effects. Chicago: University of Chicago Press; 2021. 319 p.

52. Londhe D, Chinchalkar S, Kaushik R, Prakash O. Garbha Samskar: Ayurveda Way of Epigenetic Programming. J Res Ayurvedic Sci. 2018 Jul 9(2):42–49

Transformations of the Maternal–Fetal Relationship in the Twentieth Century

From Maternal Impressions to Epigenetic States

Tatjana Buklijas

2.1 Introduction

During the 1960s and 1970s, a new understanding of the fetus emerged at the intersection of demographic changes: high fertility and reduced infant mortality in the 'baby boom' era; new medical visual technologies and the expansion of mass media; and the rise of the feminist movement and the liberalisation of abortion. These social shifts spurred scholarly and lay interest in public representations and private perceptions of the fetus [1–4], the rise of the fetus as a subject [5, 6], the politics of abortion [7], and the uses of fetal bodies in research [3, 8]. A century ago, scholars argued that the mother and the fetus were one; maternal experiences 'imprinted' the malleable fetus and maternal testimony was central to the understanding of pregnancy until the hidden fetus was revealed at birth. But starting in the nineteenth century and especially during recent decades, an increasingly visible and autonomous fetus has emerged, the mother has been erased from the picture, and the experience of pregnancy has come to be more contingent and technologically mediated.

This compelling and broad narrative glosses over subtler shifts in the way that the fetus, the mother, and, especially, the relationship between them have been conceptualised. And yet, a closer look at medical and scientific literature shows that over the course of the twentieth century, the maternal–fetal relationship has been reinterpreted and redrawn multiple times. For this chapter, I have used published sources from diverse medical and scientific disciplines, such as obstetrics, fetal physiology, evolutionary biology, developmental science, and epigenetics, to draw attention to the changing ways in which the maternal–fetal relationship has been understood. This close reading has helped me uncover underlying assumptions – shifting and competing even within a single discipline – that fed into scientific and clinical research. For example, in the 1960s, physiologists who stressed fetal autonomy when describing fetuses as lone mountaineers and astronauts also worked on questions related to the fetal control of processes within

This chapter is reprinted from T Buklijas, Transformations of the maternal–fetal relationship in the twentieth century: From maternal impressions to epigenetic states. In: U Helduser, B Dohm, eds. *Imaginations of the Unborn: Cultural Concepts of Prenatal Imprinting from the Early Modern Period to the Present.* Heidelberg, Winter, 2018; 213–234. We thank the publisher for permission to reprint it in this volume.

the fetal and maternal bodies, such as the onset of labour and fetal growth. The diverse assumptions, metaphors, and research questions tell us something about changing social views of and attitudes towards motherhood, pregnancy, and the relationship between the mother and the fetus, including and especially maternal influences on the developing organism.

Covering the long twentieth century, I have identified several key concepts and periods: the abandoning of maternal impressions, strong hereditarianism, and the fetus as the parasite in the early decades of the twentieth century, the era dominated by eugenics; the 'maternal effects' of the mid-twentieth century, when concerns over adequate nutrition and trauma of long-standing effect that emerged around the Second World War supported the idea of the 'critical' or 'sensitive' periods and revived interest in maternal influences; the autonomous fetus of the 1960s and 1970s civil rights movement era followed by the selfish fetus imagined by evolutionary biologists of later decades of the twentieth century; ending with the latest rapprochement between the mother and the fetus supported by developmental approaches and epigenetics. While it may be tempting to regard this latest development as a return of maternal impressions, I want to show that similarities are superficial: the fetal–maternal relationship was redrawn according to new rules, and it cannot be fully understood without insight into its recent history.

2.2 The Fetal Parasite

Well into the 1800s, the developing organism was seen to be malleable by external influences, and the mother was both the mediator and the source of these cues. Anything the mother ate, saw, touched, or even imagined, collectively known as maternal imagination or maternal impression, was understood to have the capacity to affect the child [9, 10]. Yet during the nineteenth century, this close bond between the mother and the fetus was broken. The concept of heredity, which reduced the mother to little more than a passive vessel transmitting elements collected from previous generations to the offspring, first appeared in the early decades of the nineteenth century and quickly gained popularity [11]. In the 1880s, the German biologist August Weismann explained how heredity worked using the tools of experimental biology [12]. According to Weismann, 'germplasm' (preserved in the germline but unfolding its potential in the body during development) was resistant to influences exerted by 'soma', so changes in somatic cells had no effect on the germline. While Weismann did allow the possibility of direct environmental influence on the germ cells, scholars who followed in his footsteps by and large reduced development to a robust pre-programmed sequence of stages. Influences received in development, unless extreme to the point of threatening maternal or fetal survival, were secondary to heredity.

Weismann's work had a major impact outside academic biology. The early twentieth century is usually seen as the high point of eugenics, a broad movement that distilled nineteenth-century concerns over rapid socio-economic change into modernist visions of society reformed through rational reproduction [13, 14]. Eugenics preceded the cellular explanation of heredity: it relied, initially, on the mid-century concept of degeneration, whereby 'organic' and social factors acted on the organism to produce a reverse evolution, cumulative over generations, taking a lineage to a downhill slope of no return [15]. Weismann's work provided it with scientific cachet.

So if we take that strong hereditarianism saw the mother as a passive vessel, rather than an active agent in the formation of the new organism and the mediator of external influences, then the appeal of the model taken from another cutting-edge scientific discipline of the period, parasitology – the relationship between a parasite and its host – begins to make sense. The parasite depended on its host for shelter and food but was also remarkably protected from the fluctuations in the host's circumstances and environment, even if the host itself suffered. Accordingly, the fetus was understood to thrive in all except the most extreme circumstances, with maternal homeostatic mechanisms maintaining environmental factors at a near-constant level and the placenta providing protection from many noxious substances [16, 17]. Yet, for the mother, the pregnancy could be precarious, as 'the increasing demands of the parasitic fetus will make the diet deficient for the mother' [18, p. 1].

There were traces of the idea of the parasitic fetus in earlier times: in the eighteenth century, Denis Diderot wrote in his *Eléments de physiologie* that 'the child is at all times an inconvenient guest for the womb' and described delivery as 'a sort of vomiting' [19, p. 406]. However, it was not until the turn of the twentieth century that the idea gained full prominence. Scientists travelled across colonial empires to study the life cycles of organisms causing frightening diseases, such as malaria and sleeping sickness, killing people, and damaging imperial economies. The idea of the parasite was engrained in public imaginations. It was also politically helpful: as civilians faced severe food shortages in the First World War, reassurances that the fetus (as well as the infant/ lactating mother) would be unaffected by maternal starvation might have been seen as comforting [20].

Yet there were voices critical of strong hereditarianism. Some came from relatively marginal movements such as prenatal culturism, associated with theosophy and drawing on the notion of prenatal impressions. It argued that heredity could be influenced by a pregnant woman's thoughts and behaviour, and thus those had to be controlled [5]. Others were mainstream physicians. They used examples of conditions such as congenital syphilis to argue against a sharp distinction between hereditary and communicable (environmentally caused) diseases [21]. The best known among them was the Edinburgh obstetrician John William Ballantyne, who gave teratology – the science of collecting and studying births with congenital abnormalities – clinical significance and reinvented it as antenatal pathology [22, 23]. For Ballantyne, the maternal body provided the immediate point of medical and research interest as 'we can only reach the unborn infant through the mother who carries him, and so the pre-natal life and the life of the woman in pregnancy are closely bound together and depend one upon the other' [24, p. x]. Indeed, he defined the relationship between the mother and the child in the following manner: 'although he [the infant] is hidden from sight in the womb of his mother, he is not beyond the influences of her environment, nay, her body is his immediate environment' [24, p. xii].

The rise of hereditarianism through the nineteenth and early twentieth centuries thus influenced the view of the maternal–fetal relationship. The concept of maternal impressions, or indeed any influences received from or through the mother, was relegated to second place, after heredity. 'The mother marks her infant, not with the fanciful imagery of birthmarks, but with the ancestral tendencies,' wrote a Chicago professor of obstetrics in this period [25]. But as the narrow notion of heredity was forged around 1900, the notion of prenatal or antenatal came into being [26]. This new concept accounted for the contingencies of conception, gestation, embryogenesis, birth, and breastfeeding, now disconnected from heredity [27].

2.3 Critical Periods

'The existence of a profusion of myths and superstitions has probably somewhat inhibited until modern times scientific thought and investigation into maternal–fetal relationships from the standpoint of how fetal development may be influenced by varying maternal factors. During the last twenty years, however, many facts and some very interesting hypotheses accumulated in the literature of various fields',

wrote the American physician Lester Sontag, who between the 1930s and 1960s studied the ways in which cues received during development – from maternal nutrition to emotional states – influenced the offspring [16, p. 996]. By the 1930s, eugenics was in retreat: in the increasingly unstable political-economic climate, the impact of environment, physical as well as social, on human health and disease could not be ignored. Genetics, an experimental discipline studying mechanisms and rules of heredity, had matured since the early 1900s, and its specialists criticised harshly what they perceived as eugenics' sloppy grasp of genetic concepts and research methods [28]. During the economic depression and in the shadow of the looming war, concerns about feeding human and animal populations in the likely conditions of severe shortage occupied politicians as well as scientists [29]. Those who subscribed to the notion of the parasitic fetus worried that poorly nourished mothers would perish under the demands of pregnancy. Others argued that in a malnourished mother, the growth and development of the fetus would suffer too. While food was seen as a prime example of outside exposures impinging upon the developing organism, other influences – microorganisms, toxins, but also maternal emotional states – came under the scrutiny of experimental and clinical scientists.

Throughout the 1930s, nutritionists and physicians, faced with deprivations caused by economic depression, studied the impact of maternal undernutrition on the offspring of cohorts of working-class women, but the results were negative or inconclusive [30, 31]. In the Second World War, however, large civilian populations suffered sieges and blockades of food shipments, providing scientists with 'natural experiments': previously well-fed women exposed to severe famines of limited duration [32]. Early findings came from the Leningrad siege, between September 1941 and January 1944, during which the urban civilian population experienced prolonged and severe famine [33]; smaller but more precise data came from Western Holland during the German siege between September 1944 and May 1945, in what became known as the Dutch Winter Famine [34]. Data showed that if the mother starved around conception, then the fetus had a greater chance of being miscarried or born malformed, and if famine struck in the last months of pregnancy, the baby was likely to be born small and light.

Wartime observations were carried forward into the lean post-war years: the British scientist Elsie Widdowson studied the birthweight of babies and milk production in hospitals, as well as the growth of children fed small and monotone food rations in orphanages in war-ravaged Germany [29]. She found that not just food but also emotions affected children's growth: children living in an orphanage directed by a strict matron lagged behind their peers raised in an institution run by a kind person [35]. Back in Cambridge laboratories, Widdowson and her collaborator Professor Robert McCance transformed clinical observations into hypotheses for experimental animal studies: they manipulated maternal nutrition and the size of the litter (which determined the amount of mother's milk received by each pup) to test how undernutrition during pregnancy and early postnatal period affects the offspring's growth and development. They found that the impact was permanent, making adult animals smaller, more prone to infections, and even changing their facial structure.

Widdowson's research supported the notion of 'critical periods' that emerged across disciplines in the 1930s and 1940s, most importantly in teratology, behavioural studies, and fetal physiology, to describe the relationship between chronological time and developmental milestones. Teratology in this period transformed from a museological discipline engaged in collecting and classifying malformed births into an experimental science that sought to explain how certain noxious agents – especially microorganisms such as the rubella virus and certain toxins – acting at well-defined developmental stages produced specific effects [36]. Other studies explored how the lack or excess of physiological substances, such as vitamins or hormones, could influence development.

Hormones offered a way to explain a problem of long-standing concern: how maternal emotional states influence the psychological set-up of the child. In the late nineteenth century, France Charles Féré had argued that external stimuli, such as loud sounds or maternal emotions, caused uterine contractions, which in turn stimulated the fetus to move [27]. Féré based his argument on the observations made on a cohort of children born to women who had suffered from 'mental shocks' while pregnant during the siege of Paris, 1870/71 [37]. In the 1940s, Lester Sontag observed a connection between increased fetal movement and fetal weight gain [38]. Heightened fetal activity, he claimed, was caused by maternal emotional states, which were then transmitted to the fetus by hormones such as adrenaline. And while loud noises and maternal fatigue did increase fetal activity, these (intermittent) factors were less significant than maternal emotional states. Sontag published cases, such as that of a mother with a 'religious and moralistic' background who during pregnancy learnt about her husband's infidelity. Her 'almost continual emotional turbulence' resulted in an 'extremely active' fetus and, finally, a short and light infant. In another case, the father developed a psychosis during the fifth month of the mother's pregnancy, causing her to live in constant apprehension of physical violence and worry about her husband's health as well as their future as a family. The infant was light for its length and 'extremely active and irritable' [38, p. 629].

While just a few decades earlier, the focus was on fetal resistance to changes in the maternal environment, the decline of eugenics, experiences of economic depression, and especially war moved the emphasis onto the ways in which the fetus was sensitive to its environment. I have argued elsewhere how broader social concerns with recovery from early trauma – nutritional, emotional, and psychological – so pertinent in post-war Europe provided the background to the idea of sensitive periods [29]. While the idea of the fetus as a parasite did not quite go away, the concept of pregnancy as a plastic, open state and the fetus in constant exchange and communication with the environment gained currency.

2.4 The Autonomous Fetus

In 1965, the prestigious Life magazine published a series of photographs by the Swedish photographer Lennart Nilsson, documenting human development over the nine months of pregnancy [39]. These photographs were hailed as the unprecedented celebration of the 'drama of life before birth'. Nilsson's images, showing the childlike fetal form floating on the 'starry sky' background, without the maternal body anywhere in sight, signalised the new status of the fetus as an autonomous being. The growing distinction between mother and fetus was evident everywhere: in the way that the fetuses were portrayed in the media, for lay audiences, but also in textbooks and research papers; in their acquisition of the status of the patient in their own right; and in the language used to talk about them. By the 1960s, society was no longer preoccupied with survival and war trauma but rather with questions of identity, subjectivity, and agency. Could it be that the severance of the umbilical cord in the representation of fetuses reflected a broader social shift?

The use of fetal images has been extensively studied in the context of feminist history (visual), politics of abortion, as well as the broader political and social history of this period [1, 2, 40]. Nilsson's photographs – the most famous and best studied – were created within a gynaecological campaign in Sweden to restrict the abortion law and published in a popular colour magazine to entertain and educate its audience; in the 1970s, they were recruited by the growing pro-life movement in the United States to teach its prospective supporters about the 'humanity' of the fetus. And in addition to Nilsson's vivid images, pro-life advocates could also draw on less attractive yet increasingly ubiquitous ultrasound scans. By the 1970s, ultrasound technology, first developed in the 1950s, had become a standard part of antenatal medicine.[1]

Historians of medicine have noted that the deployment and popularity of fetal images corresponded with the emergence of the fetus as a patient in its own right. The increased prosperity of the post-Second World War and the rise of public healthcare systems worldwide meant that more women than ever were receiving antenatal care. Yet with improved control of infectious disease and better socioeconomic conditions, both maternal and infant mortality – at least in the developed world – were falling. The medical focus now turned to relatively rare cases of congenital anomalies, prematurity, and conditions that developed in pregnancy. In this period, a leading obstetrical scientist, William Liley, pioneered a therapy targeted at the fetus to treat the hitherto incurable fetal haemolytic disease, which emerged when the mother, who did not have Rh antigen on her red blood cells, developed antibodies to the Rh antigen-bearing red blood cells of the fetus [43]. Under ultrasonic guidance, Liley performed a blood transfusion into the fetal belly – a method previously done only on children. Liley's work marked the beginning of the field of fetal medicine, which in the following decades gave rise to the highly precarious and controversial area of fetal surgery [6].

The obstetricians' increased interest in the fetus and their positioning as fetal, rather than maternal, advocates became sharply evident as the debate over the legalisation of abortion deepened in the late 1960s and 1970s. Around that time, many countries liberalised their abortion laws, but the debate continued, and obstetricians frequently stood on the 'conservative' side, against the liberal laws. Ian Donald was a prominent opponent of the legalisation of voluntary abortion and a campaigner against the 1967 Abortion Act, and he employed vivid images produced by the ultrasound technology that he had pioneered in anti-abortion campaigns. Even when his campaign failed and Britain legalised abortion, he continued to fight elsewhere, for example taking his images to Italy that in the late 1970s was in the swing of the anti-abortion debate [42, p. 243]. At the same time, alarmed by the developments in Britain, William Liley

---

[1] Roentgen was employed to visualise the fetus, but its use was limited to the skeleton and to the fetuses with sufficiently calcified skeleton to permit X-ray visualisation, so usually from the second trimester onwards. But the use of X-rays became tainted with danger, especially after Hiroshima and Nagasaki, and the final blow was a 1956 study showing that children X-rayed as fetuses had a higher risk of childhood cancer [41, 42].

launched the Society for the Protection of the Unborn Children (SPUC) in New Zealand in 1970. In contrast to most other pro-life activists, Liley was not religious but rather held a firm belief that the fetus is a being independent of its mother, 'our new individual' residing in a 'suitable host' [5, p. 114]. Yet while fetal advocacy in matters of abortion prohibition produced little in the way of results, in other areas, fetuses increasingly came to be seen as needing legal protection from the actions of their mothers [5]. From the 1970s onwards, especially in the United States, conflicts between fetal rights and the rights of women – as patients, workers, and citizens – steadily increased.

One aspect of the increasing visibility of the fetus that has hitherto been little studied is how scientists – rather than practising obstetricians – viewed the fetus. Examining their language and research topics reveals a clear shift towards the autonomous fetus. Starting from the 1960s, science books and articles no longer described the fetus as a passive parasite but rather as a fearless pioneer in extreme conditions. Metaphors drew on new technologies of ocean, space, and land exploration, calling the fetus a submarine sailor, 'a weightless astronaut in utero' [44, p. 307], or a mountaineer. At the time when Edward Hilary and Sherpa Tenzing captured the public imagination by 'conquering' Mount Everest, the fetal environment began to be described as 'Mount Everest in utero' [45]. From the 1960s until 1990, scientists met at conferences tellingly titled 'Foetal autonomy', 'The fetus and independent life', and 'Foetal autonomy and adaptation' [46–48]. Indeed, the introduction to the 1969 Foetal Autonomy Conference Proceedings said that 'it [the fetus] demonstrates its innate capacity for influencing its external and maintaining its internal environment – that is, its autonomy' [47, p. 1].

The language of fetal autonomy closely corresponded to the type of research questions that interested scientists in this period. In the 1940s and 1950s, McCance and Widdowson experimented with maternal nutrition and the size of the litter to show how the antenatal environment shaped development before and after birth. In contrast, in the 1960s and 1970s, the focus moved from external influences to the ways in which the fetus controlled its development. Research methods were developed – named chronic preparation or chronic method – that allowed precise monitoring of physiological parameters throughout the course of pregnancy, using electrodes and catheters inserted into the pregnant animal [49]. And, indeed, the fetus seemed remarkably autonomous. It could regulate its sleep patterns and its behaviour. It moved, and it appeared to breathe. It oversaw its growth through a finely balanced cascade of hormones [50]. But its agency did not stop at the boundaries of the fetal body: the fetus was also seen to 'participate in, or is responsible for, the sequence of events that ends in its birth' because 'it would be a logical feature of reproductive design if the initiation (of labour) were under fetal control, so that the other systems necessary for postnatal survival were normally mature before birth. In this sense fetal autonomy would be a necessary feature of development' [51]. Testifying before the US Congress in support of pro-life legislation, William Liley described the fetus as being 'very much in charge of the pregnancy'. The fetus, it seemed, was in control.

2.5 Neighbours at Odds

The idea of the fetus as a cosmonaut or a mountaineer implied agency and self-sufficiency. But scientists and physicians went even further: the feminist historian Ann Oakley quoted from Frank Hytten's 1976 obstetrics textbook, describing the fetus as an egoist and by no means an endearing and helpless little dependent as his [*sic*] mother may fondly think. As soon as he has plugged himself into the uterine wall, he sets out to make certain that his needs are met, regardless of any inconvenience he may cause. He does this by almost completely altering the mother's physiology, usually by fiddling with her control mechanism [41].

This 'selfish fetus' could not help itself: it was a machine governed by its selfish genes. The 1970s and 1980s were the heyday of the disciplines of sociobiology and evolutionary psychology. They explained behaviour – human and animal – using the mid-twentieth-century 'superdiscipline' of Modern Synthesis. Modern Synthesis was Darwin's theory of evolution by natural selection unified with population and experimental genetics [52]. Evolution was defined as a change in the allele (gene) frequency, and although the evolutionary environment acted upon the phenotype of the whole organism, it was the passage of the gene across generations that mattered.

And genes, as suggested persuasively in the title of Richard Dawkins' famous book, were selfish [53]. They looked after their own interests using the organism as a convenient vehicle to ferry them around, meet prospective mates, and secure survival for the next generation. One was fond of his or her parents because they shared 50 per cent of their genes but cared progressively less for his or her siblings, half-siblings, and cousins, as the percentage of shared genes dropped [54]. In 1974, the American sociobiologist Robert L. Trivers built on this concept to explain the apparent conflict over resources arising between parents and their children [55]. According to him, children demand more from their parents than the latter are willing to give because their evolutionary interests differ: individual children want all of their parents' attention (and food), yet parents have other – extant or future – children to consider. Trivers supported his hypothesis with data on the social behaviour of mammals, mostly around the time of weaning. The young aggressively demanded more food and care than their parents, who wanted to reserve their energy for other or future offspring, were willing to give.

Trivers' model met enthusiastic reception among evolutionary biologists. Steven Pinker saw the conflict as 'inherent to the human condition' [56]. Richard Dawkins described Trivers' model of parent–offspring conflict as 'brilliant' [53, p. 127]. At the same time, behavioural scientists criticised Trivers: in many species, the offspring weaned itself, while in others mothers responded to its requests. But the model remained popular. It inspired the Harvard evolutionary biologist David Haig to extend it to pregnancy and development, arguing that the mother and the child each have their own interest in mind; interests that are partially aligned (because they share 50 per cent of their genes) but substantially differ (because the remaining 50 per cent is different). Pregnancy, in Haig's view, was not a romantic alliance of 'one body and one flesh, a single harmonious unit in which conflicts of interest are impossible' – a perspective that, according to Haig, was the received view. But neither was it correct to see the mother and the fetus locked in a relationship where 'the fetus is an alien intruder within its mother's body: a parasite whose sole concern for its host is to ensure an uninterrupted supply of nutrients' [57, p. 226]. Rather, he likened this 'most intimate human relationship' to a constant negotiation, 'a tug-of-war' where 'two teams attempt to shift a flag a small distance either way, yet there is high tension in the rope and the system would collapse if either side stopped pulling' [58, p. 496].

Haig first applied the parent–offspring conflict concept to development and pregnancy to explain the phenomenon of genomic imprinting, in which for some genes only the maternal (or paternal) copy is expressed, while the copy that came from the other parent is silenced [59]. Because the mammalian mother is equally related to all of her offspring, her interests are best served by controlling resource allocation to her offspring, making sure as many survive as possible; but because the father of the fetus in the current pregnancy may not also father a future fetus or litter, it is in his interest to promote the growth of this particular fetus [60]. The hypothesis was persuasively supported by the insulin growth factor 2 (IGF2) system, in which the growth factor (promoting growth) was paternally expressed as the growth factor receptor (controlling growth) was maternally expressed. But Haig soon expanded his concept to other aspects of pregnancy, in the first place the communication between the mother and the fetus by means of chemical messages through hormones [61]. In Haig's words, this communication was a devious game played by both sides to advance their own interests: 'a response that is beneficial for a sender need not be beneficial for the responder, and vice versa' [61, p. 358]. Mothers were 'able to extract some information from placental hormones' [61, p. 374], yet placental hormones were 'fetal attempts to manipulate maternal metabolism for fetal benefit' [61, p. 357].

While Haig's hypothesis of placental hormones as tools of fetal subterfuge has remained without empirical support, the concept of maternal–fetal relationship as a state of unresolved conflict has held much attraction. For instance, clinical researchers have used it widely – moving slickly from selfish genes to selfish organisms and back – to explain various pathological phenomena of pregnancy, such as gestational hypertension and severe chronic infections [67]. The attraction of the concept may be explained by the broader social view of the maternal–fetal relationship in the last decades of the twentieth century. It was recognised that for the fetus the mother presented the immediate environment, but the idea of an autonomous fetus, whose needs and interests need not overlap with its mother's, remained in full force. Yet, the strong hereditarianism implied in the conflict model, with both the mother and the fetus seen as machines governed by their genes, left little room for considerations of environmental influences received in development [62–64].

2.6 Maternal Environment and Fetal Exposure

By the end of the twentieth century, many of the paradigms that had dominated the twentieth century came under scrutiny. As 'the century of the gene' ended with the publication of the Human Genome draft (and, a few years later, full sequence), it became obvious that the knowledge of the genome sequence was only the beginning, rather than the end, of the quest for understanding life, health, and disease [65]. The notion of the autonomous fetus was questioned too. 'We have been dazzled by the very strong control by the fetus' wrote the fetal physiologist Graham Liggins, when decades of research into the onset of birth revealed enormous interspecies variation and the fact that, in humans, the mechanism firing off labour had little direct input from the fetus [66]. The research programme studying fetal respiratory movements came to a dead end in the late 1980s. Fetal physiologists looked for inspiration elsewhere and found it in the work of David Barker, the British epidemiologist who argued that the conditions of early life – indeed, even before conception – shaped the disease risk in adulthood [48, 67]. Barker was certainly not the first to stress the importance of prenatal influences: there were studies coming from social medicine and epidemiology throughout the 1960s and 1970s, such as those by Zena Stein and Mervyn Susser [68], examining the impact of maternal nutrition on cognitive development in youth. Yet as long as the genetic paradigm and the idea of the autonomous fetus prevailed, this approach remained restricted to public health fields.

The move away from the close focus on the fetus back to the mother and the environment of the pregnancy and early life fitted well with the renewed interest in development, manifested, for example, in the return of development into evolutionary studies named 'evo-devo' [69]. It also had to do with an increased anxiety about the environment changed by human action and its impact on human health, which had been growing since the 1960s. Older research, such as the previously described work of Robert McCance and Elsie Widdowson or studies of the cohort of women who were pregnant during the Dutch Winter Famine, was reappraised and integrated into the new paradigm [70]. The reappraisal included the previously little recognised research across the Iron Curtain, by the East Berlin endocrinologist Günter Dörner, who in the 1970s compared the risk of obesity and cardiovascular diseases in the cohorts of young men born before, during, and after the Second World War [71, 72]. The difference was that, around the turn of the twenty-first century, the long-term impact of the early influences had to be expressed in molecular rather than late-nineteenth-century physiological or twentieth-century endocrinological terms.

The solution was offered by the new, rapidly growing area of biomedical research, epigenetics, which has been variously described as 'the study of mitotically or meiotically heritable changes in gene function that cannot be explained by changes in genetic sequence' or, in a less technical language, 'the molecular memory of past stimuli', the signals allowing cells to 'remember past events, such as changes in the external environment or developmental cues' [73]. Epigenetics holds the promise of explaining what genetics could not; it clarifies how, under (even slightly) different environmental influences, switching certain genes on and off may allow the same genetic code to produce different phenotypes. There seem to be many mechanisms through which genes may be turned on (and off) – some involving small RNAs and others spatial changes to the DNA–protein complex in the nucleus – but the best studied is the addition of methyl groups to promoter regions of the gene [21].

It may seem that, with developmental approaches and epigenetics, 'maternal impressions' have returned to medicine and society. Yet, while the mother was certainly brought back into the picture, her return took place in a reductionist manner, befitting the way that science operates today. The perception of the mother is evident in expressions of 'maternal effects' and 'maternal environment'. Maternal experiences are required (1) to be, or to be made, amenable to experimental, molecular approaches (2) to show a quantifiable change in parameters that may be measured using epigenetic methods.

Most research is focused on two categories of influences or exposures: nutrition and stress [21]. The impact of changes in diet is modelled in a relatively straightforward manner in animal models, by restricting nutrition or changing proportions of food groups or particular nutrients in experimental animal diets. Yet the relevance of results to human physiology has not always been obvious. There is very little 'natural' about the standardised diets fed to laboratory animals, bred in laboratory environments for generations, so the implications of experimental findings for human nutrition are not always clear. Epigenetic research has also complicated the previously established therapeutic regimens: folate, a B vitamin that has been supplemented to pregnant women to prevent neural tube deficit, is a powerful methyl-group donor, which thus changes the epigenetic state at multiple locations in the organism and possibly has widespread effects.

Even more controversial and complicated than nutritional epigenetics are the attempts to show how maternal psychological traumas and emotional states influence development. Féré once explained them with nervous reflex reaction and Sontag with hormones such as adrenaline; epigenetic research largely focuses on the expression of genes coding receptors for corticosteroid stress hormones. 'Stress' here refers to a large group of very different experiences – from parental neglect in early life to the situations where the mother is exposed to environmental stress, for example experiencing the 9/11 terrorist attack. The best-known animal model was the 'high/low licking/grooming' model. In this model, rat dams are divided into those that exhibit either frequent licking and grooming behaviour towards their offspring (thus modelling a caring mother) or opposite – infrequent licking and grooming – behaviour [74]. The caring mother is supposed to provide a positive, low-stress environment for the offspring, which in turn is understood to affect the functional activity of a group of genes involved in the production and activity of corticosteroids, stress hormones, evident in the epigenetic state of stress hormone receptors and in the level of the hormone.

In short, the new approach to the ways in which the mother modulates and transmits influences received during development is highly reductionist, made amenable to experimental physiological and molecular approaches, with very different experiences expected to produce the same chemical effect in the organism. It is thus entirely different from maternal impressions. One aspect, however, remains by and large unchanged, and that is the responsibility of the mother for the child's health – and not just in childhood, but throughout life, and even, if the transmission of epigenetic marks across generations proves true, to future generations. The way that the results of epigenetic studies are reported – by journalists but also in some cases by scientists who did the research – places the burden of guilt for a child's poor health squarely on the shoulders of the mother [75]. Maternal behaviour during pregnancy is scrutinised to an unprecedented level, with an ever-increasing list of prohibited foods, the prohibition of any alcohol, strict scrutinising of weight gain, and a growing list of medical checks. The focus on the mother may seem baffling if we know that many of the animal studies cannot be easily extrapolated to humans, that paternal effects (through the epigenetic changes in sperm cells) may play an equally important role, and that many influences are really of societal or broadly environmental nature. Yet if we keep in mind the older as well as more recent history of the maternal–fetal relationship, on the background of which these studies are conducted and results are presented, then this picture of an ambivalent association makes sense. Rather than seeing the mother and the fetus as a team, a pair working together towards a common goal, they are viewed as two parties uneasily united: the fetus requiring protection and the mother needing control.

2.7 Conclusion

In this chapter, I have argued that the focus on the maternal–fetal relationship, rather than the mother or the fetus alone, provides a richer, more instructive picture than the focus on the fetus or on the mother alone. For example, Sara Dubow's close attention to the medical and legal status of the fetus in twentieth-century America painted an image of ever-increasing autonomy and rights ascribed to the fetus, paralleled by the continuously diminishing status and control of the mother [5]. This view agrees with the older feminist critique of women's loss of authority in medicine today, for example by Barbara Duden

[4]. Yet shifting the lens slightly to capture the interaction between the two tightly connected organisms also changes, or complicates, our view of the history of the fetus, of the mother, and indeed of 'maternal impressions'. Rather than a linear process, we see an image where the importance of maternal experiences, and of influences received through the mother, periodically strengthens and weakens. These shifts tell us as much about social changes – women's position in the society, war trauma, standpoints on human identity, agency, and rights – as they do about developments in obstetrics and fetal physiology. In the era of 'hard heredity', eugenics, and the early days of genetics at the beginning of the twentieth century, the fetal parasite got what it needed from the mother to survive, but, beyond the bare minimum necessary for survival, maternal influences had no impact. But in the economic depression and political upheaval of the 1930s, which brought unprecedented civilian suffering and famines, the idea of a fetus sensitive to maternal experiences – from her diet to the psychological trauma – prevailed. By the 1960s, however, in the newly affluent society, the main concerns revolved around the issues of human rights and subjectivity. The fetus – made visible through the new technology of ultrasound and enjoying media exposure in colour magazines – was seen as an autonomous organism, able to breathe, move, and control its growth and possibly even the timing of birth. Fetal rights came to be understood as opposed to women's rights in the era of liberalisation of abortion laws; obstetricians increasingly positioned themselves as fetal rather than women's advocates. Mothers and fetuses, it seemed, were uncomfortable neighbours whose interests only partially overlapped; evolutionary biologists provided an explanation of this relationship that drew on their sharing only some of their genes. But as the genetic paradigm began to lose some of its power around the turn of the twenty-first century and concerns about the environment changed through human action strengthened, approaches emphasising the importance of environmental influences began to grow in importance. The mother is now seen as the primary environment, as well as the mediator of cues coming from the broader environment. While these approaches may be under-stood as more inclusive and accurate, they also carry the load of the recent history of maternal–fetal relationship. They imply – and sometimes explicitly state – that the mother, through her behaviour and her choices, is responsible for the health of her future child, but that she cannot be trusted and requires close supervision and control, preferably before the pregnancy has even begun. So rather than viewing the mother and the fetus as a unit, a team working towards a shared goal, their relationship remains ambivalent. Finally, while it may be tempting to see the epigenetic approach as the return of maternal impressions – with the Internet and newspapers brimming with titles such as 'you are what your mother ate' – the similarity is only superficial. The mother, in epigenetics terms, is a molecular environment, a source, and a mediator of exposures, where what matters is not the actual experience but whether it activates the gene or not.

References

1. Petchesky RP. Fetal images: The power of visual culture in the politics of reproduction. Feminist Studies 1987; 13: 263–292.

2. Jülich S. Fetal photography in the age of cool media. In: Ekström SA, Jülich FL, Wisselgren P, eds. History of Participatory Media: Politics and Publics, 1750–2000. London, Routledge, 2011; 125–141.

3. Wilson EK. Ex utero: Live human fetal research and the films of Davenport Hooker. Bulletin of the History of Medicine 2014; 88: 132–160.

4. Duden B. Disembodying Women: Perspectives on Pregnancy and the Unborn. Cambridge, MA, Harvard University Press, 1993.

5. Dubow S. Ourselves Unborn: A History of the Fetus in Modern America. Oxford, Oxford University Press, 2011.

6. Casper M. The Making of the Unborn Patient: A Social Anatomy of Fetal Surgery. New Brunswick, Rutgers University Press, 1998.

7. Reagan LJ. Dangerous Pregnancies: Mothers, Disabilities and Abortion in Modern America. Berkeley, University of California Press, 2010.

8. Pfeffer N, Kent J. Framing women, framing fetuses: How Britain regulates arrangements for the collection and use of aborted fetuses in stem cell research and therapies. BioSocieties 2007; 2: 429–447.

9. Huet MH. Monstrous Imagination. Cambridge, Cambridge University Press, 1993.

10. Shildrick M. Maternal imagination: Reconceiving first impressions. Rethinking History 2000; 4: 243–260.

11. López-Beltrán C. The medical origins of heredity. In: Müller-Wille S, Rheinberger HJ, eds. Heredity Produced: At the Crossroads of Biology, Politics and Culture, 1500–1870. Cambridge, MA: MIT Press, 2007; 105–132.

12. Müller-Wille S, Rheinberger HJ. A Cultural History of Heredity. Chicago, University of Chicago Press, 2012.

13. Levine P, Bashford A. Introduction: Eugenics and the modern world. In: Levine P, Bashford A, eds. The Oxford Handbook of the History of Eugenics. Oxford, Oxford University Press, 2010; 3–24.

14. McLaren A. Reproduction by Design: Sex, Robots, Trees and Test-Tube Babies in Interwar Britain. Chicago, University of Chicago Press, 2012.

15. Pick D. The Faces of Degeneration: A European Disorder, c. 1848–1918. Cambridge, Cambridge University Press, 1989.

16. Sontag LW. The significance of fetal environmental differences. American Journal of Obstetrics and Gynecology 1941; 42: 996–1003.

17. Martin A, Holloway K. 'Something there is that doesn't love a wall': Histories of the placental barrier. Studies in History and Philosophy of Biological and Biomedical Sciences 2014; 47: 300–310.

18. Ebbs KH, Scott WA, Tisdall FF, et al. Nutrition in pregnancy. The Canadian Medical Association Journal 1993; 46: 1–6.

19. Diderot D. Eléments de physiologie. In: Assézat J, ed. Oeuvres complètes. Vol. 9. Paris, Hachette, 1875; 236–430.

20. Members of the Department of Experimental Medicine, Cambridge, and associated workers. Studies of undernutrition, Wuppertal 1946–1949. Special Report Series 1951; 275.

21. Gluckman PD, Hanson MA, Beedle AS, Buklijas T, Felicia ML. The epigenetics of human disease. In: Hallgrímsson B, Hall BK, eds. Epigenetics: Linking Genotype and Phenotype in Development and Evolution. San Francisco, University of California Press, 2011; 398–423.

22. Al-Gailani S. 'Antenatal affairs': Maternal marking and the medical management of pregnancy in Britain around 1900. In: Helduser U, Dohm, B, eds. Imaginations of the Unborn: Cultural Concepts of Prenatal Imprinting from the Early Modern Period to the Present. Heidelberg, Winter, 2018; 153–172.

23. Al-Gailani S. Teratology and the clinic: Monsters, obstetrics and the making of antenatal life in Edinburgh, c. 1900. Unpublished PhD thesis, University of Cambridge, 2011.

24. Ballantyne JW. Expectant Motherhood: Its Supervision and Hygiene. London, Cassell, 1914.

25. Adair FL. The interrelationship of mother and fetus. Chairman's address. Journal of American Medical Association 1932; 99: 433–437.

26. Arni C. Vom Unglück des mütterlichen "Versehens' zur Biopolitik des" Pränatalen'. Aspekte einer Wissensgeschichte der maternal-fötalen Beziehung. In: Sänger E, Rödel M, eds.

Biopolitik und Geschlecht: zur Regulierung des Lebendigen. Münster, Westfälisches Dampfboot. 2012; 44–66.

27. Arni C. The prenatal: The contingencies of procreation and transmission in the nineteenth century. In: Brandt C, Müller-Wille S, eds. Heredity Explored: Between Public Domain and Experimental Science. Cambridge, MIT Press. 2016; 285–310.

28. Kevles D. In the Name of Eugenics: Genetics and the Uses of Human Heredity. New York, Knopf, 1985.

29. Buklijas T. Food, growth and time: Elsie Widdowson's and Robert McCance's research into prenatal and early postnatal growth. Studies in History and Philosophy of Biological and Biomedical Sciences 2014; 47; 267–277.

30. Sontag LW, Pyle SI, Cape J. Prenatal conditions and the status of infants at birth. American Journal of Diseases of Children 1935; 50: 337–342

31. Williams S. Relief and research: The nutrition work of the National Birthday Trust Fund, 1935–1939. In: Smith DF, ed. Nutrition in Britain: Science, Scientists and Politics in the Twentieth Century. London, Routledge. 1997; 99–122.

32. Susser M, Stein Z. Eras in Epidemiology: The Evolution of Ideas. New York, Oxford University Press. 2009; 208–210.

33. Antonov AN. Children born during the siege of Leningrad in 1942. The Journal of Pediatrics 1947; 30: 250–259.

34. Smith CA. Effects of maternal undernutrition upon the newborn infant in Holland (1944–1945). Journal of Pediatrics 1947; 30: 229–243.

35. Widdowson EM. Mental contentment and physical growth. Lancet 1951; 257: 1316–1318.

36. Kalter H. Teratology in the Twentieth century: Environmental causes of congenital malformations in humans and how they were established. Neurotoxicology and Teratology 2003; 35: 131–282.

37. Arni C. Psychischer Einfluss und generationelles Trauma. Pränatale Prägung als Problem der Transmission, oder: Die Kinder des Année terrible 1870/1871. In: Helduser U, Dohm, B, eds. Imaginations of the Unborn. Cultural Concepts of Prenatal Imprinting from the Early Modern Period to the Present. Heidelberg, Winter. 2018; 133–152.

38. Sontag LW. Effect of fetal activity on the nutritional state of the infant at birth. American Journal of Diseases of Children 1940; 60; 621–630.

39. Buklijas T, Hopwood N. 'The lonesome space traveller'. Making Visible Embryos. 2008–2010. www.sites.hps.cam.ac.uk/visibleembryos/s7_4.html (Accessed 16 June 2023.)

40. Hughes L. Burning birth certificates and atomic Tupperware parties: Antiabortion movement in the shadow of the Vietnam war. Historian 2006; 68: 541–558.

41. Oakley A. The Captured Womb: A History of the Medical Care of Pregnant Women. New York, Basil Blackwell, 1984.

42. Nicolson M, Fleming JEE. Imaging and Imagining the Fetuses: The Development of Obstetric Ultrasound. Baltimore, Johns Hopkins University Press, 2013.

43. Gluckman PD, Buklijas T. Sir Graham Collingwood (Mont) Liggins. 24 June 1926–24 August 2010. Biographical Memoirs of Fellows of the Royal Society 2013; 59: 195–214.

44. McCance RA. Summary of session I: Food reserves and food requirements of the newborn. In: Jonxis JHP, Visser HKA, Troelstra JA. Nutricia Symposium on the Adaptation of the Newborn Infant to Extra-Uterine Life. Leiden, Stenfert Kroese. 1964; 305–307.

45. Dawes GS. Foetal and Neonatal Physiology: A Comparative Studies of the Changes at Birth. Chicago, Year Book Medical Publishers, 1968.

46. Dawes GS. The fetus and independent life. Introduction. Ciba Foundation Symposium 1981; 86: 1–4.

47. Wolstenholme GEW, O'Connor M. Foetal Autonomy. London, Churchill, 1969.

48. Dawes GS, Borruto F, Zacutti A, eds. Fetal Autonomy and Adaptation. Chichester, Wiley, 1990.

49. Rudolph AM, Heymann MA. The circulation of the fetus in utero: Methods for studying distribution of blood flow, cardiac output and organ blood flow. Circulation Research 1967; 21: 163–184.

50. Gluckman PD, Liggins GC. Regulation of fetal growth. In: Beard RW, Nathanielsz PW, eds. Fetal Physiology and Medicine: The Basis of Perinatology. New York, Dekker. 1984; 511–557.

51. Dawes GS. The fetus and birth. Introduction: A historical perspective. Ciba Foundation Symposium 1977; 47: 1–4.

52. Bowler PJ. Evolution: The History of an Idea. Berkeley, University of California Press, 1984.

53. Dawkins R. The Selfish Gene. Oxford, Oxford University Press, 1976.

54. Hamilton WD. The genetical evolution of social behaviour. Journal of Theoretical Biology 1964; 7: 1–16.

55. Trivers RL. Parent–offspring conflict. American Zoologist 1974; 14: 249–264.

56. Pinker S, Bloom P. Natural language and natural selection. In: Barkow JH, Cosmides L, Tooby J, eds. The Adapted Mind: Evolutionary Psychology and the Generation of Culture. New York, Oxford University Press. 1992; 451–494.

57. Haig D. Altercation of generations: Genetic conflicts of pregnancy. American Journal of Reproductive Immunology 1996; 35: 226–232.

58. Haig D. Genetic conflicts in human pregnancy. Quarterly Review of Biology 1993; 68: 495–532.

59. Haig D. The kinship theory of genomic imprinting. Annual Review of Ecology and Systematics 2000; 31: 9–32.

60. Moore T, Haig D. Genomic imprinting in mammalian development: A parental tug-of-war. Trends in Genetics 1991, 7; 45–49.

61. Haig D. Placental hormones, genomic imprinting, and maternal–fetal communication. Journal of Evolutionary Biology 1996; 9: 357–380.

62. Abrams ET, Meshnick SR. Malaria during pregnancy in endemic areas: A lens for examining maternal-fetal conflict. American Journal of Human Biology 2009; 21: 643–650.

63. Hollegaard B, Byars SG, Lykke J, Boomsma JJ. Parent–offspring conflict and the persistence of pregnancy-induced hypertension in modern humans. PLOS One 2013; 8: e56821.

64. Muehlenbachs A, Mutabingwa TK, Edmonds S, et al. Hypertension and maternal–fetal conflict during placental malaria. PLoS Medicine 2006; 3: e446.

65. Fox Keller E. Century of the Gene. Cambridge, Harvard University Press, 2000.

66. Ciba Foundation. The fetus and birth. Final discussion. Ciba Foundation Symposium 1977; 47: 461–472.

67. Barker DJ, Osmond CD. Infant mortality, childhood nutrition, and ischaemic heart disease in England and Wales. Lancet 1986; 327: 1077–1081

68. Stein Z, Susser M. Fertility, fecundity, famine: Food rations in Dutch Famine 1944–1945 have a causal relationship to fertility, and probably to fecundity. Human Biology 1975; 47: 131–154.

69. Gilbert SF, Opitz JM, Raff RA. Resynthesizing evolutionary and developmental biology. Developmental Biology 1996; 173: 357–372.

70. Barker DJ. Developmental origins of chronic disease: The Richard Doll lecture. Public Health 2012; 126: 1–15.

71. Dörner G, Haller K, Leonhardt M. Zur möglichen Bedeutung der prä- und/oder früh postnatalen Ernährung für die Pathogenese der Arteriosklerose. Acta Biologica et Medica Germanica 1973; 31: 31–35

72. Dörner G, Rodekamp E, Plagemann A. Maternal deprivation and overnutrition in early postnatal life and their primary prevention: Historical

reminiscence of an 'ecological' experiment in Germany. Human Ontogenetics 2008; 2: 51–59.

73. Landecker H, Panofsky A. From social structure to gene regulation, and back: A critical introduction to environmental epigenetics for sociology. Annual Review of Sociology 2013; 39: 333–357.

74. Meaney MJ. Maternal care, gene expression, and the transmission of individual differences in stress reactivity across generations. Annual Review of Neuroscience 2001; 24: 1161–1192.

75. Richardson SS, Daniels CR, Gillman MW, et al. Don't blame the mothers. Nature 2014; 512: 131–132.

The First 5000 Days
Making DOHaD, 1989–2003

Mark Hanson and Tatjana Buklijas

3.1 Introduction

In June 2003, the Second World Congress on Fetal Origins of Adult Disease took place in Brighton, the UK. Alongside researchers specialising in fetal development – developmental physiologists, epidemiologists, obstetricians, and paediatricians – the meeting was addressed by a group of illustrious guests: the well-known scientists and science communicators Colin Blakemore and Lord Robert Winston; the Nobel laureate in economics Amartya Sen; and the royal patron, Princess Anne. The latter stressed the importance of this research for global health and presented a silver salver to the Southampton epidemiologist David Barker, in recognition of his pioneering work in the field [1]. At this meeting, the International Society for the Developmental Origins of Health and Disease (DOHaD) was founded, and the global ambitions of the new field were evident in its logo showing a fetus ostensibly peacefully nestled in the globe.

Yet just a decade earlier, this field had not existed. It began at a workshop at Lerici, near La Spezia in Italy, in 1989, in which David Barker presented his retrospective epidemiological research from Hertfordshire, UK, showing that low birthweight was associated with an increased risk of chronic non-communicable diseases in later life. It was at that meeting when fetal physiologists first discussed the plausibility and possible underlying mechanisms of Barker's observations [2].

This chapter, written by a founder of the field and a historian with long-term interest in DOHaD, examines this key (long) decade in the making of DOHaD, bookended by the 1989 La Spezia workshop and the 2003 Brighton Congress. It argues that, for all the attention that DOHaD has received from social and biomedical scientists, its history has not been studied in sufficient depth. Yet to understand the objectives, methods, research questions, and intellectual networks making the field of DOHaD, and the responses that it evoked and that further shaped it, we must appreciate the historical and geographical context in which it was created. For the purposes of this chapter, we focus on three key themes:

1. **Interdisciplinarity.** From its inception, DOHaD was explicitly interdisciplinary, and interdisciplinarity is a source of its intellectual dynamism and breadth. Yet this required

An early draft of this chapter was presented at a workshop in April 2022. We are grateful to the workshop participants and the volume editors for their comments. The discussion on the Acheson report has benefitted from the research conducted by Dr Salim Al-Gailani for an upcoming paper co-authored with Buklijas. Finally, we are grateful to many DOHaD researchers, only some of whom are mentioned or cited in this paper, but who collectively contributed to DOHaD's first 5000 days. Mark Hanson is grateful to the British Heart Foundation for sustained support for his research and wider work.

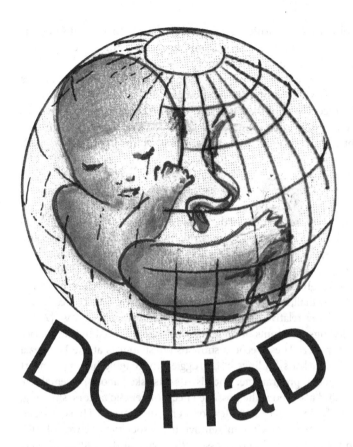

Figure 3.1 Original logo of the International DOHaD Society, created by Mark Hanson.

rendering the concepts of each collaborating discipline intelligible to all participating members [3]. As we will show, while these transformations were productive, in the process some of the context and layers of the original question were lost.

2. **Social class and health inequalities in Britain:** Barker brought to his research a concern with social inequalities in health. We briefly review its long-standing history in British science and policy and then focus on the reasons for the uptake of DOHaD by the Labour Party upon its accession to power in 1997.

3. **Globalisation and health.** DOHaD's international expansion took place during a decade of globalisation. The global interest in DOHaD has been taken for granted, but, as we show in this section, the international networks through which the field spread merit deeper investigation.

3.2 The Promises and Challenges of Interdisciplinarity

In 1989, the doyen of fetal physiology, Geoffrey Dawes, invited the epidemiologist David Barker to a meeting in Villa Marigola, a conference centre near La Spezia, Italy. The title of the conference, 'Fetal Autonomy and Adaptation', signalled both continuity and change. Twenty years earlier, Dawes chaired a meeting centred on the key idea that the fetus 'demonstrates its innate capacity for influencing its external and maintaining its internal environment – that is, its autonomy' [4]. The La Spezia meeting was intended to mark a new era in fetal physiology in which the preoccupation with the autonomous functions of the fetus would be complemented, if not replaced, with a focus on the interaction between the fetus and its broader environment [2, 5].

To inspire new thinking and draw on the views of the physiologists' collective, Dawes invited David Barker, an environmental epidemiologist from the University of Southampton. Barker had recently published a series of well-received but provocative articles. He argued that chronic non-communicable diseases were not caused (exclusively) by adult lifestyles but by the conditions of early life that set the organism on a path that increased, or reduced, the later disease risk [6, 7].

Barker built his hypothesis by linking historical with contemporary demographic and epidemiological data. His first studies took an 'ecological' approach, by demonstrating a geographical correlation between high infant mortality in the early twentieth century and high morbidity from cardiovascular disease (in men) in the period 1968–1978. The causal link, he proposed, was poor early-life nutrition, caused by maternal malnutrition and poor health, infectious diseases in infancy, and artificial feeding practices. Ecological studies were followed by a retrospective cohort study on a group of men born in Hertfordshire around 1920, whose records of birth and infant weight were, unusually, preserved. Their matched mortality records showed that those born small, and especially those whose growth failed to 'catch up' in the first year of life, had a higher relative risk of death from cardiovascular disease [7].

In the conference proceedings, printouts of presentations were followed by summaries of the discussions after each paper. These records show us physiologists at the La Spezia conference were intrigued by Barker's findings but struggled to imagine how to convert them into a workable experimental programme. The discussants asked about placental size and gestational age at birth, and also about the possible effects of genetic factors, smoking, and breastfeeding. Significantly, in view of later developments in DOHaD, Hanson asked Barker whether correcting for social class might remove the association between birthweight and later disease, in view of the well-known association with cardiovascular disease, which we will discuss in the next section. This correction might distinguish between an underlying mechanism and merely an association. Barker replied that 'Hertfordshire *at the time in question* [emphasis original] was a rural county in which social class was relatively unrelated to health' [2, p. 35]. While Barker noted that future data on social class and early life would become available, the fetal physiologists left with the resolve to devise studies in animal models to investigate possible fundamental mechanisms.

Hanson's group provides an example of such early physiological, animal DOHaD work. When they moved to University College London in 1990, they secured funding to investigate the effect of small reductions in the food intake of ewes during early pregnancy. These reductions were not large enough to produce a sustained reduction in maternal body weight or lambs' birthweight but did produce effects on fetal and neonatal cardiovascular and endocrine function. This experiment, they argued, distinguished between a physiological ('normal') adaptive process, albeit with possible later health consequences, and a pathophysiological process in utero. The physiological proposition was indeed confirmed, although the misconception that developmental processes 'harm' the fetus has been persistent [8, 9]. Barker and researchers investigating the effects of moderate to severe challenges such as the Dutch Hunger Winter imagined the environment of early human development as a complex web of social and economic forces ultimately manifested as the food available to women and girls. Physiologists, in contrast, had in mind specific graded and quantifiable changes in physiological parameters such as blood pressure, oxygen level, or concentration of nutrients that could be registered by receptors and which then altered development through plasticity [10].

Experimentalists initially turned to the animals – namely, sheep – that had been traditionally used to model human pregnancy. Indeed, their confidence in this animal model was validated when ultrasound, a technology introduced in the 1960s, confirmed similarities between ovine and human fetal development [8, 11]. But studies testing the effects of specific nutritional modification on developing offspring required larger numbers of animals than pregnancy research. Sheep were expensive, slow to reproduce, and difficult to manipulate nutritionally for such studies. At the same time, animal experimental regulations were becoming much more stringent. DOHaD scientists replaced sheep with smaller animal 'models' – rats, mice, and guinea pigs – that had the advantage of rapid reproductive cycles, lower cost, and simpler regulatory approval. Yet with their large litters and fast development, much of which occurred after birth, they had far less in common with human fetal development. While the replacement of the sheep with small animals was a pragmatic decision, the transferability of observations from small experimental animals to humans was uncertain.

These regulatory and economic pressures on experimental physiology were happening simultaneously with the rise of genomics, which culminated with the publication of the human genome at the end of our examined period (2000, officially in 2003) [12, 13]. This co-occurrence was not coincidental but the result of the economic and policy shift in the UK through the 1970s and 1980s. The political pressures to cut costs and modernise science were translated into support for certain scientific fields, while other fields lost funding, institutional footing, and political advocacy. In agriculture, traditional animal genetics that relied on long-term follow-up of generations of farm animals was defunded in favour of genomic biotechnology [14, 15]. Fetal physiology, also using large farm animals, saw funding cuts too. Through the 1980s and 1990s, the spotlight on novel animal 'disease models' developed in genomics laboratories – animal strains genetically modified to carry mutant genes predisposing them to specific diseases – and the first successful experiment in cloning a mammalian organism further increased public concern about animal rights [16].

DOHaD, with its focus on the environment–organism relationship, had no interest in genomics at first; however, the overarching push away from experimental physiology and towards genomics was likely the key reason for DOHaD's entrance into epigenetics in the early 2000s [17]. This disciplinary relationship was mutually beneficial: while epigenetics provided molecular evidence to DOHaD, DOHaD secured policy relevance for epigenetics [18]. This disciplinary relationship between DOHaD and (environmental) epigenetics is so close that many see it as the same field [9]. Yet it is important to note that each field began on its own, roughly simultaneously in the late 1980s, and had over 15 years of independent development [19]. Many scientists who have used epigenetics to explain intergenerational transmission of disease, or, more broadly, inheritance of phenotypic traits, do not see themselves as members of the DOHaD community. Similarly, for many in the DOHaD community, epigenetics is not a core element of the field but rather one of the tools to address the question of 'developmental origins'. As this chapter stops in 2003, the DOHaD–epigenetics relationship is beyond its scope.

A field of particular interest to the emerging DOHaD community was human medicine. Here we must distinguish between epidemiologists and nutrition scientists working inside medical institutions and research groups, who had been interested in

'Barker's hypothesis' throughout, from practicing clinicians. In particular, specialists in internal medicine – cardiologists, diabetologists, and endocrinologists – who treated adults, and, increasingly, elderly patients, and whose primary objective was treatment rather than early prevention of chronic disease showed little interest in DOHaD [20, p. 47]. In terms of elucidating mechanisms of cardiovascular and metabolic disease, they placed greater trust in genomics, which promised to reveal the basis of risk of disease at the individual level; a promise later captured in the term 'personalised medicine' [21]. In contrast, obstetricians and paediatricians, communities that had already collaborated closely with experimental physiologists in the fields of fetal and neonatal physiology, joined DOHaD in larger numbers. So, while the field was meant to bridge two opposite ends of the human lifespan, in practice, clinical disciplines studying life's beginning took up more space in the field than those at the other end, and this influenced DOHaD's direction. Probably the most significant criticisms came from Barker's own discipline. Epidemiologists argued that his observations were artefacts arising from over-controlling for variables such as BMI and other confounders. They lacked confirmation in studies of cohorts where birthweight was smaller such as twins. The potentially underestimated importance of social factors was also emphasised [22, 23].

The retrospective nature of the early studies made it difficult if not impossible to resolve such issues, and epidemiologists began to use case-control and cohort studies to clarify the causal links [24, 25]. The Southampton group established the Southampton Women's Survey (SWS) between 1998 and 2002 [26]. With the help of general practitioners in the city, researchers recruited women and then followed up the pregnancies and children of those who conceived. The SWS collected rich data, produced many papers, and confirmed and extended DOHaD thinking in many ways.

Through the early 1990s, we can track the process of disciplinary expansion, to incorporate new knowledge, and then its translation. *Mothers, babies and disease* – a 1994 book-length explanation of the 'Barker's hypothesis' – combined Barker's own historical epidemiological studies with a summary of research investigating adult risk factors of chronic disease; animal studies of the long-term impact of nutritional modifications, especially during so-called 'sensitive periods'; and existing clinical data [27]. Although the idea itself was not necessarily new, the disciplinary collaboration was novel, and Barker, with his team, was its tireless champion.

Yet in this interdisciplinary translation and expansion that required 'telescoping' from social conditions to dietary components and then specific molecular pathways, the link with the broader social environment became difficult to maintain. Social scientists have critiqued the ways in which social class, gender, and race are ostensibly erased in DOHaD research [9, 28]. We borrow the term 'telescoping' from Warin and colleagues who criticised the shift from the long-term impact of early-life undernutrition to overnutrition as the key question in the field [29]. In their view, this also meant a move from concerns over social determinants of health to assumptions about individual women's bodies [32]. Here we want to add another meaning: the entrance of experimental and molecular fields and the pressures of interdisciplinarity. This disciplinary structure of DOHaD as a biomedical field – rather than being situated within social medicine or even epidemiology – has profound consequences. As a recent ethnographic study of DOHaD science argued, while researchers are aware of the importance of understanding the structural reasons underlying different early life conditions, current DOHaD studies, with their focus on individual behaviour and measurement of a limited set of variables, make these connections difficult [30].

3.3 Social Class, Health Inequalities, and Government Policy in the UK

The relationship between social class and health has long been a key preoccupation of British scientists and policymakers. Francis Galton's eugenic ideas were a defence of the existing social order based on innate and fixed biological characteristics [31]. Yet by the interwar period the practitioners of the new discipline of genetics began to insist on the precise delineation and description of heritable traits and to criticise the ambiguity of eugenics. Studies such as Lionel Penrose's Colchester Survey, which examined the heritability of 'mental retardation', pointed to a range of congenital (i.e. associated with birth or pregnancy), but not heritable, factors influencing the characteristics of the new individual [32]. The economic depression of the 1930s further exposed problems with the eugenic argument, showing that poverty rather than heritable traits was the main cause of many diseases. Soon thereafter, the Second World War strengthened social and political support for the emerging welfare state. Simultaneously, eugenics was replaced by social medicine – a new field that joined together the commitment to redistributive economic policies, public health concerns with living conditions, and the interest in 'lifestyles' [33].

Between the 1940s and 1960s, social medicine flourished at British universities [34, 35]. David Barker received his PhD in 1967 under one of the leaders of the field, Professor Thomas McKeown at the University of Birmingham. McKeown's research programme investigated the relationship between human reproduction, social conditions, and mental health [36]. Even though Barker subsequently worked in or led departments of epidemiology rather than social medicine, his methodology resembled McKeown's in its blending of historical with contemporary epidemiological data and his enduring preoccupation with social inequalities.

Barker collaborated with epidemiologists who studied links between social class and disease. He worked with Geoffrey Rose, a lead investigator in the longitudinal 'Whitehall Study' that interpreted coronary heart disease as an outcome of class-based inequalities rather than a disease of 'affluent lifestyles' [37]. Barker participated in the debate on health inequalities through his series of investigations into the links between contemporary geographical distributions of chronic diseases and the patterns of predisposing factors in earlier generations. In the 1970s, he mapped the occurrence of Paget's disease (of the bone) in the elderly onto the incidence of childhood rickets in earlier generations. This research can be understood as a precursor to his more famous 1980s studies [38]. But in contrast to McKeown, Barker was operating not in the context of a rising welfare state but in the neoliberal response to the 1970s economic crisis: a political and economic environment in which the elements of the 'welfare state' were progressively eroded.

An explicit contribution to the debate was written in 1987, when Barker quoted the report on inequalities in health by the committee led by Sir Douglas Black – a report commissioned by the Labour government but issued by the new Conservative government under Margaret Thatcher in 1980 – which explained inequalities as 'the more diffuse consequences of the class structure' [39, 40]. Barker argued that 'specific explanations may be found in the environmental influences that determined past differences in child development. These explanations may allow a national strategy for reducing inequalities in health to be developed' [39].

This quote, Barker's intellectual networks, and his epidemiological research indicate that a contribution to policymaking aimed at reducing health inequalities had long been one of his objectives, although perhaps out of reach through the 1980s under the Thatcher government. But by the early 1990s, conditions for health and social policy in the UK started to change. In his 1994 book *Mothers, Babies and Disease in Later Life*, Barker stressed the profound implications of emerging interdisciplinary research – his earlier epidemiological work and the incipient physiological and clinical research on 'Barker's hypothesis' – for government policy [27, pp. 170–171]. He referred to the UK's *Health of the Nation* strategy, based on the WHO's *Health for All* (1978) and launched in 1992 as 'the first attempt by a British government to develop a strategy explicitly to improve the health of the population' [41]. Yet although broadly welcomed, this strategy was also criticised, both for its disease-based model and, importantly, for not considering the socio-economic determinants of health [41, p. 4].

The Labour Party's historic accession to power in 1997, after 18 years in opposition, meant a renewed focus on socio-economic determinants of health, within a broader commitment to marshalling scientific evidence into public policy. The new government immediately commissioned a report on 'inequalities of health', with the objective of identifying priority areas for policies to 'develop beneficial, cost effective and affordable interventions to reduce health inequalities' [42]. Chaired by Donald Acheson, Barker's predecessor as Director of the MRC Environmental Epidemiology Unit in Southampton who was then appointed Chief Medical Officer of the UK, the working group included scholars who would become synonymous with research into inequalities and health, namely the epidemiologist Michael Marmot and the sociologist Hilary Graham, along-side David Barker.

DOHaD influenced the report and the British policy. Both nutrition and gender would have likely received attention, with or without DOHaD. But the explicit statement on the nutrition of women before and during pregnancy, influencing the long-term health of the next generation, and an entire discussion on the risks of reduced fetal growth, referenced by the recent work of the Southampton group, were most likely contributed by Barker [42]. Correspondence kept in the National Archives confirms this hypothesis: in a letter to Acheson dated 4 September 1997, Barker explained the policy implications of inequalities in fetal growth, and Acheson wrote on the margins, 'Thank you very much for your interesting and important letter which will be duly fed into our process.'

An early outcome of the report's – and DOHaD's– impact on British policy may be the cross-departmental programme Sure Start, which brought together social services, health, early childhood and primary education, and social justice, to improve the 'physical, social, emotional and intellectual status of children' [43]. While the original remit was children under seven years of age, as the review developed 'there was an accumulation of evidence that successful intervention in the earliest years offered the greatest potential for making a difference' [43, p. 260]. This text did not explicitly reference Barker or Acheson, but it named the Health Secretary Tessa Jowell who oversaw both the Acheson Report and Sure Start and who steered the 1997 Comprehensive Spending Review in which the Sure Start programme originated 'towards services for families and their children aged nought to three, including the pre-natal period' [43, p. 260].

In conclusion, although the reception of DOHaD in the science community in the late 1990s was not fully settled, the historical moment in British politics, with the election of a party explicitly committed to using the latest evidence to reform social and health policy, created the conditions for DOHaD to enter public policy early in the history of the field.

3.4 Developmental Origins in the Era of Globalisation and Global Health

DOHaD began in the UK, indeed in England: at Barker's home institution, Southampton; at University College London, where Hanson led a fetal physiology group; with Alan Lucas' research team at the Childhood Nutrition Centre of the Institute of Child Health in London; and in Cambridge where Nicholas Hales' group studied clinical biochemistry and metabolism. But the field almost immediately began to expand internationally. In this section, we show how early collaborative networks were created along the established intellectual networks in the British Commonwealth. Then we show how multilateral global organisations became key proponents and advocates of DOHaD.

In 1994, Barker published a report of the 'first international study group' meeting in Sydney in October 1994, bringing together scientists from the UK, Australia, Canada, and New Zealand [44]. The geographical location is significant as it maps onto the leading centres of fetal physiology and medicine. And while these were relatively new fields, launched in the mid-twentieth century, they built on the long-standing networks of research and practice of agriculture, and especially sheep breeding, in the British Empire [45–47]. These scholarly communities had been studying animal growth for decades; they had developed sophisticated research methodologies and had easy access to animals. DOHaD provided a new framework for their research, by putting the emphasis on environmental (nutritional) influences on fetal growth, and new relevance, by linking their work to adult clinical medicine. In turn, these research communities responded enthusiastically. DOHaD groups sprung up in the UK beyond the southeast: in Bristol, Nottingham, Aberdeen, and Edinburgh; in Toronto, Adelaide, and Auckland; and in US centres with a strong tradition of animal agricultural research – Cornell and Portland, Oregon [48].

But it was human studies in the Global South that provided the key missing piece. As the previous section discussed, human prospective studies were central to the confirmation of the DOHaD hypothesis developed on retrospective historical data. And while the Southampton Women's Study was important for its rich insight into the everyday lives of 'Western' women – now conceptualised as developmental environments – prospective human studies in the Global South were important for three reasons. At least since the 1950s, biomedical scientists trying to explain and predict the impact of a rapidly changing environment upon humankind have taken the Global South populations – more likely to subsist on sparser diets than the late twentieth-century people of Europe and North America – as a window into the recent global past [49, 50]. DOHaD researchers further wanted to understand differences between human populations: do they all respond to developmental nutritional fluctuations in the same manner? Are the risks of cardiovascular and metabolic diseases the same for all? Finally, the 1990s were the heyday of the economic, cultural, and technological transformation termed 'globalisation', which helped spread the 'nutritional transition' – a shift to a diet high in ultra-processed, high-fat, and high-sugar foods – from the Global North to the South [51, 52]. By launching human studies in the Global South just as this transition was starting, DOHaD researchers hoped to capture this fleeting moment, when generations raised under 'old' nutritional regimes were bearing children into new ones.

The new DOHaD human medicine centres in the Global South were established through Commonwealth networks too, but in former British colonies rather than settler societies. An early and highly significant collaboration flourished between Southampton and Chittaranjan Yajnik who set up the Pune Maternal Nutrition Study in 1994. The aim was to study the long-term, especially metabolic, effect of maternal malnutrition on children born to women in villages around Pune, in the hope of explaining the much higher risk of insulin resistance and diabetes mellitus among the subcontinent's population [53, 54]. Similarly, a study in Jamaica led by Terrence Forester linked birthweight with the later response to famine: children who were born small tended to respond with the wasting illness, marasmus, and those born larger were more likely to develop the more life-threatening kwashiorkor [55]. At the Medical Research Council Unit in The Gambia, DOHaD research was integrated into an existing programme of human nutrition research in West Africa [56].

DOHaD was new, but, as we show in this section, it built upon the existing disciplinary and institutional networks largely within the British Commonwealth, with histories dating back to the British Empire. Whether these were fetal physiologists whose animal models and research methodologies built upon the structures of settler agriculture, or medical institutions and knowledge networks that traditionally prioritised diseases of greatest economic significance to the empire, their legacies and assumptions influenced the new field of DOHaD. Further research is needed – and in particular case studies focusing on specific countries or research fields and institutions – to elucidate the specific forms and impacts of these influences.

3.5 Conclusions

The field that became DOHaD started in the intimate environment of an academic workshop, but just over a decade later it had sufficient appeal and reputation to hold a world congress bringing together the research community with celebrity scholars and royalty. This chapter argued that to understand this trajectory we must situate the field in the geographical and historical context in which it was created and flourished. We then identified three key themes to help us explain both its success and the controversies: effective interdisciplinarity; ability to offer a new solution to the long-standing problem of social class in Britain; and the ability to recruit existing international knowledge and institutional networks to build a novel approach to emerging global health problems. We summarise our argument in the following way:

First, the interdisciplinarity of DOHaD was its central feature from the start: a source of innovation, intellectual richness, and an effective way to broaden the field's appeal and recognition. Yet at the same time it was a source of challenges and controversies, with the field having to reconcile diverse methodologies and data types and also respond to criticisms from different disciplinary corners. Furthermore, for all its rapid global spread, DOHaD was deeply marked by its British origins. The long-standing concern with the effect of social class on health not only influenced Barker in the formulation of his original hypothesis but also provided the opportunity and context for DOHaD to influence public policy relatively early in its history. This track record in British social and health policy, right at the time when the New Labour government was gaining international interest for its conscious attention to scientific evidence in policymaking, became important in the twentieth century [57]. This period marked the entrance of DOHaD into global health policy, at first through the established scientific connections of the former British Empire. While this could have sounded its death knell in times of wider recognition of the harmful legacy of this past, in fact it gave DOHaD new life as the realisation grew in the early years of the current millennium that inequalities in health affect all societies, and none more so than those passing through the nutritional and economic transitions associated with globalisation.

References

1. Hanson M, Gluckman P, Bier D, Challis J, Fleming T, Forrester T, et al. Report on the 2nd World Congress on Fetal Origins of Adult Disease, Brighton, UK, June 7–10, 2003. Pediatric Research 2004; 55: 894–897.

2. Dawes GS, Borruto F, Zacutti A, Zacutti A Jr. (eds). Fetal Autonomy and Adaptation. Chichester, UK: Wiley; 1990.

3. Kluger MO & Bartzke G. A practical guide how to tackle interdisciplinarity: A synthesis from a postgraduate group. Humanities and Social Sciences Communications 2020; 7: 47.

4. Wolstenholme G & O'Connor (eds). Fetal Autonomy. Basel: CIBA Foundation; 1968.

5. Buklijas T & Al Gailani S. A fetus in the world: Autonomy and environment in the making of fetal origins of adult disease. History and Philosophy of the Life Sciences [accepted].

6. Barker DJP & Osmond C. Infant mortality, childhood nutrition, and ischaemic heart disease in England and Wales. Lancet 1986; i: 1077–1081

7. Barker DJP, Winter PD, Osmond, C, Margetts B, & Simmonds SJ. Weight in infancy and death from ischaemic heart disease. Lancet 1989; ii: 577–580.

8. Hawkins P, Steyn C, McGarrigle HH, Calder NA, Saito T, Stratford LL et al. Cardiovascular and hypothalamic-pituitary-adrenal axis development in late gestation fetal sheep and young lambs following modest maternal nutrient restriction in early gestation. Reproduction Fertility and Development 2000; 12(8): 443–464.

9. Richardson S. The Maternal Imprint: The Contested Science of Maternal-fetal Effects. Chicago: University of Chicago Press; 2021.

10. Hanson M. 1990. Fetal baroreflexes and chemoreflexes: Adaptation and autonomy. In Dawes GS, Borruto F, Zacutti A, Zacutti A Jr, eds. Fetal Autonomy and Adaptation. Wiley, pp. 5–13.

11. Nicolson M & Fleming JEE. Imaging and Imagining the Fetus. Baltimore: Johns Hopkins University Press; 2013.

12. Fox Keller E. The Century of the Gene. Cambridge, MA: Harvard University Press; 2000.

13. Hood L & Kevles E (eds). The Code of Codes: Scientific and Social Issues in the Human Genome Project. Cambridge, MA: Harvard University Press; 1993.

14. García-Sancho M. 2015. Animal breeding in the age of biotechnology: The investigative pathway behind the cloning of Dolly the sheep. History and Philosophy of the Life Sciences 2015; 37 (3): 282–304

15. Myelnikov D. Cuts and the cutting edge: British science funding and the making of animal biotechnology in 1980s Edinburgh. British Journal of History of Science 2017; 50(4): 701–728.

16. Balls M. The ethics of research involving animals: the report of the Nuffield Council on Bioethics. Alternatives to Laboratory Animals 2005;33(6): 649–649.

17. Brawley L, Poston L, & Hanson MA. Mechanisms underlying the programming of small artery dysfunction: review of the model using low protein diet in pregnancy in the rat. Archives of Physiology and Biochemistry 2003 Jan; 111(1): 23–35.

18. Kenney M, & Müller R. Of rats and women: Narratives of motherhood in environmental epigenetics. BioSocieties 2017; 12(1): 23–46

19. Buklijas T. Histories and meanings of epigenetics. In: Meloni M, Lloyd S, Fitzgerald D, Cromby J, eds. Handbook of

Biology and Society. London: Palgrave; 2018, pp. 167–187.

20. Reynolds LA & Tansey AM. Cholesterol, Atherosclerosis and Coronary Disease in the United Kingdom, 1950–2000. London: Wellcome Witness Seminar; 2005, no. 27.

21. Prainsack B. Personalized Medicine: Empowering Patients in the 21st Century. Cambridge, New York: New York Press; 2017.

22. Paneth N & Susser M. Early origin of coronary heart disease (the 'Barker hypothesis'). BMJ. 1995, 18 Feb ;310 (6977): 411–412.

23. Rich-Edwards JW & Gillman MW. Commentary: A hypothesis challenged. BMJ. 1997, 22 Nov;315(7119): 1348–1349.

24. Elford J, Shaper AG, & Whincup P. Early life experience and cardiovascular disease. Ecological Studies. Journal of Epidemiology and Community Health 1992; 46(1): 1–8.

25. Elford J, Whincup P, & Shaper AG. Early life experience and adult cardiovascular disease: Longitudinal and case-control studies. International Journal of Epidemiology 1991; 20(4): 833–844.

26. Inskip HM, Godfrey KM, Robinson SM, Law CM, Barker DJ, Cooper C. Cohort profile: The Southampton women's survey. International Journal of Epidemiology. 2006 Feb 1;35(1): 42–48.

27. Barker DJP. Mothers, Babies and Disease in Later Life. London: BMJ Publishing Group; 1994.

28. Valdez, N. Weighing the Future: Race, Science, and Pregnancy Trials in the Postgenomic Era. Berkeley: University of California Press; 2021.

29. Warin M, Moore V, Zivkovic T & Davies MJ. Telescoping the origins of obesity to women's bodies: How gender inequalities are being squeezed out of Barker's hypothesis. Annals of Human Biology 2011; 38(4): 453–460

30. Penkler M. Caring for biosocial complexity. Articulations of the environment in research on the Developmental origins of health and disease. Studies in History and Philosophy of Science 2022 Jun; 93: 1–10.

31. Bland L & Hall L. Eugenics in Britain: The view from the metropole. In: Bashford A, Levine P, eds. The Oxford Handbook of the History of Eugenics. Oxford, UK: Oxford University Press; 2012, pp. 212–227.

32. Kevles, D. In the Name of Eugenics: Genetics and the Uses of Human Heredity. Cambridge, MA: Harvard University Press; 1985.

33. Oakley A. Eugenics, social medicine and the career of Richard Titmuss in Britain 1935–50. The British Journal of Sociology 1991; 42(2): 165–194.

34. Porter D. Social medicine and the new society. Medicine and the scientific humanism in mid-twentieth century Britain. Journal of Historical Sociology 1996; 9(2): 168–187.

35. Porter D. The decline of social medicine in the 1960s. In: Porter D, ed. Social Medicine and Medical Sociology in the 20th Century. Amsterdam: Rodopi; 1997, pp. 97–119.

36. McKeown LI. Record and the epidemiology of malformations. Paediatric and Perinatal Epidemiology 1996; 10(1): 2–16.

37. Clark P. "What else can you expect from class-ridden Britain?": The Whitehall studies and health inequalities, 1968 to c. 2010. Contemporary British History 2021; 35(2): 235–257.

38. Barker DJP & Gardner MJ. Distribution of Paget's disease in England, Wales and Scotland and a possible relationship with vitamin D deficiency in childhood. British Journal of Preventive & Social Medicine 1974; 28(4): 226–232.

39. Barker DJP & Osmond C. Inequalities in health in Britain: Specific explanations in three Lancashire towns. BMJ 1987; 294: 749–752.

40. Black D. Report of the Working Group on Inequalities in Health. London:

Department of Health and Social Security; 1980.

41. Hunter DJ, Fulop N, & Warner M. From "Health of the Nation" to "Our Healthier Nation". Policy Learning Curve Series No 2. Copenhagen: Regional Office or Europe, WHO; 2000.

42. Acheson D. Independent Inquiry into Inequalities in Health: Report. London, UK: The Stationery Office; 1997.

43. Glass N. Sure Start: The development of an early intervention programme for young children in the United Kingdom. Children & Society 1999; 13: 257–264.

44. Barker DJP, Gluckman PD & Robinson JS. Conference report: Fetal origins of adult disease – report of the First International Study Group, Sydney, 29–30 October 1994. Placenta 1995; 16 (3): 317–320.

45. Franklin S. Dolly Mixtures: The Remaking of Genealogy. Durham, NC: Duke University Press; 2007.

46. Buklijas T. Food, growth and time: Elsie Widdowson's and Robert McCance's research into prenatal and early postnatal growth. Studies in History and Philosophy of Science Part C 2014; 47: 267–277.

47. Gluckman PD & Buklijas T. Sir Graham Collingwood (Mont) Liggins. 24 June 1926–24 August 2010. Biographical Memoirs of the Royal Society 2013; 59: 193–214.

48. Fall C & Osmond C. Commentary: The developmental origins of health and disease: An appreciation of the life and work of Professor David J. P. Barker, 1938–2013. International Journal of Epidemiology 2013; 42(5): 1231–1232.

49. Ventura Santos R, Lindee S, & Sebastião de Souza V. Varieties of the primitive: Human biological diversity studies in Cold War Brazil (1962–1970). American Anthropologist. 2014 Dec;116(4): 723–735.

50. Santos RV, Coimbra Jr CE, & Radin J. 'Why Did They Die?' Biomedical narratives of epidemics and mortality among Amazonian indigenous populations in sociohistorical and anthropological contexts. Current Anthropology. 2020 Aug 1;61(4): 441–470.

51. Popkin B. Nutritional patterns and transitions. Population and Development Review 1993; 19(1): 138–157.

52. Labonté R, Mohindra K, Schrecker T. The growing impact of globalization for health and public health practice. Annual Review of Public Health 2011; 32: 263–283.

53. MRC Lifecourse Epidemiology Unit. The Pune Maternal Nutrition Study [Internet]. Southampton: University of Southampton [Cited 2022 November 1]. Available from: www.mrc.soton.ac.uk/web2/cohorts/studies-in-india/the-pune-maternal-nutrition-study/

54. Metabolic Health Digest. Q & Session with Dr. C. S. Jaynik: the one who coined the term "thin-fat" [Internet]. [Cited 2022 November 1] Available from: www.metabolichealthdigest.com/q-a-session-with-dr-c-s-yajnik-the-one-who-coined-the-term-thin-fat/.

55. Forrester TE, Badaloo AV, Boyne MS, Osmond C, Thompson D et al. Prenatal factors contribute to the emergence of kwashiorkor or marasmus in severe undernutrition: Evidence for the predictive adaptation model. PLoS One 2012; 7(4): e35907.

56. Green A. A new paradigm of the MRC units in The Gambia and Uganda. The Lancet 2018, 3 Feb; 391(10119): P418.

57. Wells P. New Labour and evidence-based policy making: 1997–2007. People, Place & Policy Online 2007; 1(1): 22–29.

Chapter

4

A Biosocial Return to Race? Racial Differences in DOHaD and Environmental Epigenetics

Maurizio Meloni, Christopher Kuzawa, Ayuba Issaka, and Tessa Moll

4.1 Introduction

The growth of research within the Development Origins of Health and Disease (DOHaD) and related environmental epigenetics fields has catalysed a shift in the understanding of how genes and environments shape phenotypes. The attention to embryonic and fetal development as critical periods with important long-term health effects has led to a focus on the gestational environment and maternal experiences like nutrition and stress, as *intergenerational* determinants of health [1–3]. This emerging science has inspired claims that social exposures, including race-related inequalities, can drive physiological, developmental, and epigenetic processes operating in utero and during early postnatal life, becoming 'embodied' as relatively durable, albeit in principle modifiable, biological differences [4–6].

By eschewing fixed genetic differences, 'biosocial' perspectives on race have brought with them a renewed hope for a focus on the social, historical, and political bases of contemporary health disparities [7]. This emerging understanding of the role of environment-driven phenotypic and epigenetic plasticity is often viewed as aligning with progressive policy goals because it demonstrates newly appreciated pathways by which major health differentials might be reversed by timely intervention. This is reflected, for instance, in the emphasis on the 'first 1000 days' in global health initiatives [8, 9] and a vibrant area of economics that harnesses DOHaD frameworks to promote investments in maternal and child health [10, 11].

However, despite the promise of DOHaD and environmental epigenetics to set out modifiable and plastic models of biological inheritance, social scientists have illustrated how enduring forms of 'environmental determinism' [12] may become intertwined with local conceptions of racial difference. As one example, one thread of research has argued that environmental exposure to poverty (which is highly racialised in many contexts) could impair early brain development and determine children's lifelong potential [13]. Indeed, a growing number of scholars, in studies from microbiomics to brain development, have raised critiques of what could be characterised as a postgenomic reinstantia-

An extended version of this chapter has originally appeared as an article in the American Journal of Human Biology. Ref: Meloni, M., Moll, T., Issaka, A., & Kuzawa, C. W. (2022). A biosocial return to race? A cautionary view for the postgenomic era. American Journal of Human Biology, 34(7), e23742. https://onlinelibrary.wiley.com/doi/full/10.1002/ajhb.23742 This article was originally published under a CC-BY License (https://creativecommons.org/licenses/by/4.0/). It is re-printed here, with a modified title, under the same license.

tion of race [14–18].[1] As sociologist Dorothy Roberts has warned, 'When scientists write that epigenetic effects of racial discrimination are durable across generations, it sounds perilously close to biological theories of race' [18, p. 143].

As epigenetic and DOHaD analyses of racial/ethnic health disparities expand significantly in scope and impact, we echo others in urging caution in the collection and interpretation of these new data. We recognise that much of this growing work has gravitated to biosocial understandings of health disparities in part because these understandings both avoid reductionist genetic explanations and offer new explanations that can hopefully be harnessed to foster positive social change, such as making links between current health differentials and past injustices [20–22].

Our cautionary view stems from two arguments that we will lay out in the following: in the first, we seek to undermine the assumption that environmentally driven effects are always inherently progressive. Not unlike gene-centric models of race, environmentally driven models are similarly capable of being abused and used to promote racial hierarchies, as evidenced by work on race in Latin America [23]. Here, we explore a lengthy history of proto-racism that traces presumed inherent group differences to environments, not genes. In the second, we explore the results of a review of current literature on racial health disparities in DOHaD and environmental epigenetics. This review demonstrates the enduring problems of reductionism and typological thinking in contemporary research. We believe that ongoing interdisciplinary work between social and biological scientists is key to correcting these creeping trends and strengthening this research in service of the goals of social justice. Towards these ends, we suggest various tools, such as community participation in all stages of research and moderation in reporting results, that can help avoid a potential reification of racial typologies in DOHaD research.

4.2 On the Long History of Biological Determinism and Racialisation

4.2.1 Genetic Determinism and Its Counterparts

For many contemporary researchers who grapple with debates about biological race, the modern concept that humans can be arranged into hierarchical typologies is often a starting point for discussion [24, 25]. In the eighteenth century, the Linnaean system of classifying living things, including humans [26], became the template for later anthropological work that assumed that humans could be ordered into distinct, indelible types that varied in level of sophistication as a matter of inborn potential. Modern racial science, grounded in assumptions of permanent psychophysical differences, experienced new legitimation in simplified understandings of Mendelism and early twentieth-century anthropology and eugenics. The crux of the argument was that genetic differences, assumed to determine phenotypes in a direct fashion, rendered environmental exposures or habits insignificant when considering racial characteristics: human types, now conceptualised as clustering of genes within geographically bounded groups, were viewed as fundamentally unchangeable at least within certain geographic clusters [27].

---

[1] Postgenomics is an increasingly common umbrella term that covers all research on the complex molecular architecture that connects genomic sequences to the phenotype, inclusive of a new set of approaches dubbed the '-omics' (e.g. epigenomics, microbiomics, and transcriptomics [19][20]).

Genetic determinism – 'the idea that genes alone have the power to shape both bodies and behaviors' – enjoyed a remarkable albeit controversial success during the twentieth century [28]. The assumption that diverse groups of people can be characterised and essentialised based on presumed, immutable genetic characteristics has been evoked to naturalise the social, political, and historical underpinnings of inequality. As obvious examples of these dangers, during the twentieth century, research on human genetics and hard hereditarianism helped justify scourges like forced sterilisations in the USA and the Holocaust in Nazi Germany. More recently, widely discussed and controversial books have argued for a genetic basis to intelligence and a need to temper public investments in education [29], joining a long tradition of hard hereditarians that considered public welfare a wasted or misguided form of sentimentalism – a classical eugenic trope since the time of Galton (1822–1911).

As a response to the twentieth-century abuses of genetic determinism, the idea that human differences are tied to environmental influences and nurture has maintained an allure of progressivism [30], especially in the social sciences and humanities [31]. This is particularly obvious in Northern Europe and North America where most of the eugenics movement drew from theories and practices of genetic determinism. This means that the historical prominence of environments as determinants of racial typologies remains hidden. Focusing on a longer history, *spanning two millennia rather than three centuries*, demonstrates the potential for hierarchy and discrimination to be grounded in, and justified by, patterns of human difference tracing *to shared environments and experiences* (food, climate, and habits) rather than genetic or innate factors.

This ancient proto-racism reflected a persistent tendency at least since Graeco-Roman antiquity (where the most ancient evidence can be found) to refer to a range of sciences, prominently including humoralist medicine and geography, to express prejudices and a hierarchy of values among different populations, often in the context of imperial or military arguments [32]. We argue that a re-emergence of conceptual-isations of body and race as open and malleable rather than fixed could lead to the subtle but gradual replication of biological race in contemporary postgenomic and biosocial developments, at a time when biology is moving away from the presumed centrality of DNA sequences as masters of phenotypic development. In what follows, we provide a concise summary of a lengthy history of pre-modern essentialism, in which intrinsic group-level human differences were viewed as an output of environmental mechanisms.

4.2.2 The Power of the Environment Before the Gene

Although this was not the only way to construct racial hierarchies in pre-modern times, the tendency to view people as deeply shaped by the places where they lived or the food they ate was a powerful intellectual device to assert the superiority of certain human groups [32, 33]. Often combined with a strong moralistic flavour, arguments about racial differences acquired through the embodiment of different environments were used to condemn whole human groups to inferiority because of the unfavourable places where they were born or, more subtly, by claiming that their placement in particularly unfavourable settings was a sign of their subordinate nature [34]. Nations were viewed as fit or unfit to rule not because of innate deficiencies but because of the power of the outside, such as the persisting effects of climate or habits on their bodies and minds. This framework has shaped pre-modern ideas of racial inferiority for centuries, connecting, with different nuances, Greek and Roman views of the East, to Columbus' interpretation of the tropics as inhabited by people unfit to 'exercise power' [35].

In Classical Antiquity, grouping physical and moral traits of different populations and relating them to various environments – the geography of the places they lived, the climate in those areas, or the food they ate – was a common tool in developing the tropes and hierarchies of differing populations [32, 33, 37]. This is clearly seen in Hippocrates' *Airs, Waters and Places* (fifth century BCE), a medical treatise written as a guide for travelling doctors, in which Asians are described as 'more gentle and affectionate' than Greeks as they live in a land where the weather is uniform and everything grows 'more beautifully'. *Airs, Waters and Places*, while often overlooked in histories of proto-racism, was a widely influential text and translated for centuries through Pagan Antiquity, Latin and Oriental Christendom, and the Muslim world. It is considered a foundational text for theories of health, ecology, and geography of disease, and further one of the first scientific texts to establish 'the greatest and most marked differences' between Europeans and Asians.

A generation after Hippocrates, Aristotle built on these ideas to justify political differences within a wider imperial framework. People of Asia were now described as 'intelligent and skilled but cowardly. Thus, they are in a perpetual state of subjection and *enslavement*' (350 BCE: *Politics*, 7.5.6.1327b our emphasis; translation in [37, p. 44]. Filled with references to eugenic topics, the seventh book of the *Politics* (available in the West since 1260) went on to decisively influence early modern debates in the Spanish, French, and British colonies. There, the Greek/Asian dichotomy was replaced by one between temperate and tropical weather, leading to a climatological distinction between master races and naturally born slaves sealed by the authority of Aristotelian natural philosophy [38].

The Roman world continued and expanded the climatological tradition. Roman military treatises developed similar theories to maintain, for instance, that Orientals were naturally prone to slavery (from the ancient Roman historian Livy 36.17), to distinguish between the environment and hence 'innate' characters of different troops to favour a more rational process of recruiting militias (late-Roman writer Vegetius), or to avoid the risk of dangerous environmental influences in foreign areas [32]. We also see the appearance of a certain asymmetry in how negative and positive environmental effects are perceived as impacting populations, which foreshadow later doctrines of racial purity: with Roman historians like Tacitus or Livy, men transplanted from Rome into 'inferior' locales 'acquire the degenerate characteristics of the alien environment' but the reverse is only rarely mentioned [33, 37, p. 33].

While the Middle Ages are often overlooked in histories of racialisation based on environments, this period's influence on the mental cartography of early modern European colonialism and political theory was immense [39, 40]. From the twelfth century onwards, the Middle Ages saw an increasing tendency to essentialise biological differences in humoral composition based on emerging ideas of human nature, heredity, or religious affiliation. Not only were people seen as a mirror of where they lived, but human groups who differed by 'blood' were often thought to inherit the same traits if living 'under the same sky'. However, factors that could potentially alter the *innate but changeable* complexion of human groups were incorporated into medical and geographical treatises of the time. Hippocratic-Galenic ideas of environmental effects on *humours* led to concerns about the 'transplantation' of human groups into new soils and under new stars that 'would affect not only themselves but their descendants' [41], deeply shaping anxieties surrounding the first colonial expansions and lasting well into the European Renaissance and Elizabethan England [42]. Hence, colonies became places where the coloniser could be 're-raced' [42, p. 19], spurring anxieties around the potential degeneration of a nobler European 'stock' under new environmental conditions [14].

As colonial expansion continued, and migration became increasingly common, racial science began to intermingle fixed and malleable characteristics strategically. For instance, this included the growing colonial anxiety that white settlers could degenerate in hot climates. Some historians have argued that it was precisely this fear of changeability under new environmental conditions, and the tendency of these ideas to potentially hinder colonial projects, that incentivised their replacement by notions of race as innate and immune to such environmental effects [43]. Lamarckian thinking, melded with rising social stratification and inequality, fuelled concerns about decay and degeneration in the European metropoles [44]. At the very foundation of the Enlightenment in the eighteenth century, we find a strong presence of environmental and climatological explanations of race differences. It would therefore be somewhat artificial to view the history of racism as the sole brainchild of the Enlightenment, overlooking the reality that Enlightenment intellectuals themselves wittingly inherited their ideas from Greek and Roman sources.

4.2.3 Historical Lessons for Current Work in DOHaD and Epigenetics

Our historical review highlights that the emphasis on immutable characteristics as essential to differentiating and hierarchising populations is a relatively recent phenomenon, and one influenced by the much lengthier prior history of differentiating groups based on shared environments. Without flattening different historical contexts into a simplified continuity or denying the distinct implications of environmental determinism with regard to contemporary political, legal, and economic formations, we suggest that it is possible to highlight a number of recurring characteristics in models of environmentally patterned human difference. Firstly, there is a predominance of *typological* models based on the causal power of the environment where common biological essences are viewed as being directly established by environmental effects and ignoring within-group variability. Secondly, *binary thinking* manifests in several ways. Environments were divided into categories of normal (that of the observer) and abnormal/pathological (that of the colonial subject or 'other'), and 'exposures' were similarly viewed as having effects that were either present or absent, ignoring the possibility of a spectrum of phenotypic outcomes. Thirdly, there was a tendency to establish an asymmetry between *negative* and *positive* environmental effects, with the former more common and used to characterise the developmental trajectory of non-Western or subordinated groups. Fourthly, this work often assumed that environmental and social disturbances were transferred directly to individual bodies, which are portrayed as passive recipients of external forces: damaged environments (or non-European ones) were viewed as becoming *ipso facto* damaged bodies, thus eliding a wider focus on underlying causes. Finally, it was common to argue that environmental factors can *cause loops* that are difficult to break, with whole groups being stuck in social or cultural inertia because of acquired environmental insults.

Of course, even when based on environmental models, contemporary expressions of environmentally or socially patterned race and biology do not extrapolate seamlessly from these recurring patterns and historical examples. Our point is simply that environments are neither an innocent nor an inherently more progressive factor in explaining racial health disparities. Clearly, current postgenomic work around race and embodiment has overwhelmingly good intentions – of clarifying pathways, reducing societal impacts, and addressing the unequal distribution of ill health. However, some of the conventions of biomedical research may create openings to unwittingly recapitulate typological and essentialised thinking [18, 45]. We thus set out to investigate the literature and findings in DOHaD and environmental epigenetics that address the role of race/ethnicity in human health.

4.3 Current Work in DOHaD, Environmental Epigenetics, and Race

How common are essentialised and typological notions of environment-driven race and human difference in the DOHaD and environmental epigenetics literature? While an important catalyst for studies of developmental plasticity, DOHaD remains a niche in a wider trend exploring relationships between epigenetic changes, particularly DNA methylation (DNAm), and racial/ethnic differences. Within this broader field, do we see an emphasis on environmental determinism, a focus on negative environments understood as leading to permanent scarring, or perspectives that foster binary inter-pretations of exposures and outcomes?

Before we look specifically at research that addresses race and ethnic health disparities, there are some common practices within research design in the field generally that are worth noting for their potential to contribute to a reductionist portrait. For one, some DOHaD or epigenetic studies use observational and population-based case-control designs; these have a high potential for confounding because key influences on health, such as environmental stressors, diet, or activity levels, tend to cluster as a result of influences like socio-economic status, ethnicity, class, or gender [46]. Other studies have harnessed natural or quasi-experimental designs, using 'exogenous' stressors such as a war-imposed famine, terrorist attack, global pandemic, or earthquake (for instance, [47]) to evaluate the impacts of maternal exposure during pregnancy. Because this work approximates a randomised exposure, it achieves a stronger basis for causal inference; however, it does so at the expense of studying severe shocks and stressors, which are not effective targets for intervention. (See Pentecost et al. in this volume on the move in DOHaD to preconception interven-tion trials.) Such 'shock' focused research is not capable of assessing more subtle exposures that reflect typical lived experience, let alone potentially beneficial or favourable exposures. On a similar note, experimental animal model research, which represents the 'gold standard' of causal evidence in this field, often imposes extreme prenatal nutritional stress on species with far less maternal capacity for fetal nutritional buffering than humans [3, 5]. In addition to using models of severe stress, relatively little DOHaD work to date has been explicitly designed to clarify the potential revers-ibility of early life effects (see Lloyd et al. in this volume). This creates a default assumption that any effects induced by these (again, severe) exposures are also per-manent. This simplified picture of permanent scarring may be further reinforced by the common convention in biomedical research of reporting relationships in a binary fashion, as being present or absent, depending on whether a threshold for statistical significance has been reached [48] (see also Sigurdadottir and Ayis in this volume).

As many of these observations apply to population-based health research more generally, we sought to offer a specific analysis of the use of the race concept in DOHaD and environmental epigenetics. We conducted a scoping review of studies within the fields of DOHaD and environmental epigenetics that address racial health inequities. We limited our review to empirical human studies that focused on race and ethnicity in health and related to epigenetics within a DOHaD framework. We reviewed 49 studies in total as they met all inclusion and exclusion criteria (see [49] for a full description of our methodology).

Given the largely biomedical nature of the reviewed literature, an emphasis on pathology is predominant, and exposures are generally understood exclusively in the negative, that is, as a source of risk for chronic disease and mortality and dysfunction of biological processes. Populations emerging from often self-reported categories are reframed as aligning through differences in methylation level, for instance, from our sample: 'African American adults', 'African American children', 'black women', 'black ethnicity', 'Hispanic ethnicity', and 'Native Hawaiians'. All these groups are defined as at-risk populations mostly via reference to abnormal methylation levels, even in instances when the data do not fit with this account (e.g. higher global methylation levels, suggesting reduced cancer risk in African American children). Intra-group variability in biological responses to environmental exposures is rarely given credence, and often differences – such as immigration status or the wide array of meanings, countries, and backgrounds coalescing under 'Hispanic' in the USA – are flattened into typological race categories.

Many social scientists have urged researchers to reframe their discussions and suggestions for policy towards structural factors – namely enduring systems of racism, widespread income inequality, and the historical legacies of colonialism (see Kenney and Müller, Keaney et al., and Karpin in this volume). In our review, we found that only three articles (6 per cent) mention or recognise the importance of wider socio-structural factors as 'drivers of racial health differences' [50]. Similarly, reversibility is explicitly mentioned by 14 articles (28 per cent), but most discussions of this are brief and often limited to the conclusion.

Only a limited number of studies are self-reflective about the uncritical usage of racial categories (e.g., [50]). A few go in the opposite direction and suggest that methylation markers differ significantly by race [51], and one claims that it is possible to separate distinct populations (Caucasian American, African American, and Han Chinese American) by using differences in methylation [52]. One study is explicit about the importance of having one basal methylome map for each population and the potential value of epigenetic marks as distinct criteria for racial classification beyond and sometimes in contrast to genetic findings ([53], see [49] for further details).

A final significant finding in our sample is the application of epigenetic clock studies, which use methylation to gauge the pace of biological ageing, to explain racial or ethnic differences in health outcomes. In a highly cited article in our sample, the authors remain cautious about the mechanisms by which 'race/ethnicity and sex affect molecular markers of aging' [53]. At the same time, the study uses several conventions that reify typological thinking around human population variation. As one example, the authors describe differences across these groups in largely typological terms, without devoting space to intra-population heterogeneities (e.g. 'African Americans have been shown to have longer telomere lengths than Caucasians'; 'Hispanics have a consistently lower IEAA (i.e. intrinsic epigenetic *age* acceleration) compared to Caucasians'; 'Tsimane have a lower intrinsic aging rate than Caucasians') [53, p. 170].

4.4 Fostering a Balanced Approach in Postgenomic Treatments of Race

Echoing a growing number of scholars [12–18], we believe it is important to interrogate practices within DOHaD and environmental epigenetics that run the risk of reinstantiating new forms of biological race. For one, we believe it important to remain vigilant against 'damage-centred research', a term coined by Indigenous academic Eve Tuck [54] to describe research that catalogues harms endured in a marginalised community with the intention of producing change, yet in practice rarely alters the social, material, or political causes of those harms and leaves populations labelled as 'damaged'. Yet, we do not want to convey only criticism: these fields are stimulating crucial new understandings of the social and historical pathways underlying health inequalities, and many communities are leveraging this research to advance agendas of social justice and community resilience ([22, 55]; Keaney et al. in this volume). In the spirit of moving beyond critique, we end with recommendations for ways that researchers can help ensure that their work benefits communities while avoiding any unintended stigma or repetition of the simplifications and pitfalls of the past.

As noted in many of our above points, there are practices across biomedical research that may contribute to reductionist, simplified, and potentially stigmatising portraits of marginalised communities. The predominant focus in DOHaD research on documenting exposure–disease relationships that are characterised in such a *de facto* binary fashion (present or absent) can reinforce the idea that populations faced with early life adversity and stress *necessarily* carry negative biological baggage because of those experiences. These binary assessments can often also fail to find evidence of an effect simply due to a small sample size or, conversely, can find evidence that biologically trivial effects are significant if sample sizes are large enough [48]. Publication bias, as Non [56] points out, also contributes to foregrounding research that shows dramatic methylation differences, but that may not translate into phenotypic differences.

This convention in reporting and discussing findings leads to a form of binary thinking in which effects are either present or not, and the magnitude of effect, or biological importance in a typical human population, often receives comparably little attention. Thus, we support the efforts in fields like statistics and epidemiology to do away with this focus on binary or 'bright line' assessments of the significance of findings [57]. Furthermore, we identify practices that could prevent stigmatising groups: (1) moving away from interpretations of data that reinforce simplified cause-effect models, (2) avoiding characterisation of outcomes as present or absent, and (3) avoiding the generalisation of pathologies to entire groups without considering the magnitude, heterogeneity, or reversibility of these effects.

Non's [56] recent review also points to other conventional practices in biomedical research that may contribute, for instance, to sampling biases favouring white populations (which perhaps feeds into the use of white populations as the norm from which other groups are seen as differing as we have detailed in our sample, see above). This type of practice, which we have documented in our sample (see for wider materials [49]), runs the risk of ascribing abnormality to marginalised communities ([45]; see also [58]). Researchers should consider the implication of their samples and the implicit racial 'narratives' (see Kenney and Müller's chapter on narrative choreographies) that may emerge as a result.

Finally, we both echo the calls of communities involved in DOHaD research to study resilience and amelioration from early life adversity and reiterate alongside other chapters within this volume (Tu'akoi et al., Bourke, and Lovett) that future research needs greater collaboration with communities on DOHaD research. In the first, our review demonstrated an overwhelming, though not surprisingly, focus on pathology and ill heath arising from early life events. But DOHaD research cannot be limited to this. Future work should also explore the development of resilience from early adversity and the capacity for reversibility or amelioration of early life effects in response to later favourable experiences or other interventions. When reversibility is not explored, the default of permanence may often be assumed, thus increasing the potential for stigmatisation.

In the second, our point regarding reversibility has in fact been made by many communities that are the subject of DOHaD research, demonstrating the emergence of 'bottom-up' demand for research into practices that build resilience [55]. This demand points to the need for researchers to conduct future work in ways that are aligned with the interests of affected communities, including requests for reparation. This will require meaningful engagement with participants across the research cycle. (See Tu'akoi et al. and Saulnier et al. in this volume.)

Collaborative and interdisciplinary endeavours will continue to prove essential to any future efforts to improve the production, interpretation, and consumption of epigenetic and DOHaD knowledge. This volume is a testament to the growing embrace, challenges, and value of interdisciplinary work in DOHaD. If we can apply the metaphors from this field to its development, early exposure to cross-disciplinary collaboration – from inception, funding, and through the research cycle – should also foster introspection and a stronger mature science.

References

1. Kuzawa CW. Fetal origins of developmental plasticity: Are fetal cues reliable predictors of future nutritional environments? *American Journal of Human Biology.* 2005; 17(1): 5–21.

2. Kuzawa CW. Pregnancy as an intergenerational conduit of adversity: How nutritional and psychosocial stressors reflect different historical timescales of maternal experience. *Current Opinion in Behavioral Sciences.* 2020; 36: 42–47.

3. Thayer ZM, Rutherford J, Kuzawa CW. The maternal nutritional buffering model: An evolutionary framework for pregnancy nutritional intervention. *Evolution, Medicine, and Public Health.* 2020; 1: 14–27.

4. Kuzawa CW, Sweet E. Epigenetics and the embodiment of race: Developmental origins of US racial disparities in cardiovascular health. *American Journal of Human Biology.* 2009; 21(1):2–15.

5. Kuzawa CW, Thayer ZM. Toppling typologies: Developmental plasticity and the environmental origins of human biological variation: Genes, biology, and culture. In: Hartigan, J. (ed.) *Anthropology of Race: Genes, Biology, and Culture.* Sante Fe, NM: SAR Press; 2013. pp. 43–56.

6. Gravlee CC. How race becomes biology: Embodiment of social inequality. *American Journal of Physical Anthropology.* 2009; 139(1):47–57.

7. Landecker H, Panofsky A. From social structure to gene regulation, and back: A critical introduction to environmental epigenetics for sociology. *Annual Review of Sociology.* 2013; 39: 333–357.

8. Victora CG, Adair L, Fall C, Hallal PC, Martorell R, Richter L, et al. Maternal and

child undernutrition: Consequences for adult health and human capital. *The Lancet.* 2008; 371(9609): 340–357.

9. Martorell R. Improved nutrition in the first 1000 days and adult human capital and health. *American Journal of Human Biology.* 2017; 29(2): 1–12.

10. Heckman JJ. The developmental origins of health. *Health Economy.* 2012; 21(1): 24–29.

11. Almond D, Currie J. Killing me softly: The fetal origins hypothesis. *Journal of Economic Perspectives.* 2011; 25(3): 153–172.

12. Saldaña-Tejeda A, Wade P. Eugenics, epigenetics, and obesity predisposition among Mexican Mestizos. *Medical Anthropology.* 2019, 24 Apr; 38(8): 1–16.

13. Pitts-Taylor V. Neurobiologically poor? Brain phenotypes, inequality, and biosocial determinism. *Science, Technology, & Human Values.* 2019, 4 Jun; 44(4): 660–685.

14. Baedke J, Delgado AN. Race and nutrition in the New World: Colonial shadows in the age of epigenetics. *Studies in History and Philosophy of Biology & Biomedical Science.* 2019, 1 Aug; 76: 101175.

15. Duster T. A post-genomic surprise. The molecular reinscription of race in science, law and medicine. *The British Journal of Sociology.* 201, 18 Mar; 66(1): 1–27.

16. Meloni M. Race in an epigenetic time: thinking biology in the plural. *The British Journal of Sociology.* 2017; 68(3): 389–409.

17. Saulnier KM, Dupras C. Race in the postgenomic era: Social epigenetics calling for interdisciplinary ethical safeguards. *American Journal of Bioethics.* 2017; 17(9): 58–60.

18. Roberts D. *Fatal Invention: How Science, Politics, and Big Business Re-create Race in the Twenty-first Century.* 2011. New York: The New Press.

19. Richardson S, Stevens H. (eds.). *Postgenomics.* 2015. Durham, NC: Duke University Press.

20. Nelson A. *The Social Life of DNA: Race, Reparations, and Reconciliation after the Genome.* 2016. Boston, MA: Beacon Press.

21. Davis D-A. *Reproductive Injustice: Racism, Pregnancy, and Premature Birth.* 2019. New York: New York University Press.

22. Warin M, Keaney J, Kowal E, Byrne H. Circuits of time: Enacting postgenomics in Indigenous Australia. *Body & Society.* 2023; 29(2): 20–48.

23. Stepan N. '*The Hour of Eugenics': Race, Gender, and Nation in Latin America.* 1991. Ithaca, NY: Cornell University Press.

24. Biddiss MD. Toward a history of European racism. *Ethnic and Racial Studies.* 1979; 2(4): 508–513.

25. Stocking G. *Victorian Anthropology.* 1987. New York: The Free Press.

26. Sloan PR. The gaze of natural history. In Fox C. et al. (eds.) *Inventing Human Science: Eighteenth-century Domains.* Berkeley: University of California Press; 1995. pp. 112–151.

27. Weiss S. *The Nazi Symbiosis: Human Genetics and Politics in the Third Reich.* 2010. Chicago, IL: University of Chicago Press.

28. Esposito M. Expectation and futurity: The remarkable success of genetic determinism. *Studies in History and Philosophy of Science Part C: Studies in History and Philosophy of Biological and Biomedical Sciences.* 2017; 62: 1–9.

29. Herrnstein RJ, Murray C. *The Bell Curve: Intelligence and Class Structure in American Life.* 2010 May 11. New York: Simon & Schuster.

30. Degler C. *In Search of Human Nature: The Decline and Revival of Darwinism in American Social Thought.* 1991. Oxford: Oxford University Press.

31. Meloni M. *Political Biology: Science and Social Values in Human Heredity from Eugenics to Epigenetics.* 2016. London: Springer.

32. Isaac B. Proto-racism in Graeco-Roman antiquity. *World Archaeology*. 2006; 38 (1): 32–47.

33. Isaac B. *Empire and Ideology in the Graeco-Roman World: Selected Papers*. 2017. Cambridge, UK: Cambridge University Press.

34. Livingstone DN. The moral discourse of climate: Historical considerations on race, place and virtue. *Journal of Historical Geography*. 1991; 17(4): 413–434.

35. Wey-Gomez N. *The Tropics of Empire: Why Columbus Sailed South to the Indies*. 2008. Cambridge, MA: MIT Press.

36. Eliav-Feldon M, Isaac BH, Ziegler J. (eds.). *The Origins of Racism in the West*. 2009. Cambridge, UK: Cambridge University Press.

37. Kennedy RF. *Race and Ethnicity in the Classical World: An Anthology of Primary Sources in Translation*. 2013. Indianapolis, IN: Hackett Publishing.

38. Huxley GL. *Aristotle, Las Casas and the American Indians*. Proceedings of the Royal Irish Academy. Section C: Archaeology, Celtic Studies, History, Linguistics, Literature, 57–68. 1980.

39. Bartlett R. Medieval and modern concepts of race and ethnicity. *Journal of Medieval and Early Modern Studies*. 2001; 31(1): 39–56.

40. Weeda C. Geographical determinism, ethnicity and religion c. 1100–1300 ce. In Kennedy, R. F. & Jones-Lewis, M. (eds.) *The Routledge Handbook of Identity and the Environment in the Classical and Medieval Worlds*. London and New York: Routledge; 2016. pp. 67–92

41. Feerick J. *Strangers in Blood*. University of Toronto Press; Fields KE, Fields BJ. *Racecraft: The Soul of Inequality in American Life*. 2012. London: Verso Books.

42. Floyd-Wilson M. *English Ethnicity and Race in Early Modern Drama*. 2003. Cambridge, UK: Cambridge University Press.

43. Braude B. How racism arose in Europe and why it did not in the near east. In Berg M. & Wendt S. (eds.) *Racism in the Modern World: Historical Perspectives on Cultural Transfer and Adaptation*. New York: Berghahn Books; 2011. pp. 41–61.

44. Pick D. *Faces of Degeneration: A European Disorder*. 1993. Cambridge: Cambridge University Press.

45. Mansfield B, Guthman, J. Epigenetic life: Biological plasticity, abnormality, and new configurations of race and reproduction. *Cultural Geographies*. 2015; 22(1): 3–20.

46. Hernan MA. The C-Word: Scientific euphemisms do not improve causal inference from observational data. *American Journal of Public Health*. 2018; 108(5): 616–619.

47. Roseboom T, de Rooij S, Painter R. The Dutch famine and its long-term consequences for adult health. *Early Human Development*. 2006; 82(8): 485–491.

48. Wasserstein RL, Lazar NA. The ASA statement on p-values: Context, process, and purpose. *The American Statistician*. 2016; 70(2): 129–133.

49. Meloni M, Moll T, Issaka A, Kuzawa C. A biosocial return to race? A cautionary view for the postgenomic era. *American Journal of Human Biology*. 2022; 34(7): e23742.

50. Pepin ME, Ha CM, Potter LA, Bakshi S, Barchue JP, Asaad AH. et al. Racial and socioeconomic disparity associates with differences in cardiac DNA methylation among men with end-stage heart failure. *American Journal of Physiology - Heart and Circulatory Physiology*. 2021; 320(5): 2066–2079.

51. Giri AK, Bharadwaj S, Banerjee P, Chakraborty S, Parekatt V, Rajashekar D et al. DNA methylation profiling reveals the presence of population-specific signatures correlating with phenotypic characteristics. *Molecular Genetics and Genomics*. 2017; 292(3): 655–662.

52. Heyn H, Moran S, Hernando-Herraez I, Sayols S, Gomez A, Sandoval J. et al. DNA methylation contributes to natural human variation. *Genome Research*. 2013; 23(9): 1363–1372.

53. Horvath S, Gurven M, Levine ME, Trumble BC, Kaplan H, Allayee H. et al. An epigenetic clock analysis of race/ethnicity, sex, and coronary heart disease. *Genome Biology*. 2016; 17(1): 171.

54. Tuck E. Suspending damage: A letter to communities. *American Journal of Physiology - Heart and Circulatory Physiology*. 2009; 79(3): 409–427.

55. Müller R, Kenney M. A science of hope? Tracing emergent entanglements between the biology of early life adversity, trauma-informed care, and restorative justice. *Science Technology and Human Values*. 2021; 46(6): 1230–1260.

56. Non AL. Social epigenomics: Are we at an impasse? *Epigenomics*. 2021; 13(21): 1747–1759.

57. Cummins KM, Marks C. Farewell to Bright-Line: A guide to reporting quantitative results without the S-Word. *Frontiers in Psychology*. 2020, 13 May; 11: 1–7.

58. Wiley AS. Pearl lecture: Biological normalcy: A new framework for biocultural analysis of human population variation. *American Journal of Human Biology*. 2021; 33(5): e23563.

The Promise and Treachery of Nutrition in DOHaD

Science, Biopolitics, and Gender

Vivienne Moore and Megan Warin

5.1 Introduction

In this chapter, we explore how and why the application of Developmental Origins of Adult Health and Disease (DOHaD) theory has not led to social change and improved reproductive justice. We draw upon the framework of reproductive justice, paying homage to the work of feminist scholars of colour who argued that concepts of reproductive rights were too narrow in their focus on autonomy, choice, and abortion [1, 2]. In combining 'reproductive rights' with 'social justice', the concept of reproductive justice encompasses much broader aspects of social life that intersect with reproduction, including family relations, conditions of work, housing, and welfare arrangements. Reproductive justice invites us to envisage DOHaD in a broader political field that takes account of how these social and structural inequalities profoundly shape the reproductive experiences of women.

In previous work, we have examined how DOHaD ideas can lead to blaming of mothers when health is seen as an individual responsibility, rather than socially determined. In this present piece, we try to understand more about the unfulfilled promise of addressing health inequities relating to food, gender, and reproductive justice. We suggest it is not just the tenacity of neoliberal ideas that gained prominence in the 1980s, foregrounding individual choice and responsibility while curtailing public services and welfare provisions (see [3]). We argue that older entangled histories of nutrition and militarism as well as neoliberal politics have enabled a particular understanding, positioning, and uptake of nutrition within DOHaD.

We build on the arguments of others that the field of nutrition and health has long been dominated by a narrow mode of thinking that has been termed 'hegemonic nutrition' [4]; this is characterised by standardisation and reductionism, in which food is reduced to its constituents and bodies are decontextualised [4, 5]. In the United Kingdom (UK), as we will explain, this ideology resonates with a celebrated history of nutritional research from the early twentieth century that identified the causes of common, intractable diseases and enabled improvements to be achieved by simple means. The approach was only slightly modified when dietary imbalance and energy excess came to the fore as the nutritional problems of the second half of the twentieth century, with dietary advice now the remedy.

Drawing on Foucault's concept of biopolitics and approaches used in the field of feminist science and technology studies (STS), we critically explore the deeply embedded logic of hegemonic nutrition, pointing to an assemblage of taken-for-granted politics and practices that work towards efficiency, bodies fit for purpose, and 'proper' moral conduct (long before the present neoliberal era). We trace this history and argue that this mode of thinking pervades the research that was undertaken to advance DOHaD ideas and the dominant interventions that were then devised. This stance continues to reproduce universal views of food and women's bodies that render invisible the complex realities of daily lives.

5.2 A Feminist Science and Technology Studies Approach

We come to the field of DOHaD from our respective disciplines of social epidemiology and social anthropology, with central interests in health inequalities, gender, and feminist STS. Science and technology studies sees science and society as inextricably intertwined. The analytic approach entails tracing the histories that are written into scientific practice, of how 'particular knowers, were embedded in, and influenced by, their religious, political, or gendered convictions, about how they could know depended on the people around them, the time and place, their class, and their own identities and interests' [6, p. 161]. While there are many different approaches within STS, a feminist STS approach draws attention to gender and its intersections with other relations of power and how these are smuggled into a science that is often presented as value free.

As feminist STS scholars, we actively interrogate disciplinary knowledge (including our own), their boundaries, and unequal power relations, reflecting on the taken-for-granted assumptions that underpin common-sense understandings of women's biosocial lives in DOHaD. We attend to matters of power within DOHaD and where it is vested – manifest in the conference arrangements, the keynote speakers, the websites, the reviews, and special issues. We notice who and what gets funded; how calls for new grants are framed and specified. We notice what sort of research receives accolades. We notice what is marginalised or left out. We think about how this is the result of much larger historical and political agendas and the continued dominance of biomedicine [7].

We are attuned to the boundary work that defines the fields of nutrition and DOHaD, and how nutrition has been discursively constructed to align with the 'epistemic authority of science' [8, p. 12], that is, the biomedical model. Such 'legitimation of knowledge claims [are] intimately tied to networks of domination and exclusion' [9, p. 1], which are themselves tied to structural systems of inequality.

We know that many DOHaD researchers will not be familiar with the above ideas. More simply, but with much loss of nuance, we think about which disciplines are seen as authorities on women's health and the implications of this view. When social conditions lead to health problems, surely this would invite social research and responses. Instead, what occurs is biomedical research and responses, and we seek to understand and critique this.

5.3 Social Inequalities in Health and the Promise of DOHaD

In 1980, the UK Working Group on Inequalities in Health reported that inequalities in health had widened since the National Health Service was established in 1948; this was attributed to various aspects of daily life and work, with implications for social policy [10]. Shunned by the Thatcher government, the 'Black report' (named after the chair of the Working Group) nevertheless received international attention and renewed research and advocacy around the social determinants of health.

Against this backdrop, within a decade, the theory that growth and development before birth influenced a person's health over the life course was proposed by David

Barker and his colleagues. It suggested a new mechanism for the link between social position and health [11], expanding the reach and relevance of ideas about the social determinants of health. With the accumulation of evidence and growing acceptance of DOHaD ideas, action to address social determinants seemed imminent with the 1998 Independent Inquiry into Inequalities in Health [12].

Yet social inequalities have continued to widen, in the UK and elsewhere, accompanied by an increase in economic insecurity [13, 14]. In Western countries, DOHaD ideas have not led to improvements in the social determinants of health of women and infants. Instead, a narrow view of nutrition and its role in the first 1,000 days has taken hold [15].

5.4 Developmental Origins of Adult Disease and Maternal Nutrition

The cohort studies undertaken by Barker and his colleagues in the UK in the late 1980s showed that an individual's weight at birth was associated with the risk of death from cardiovascular disease many decades later. Extended work pointed to problems with nutritional supply in fetal life. This understanding was consolidated in discussions with specialists in fetal physiology and placental development in the UK, Australia, and New Zealand [16].

Barker had been thinking about intergenerational nutrition for many years. In 1966, he published three papers from his PhD on prenatal factors and 'subnormal intelligence'. He noted an excess of children with an intelligence quotient between 65 and 74 in the two lowest social classes and suggested this might be explained by poor maternal diet or physique (with short stature reflecting stunting). In subsequent research, he considered a wide range of explanations for geographic variations in disease (such as gout and gallstones) within Britain, including occupational exposures and trace elements in drinking water [17]. However, he is said to have been most interested in adult diseases as possible consequences of nutritional conditions or infections in early life, evident in the studies that commenced when he became director of the Medical Research Council (MRC) Environmental Epidemiology Unit at Southampton University in 1984.

Research on disease aetiology, as upheld in biomedicine, is inevitably reductionist through the emphasis on identifying mechanisms and insisting that causation is only convincingly demonstrated by the experimental manipulation of specific factors [18]. Thus, despite the appreciation by Barker and his colleagues of the relevance of social circumstances and structural factors [19], wider environments were erased in the laboratory experiments and clinical studies required to provide the proof that maternal nutrition has effects on fetal growth and development. Not only has this logic directed vast attention to the physiology (and later, epigenetics) of the fetus and placenta, but it has also heavily influenced ideas about how to respond to nutrition as a cause of poor health.

Research motivated by the DOHaD theory concerning women's diets, pregnancy, and fetal growth indicated that the problem did not lie in specific nutrient deficiencies or in a specific condition such as anaemia. Historical and contemporary cohort studies of pregnant women suggested dietary imbalance or quality might be relevant, but also body composition (see [20]). Women's diets in pregnancy are usually a continuation of their established dietary patterns, and older work had already suggested that cumulative nutritional status before pregnancy influenced fetal growth more than dietary intake during pregnancy [21].

By the early 2000s, the focus had shifted to body size and women classified as obese, partly in response to concerns about gestational diabetes and obesity in children [22]. DOHaD researchers and practitioners might have emphasised the connections between obesity and stress and hardship [23]. Instead, they largely succumbed to what Scrinis [24] has called 'nutritionism', where individuals are provided with advice and detailed information on the constituents of food and induced to think in microbiological terms. This is an approach to problems involving nutrition that harks back to early-twentieth-century ways to address nutritional deficiencies. Excess body weight does not arise from a nutritional deficiency, but it is cast as a deficiency of information and willpower that is squarely located within 'non-normative' bodies [25].

5.5 The Treachery of Nutrition

We suggest that identifying nutrition as a cause of poor health invokes modes of research and institutional responses that do not involve social or structural change. As we will explore, nutritional causes of poor health are widely seen to require detailed biomedical analysis, translated into 'lifestyle' advice for individuals. This template does not attend to eco-social causes [26]; thus class and racial/racist inequalities are unacknowledged and undisturbed. We refer to this as the treachery of nutrition. This epistemic privileging of biomedical sciences renders other disciplines (such as social sciences) marginal to DOHaD knowledge and acceptance and constrains possibilities: for multiple knowledge (including lay knowledge); for inclusive funding for different research questions, methods, and interventions; and for new policy agendas.

At the core of the treachery of nutrition are its historical roots in biochemistry and physiology and the biomedical model. This disciplinary alliance and approach were remarkably successful in addressing deficiency diseases (such as rickets) in the early twentieth century, as will be outlined. However, the nature of the pressing problems changed to dietary imbalances and over-consumption. The old emphasis on micronutrients and the need to instruct people to consume unpalatable substances (such as cod liver oil) was carried forward. The approach was renovated as profiling of nutrients in foods and diets and providing people with instructions around this, despite the fact that lack of knowledge was hardly the problem it had been. Others have criticised the reductionist approach that dominates thinking about nutrition and health, in general, and the narrow responses this offers [4, 24, 27]. Here we take this up specifically in relation to DOHaD, which has become a site for the reproduction of hegemonic nutrition and a means for its proliferation in healthcare and popular media.

The expectations of nutrition as a means to improve public health rest on portable, insertable solutions: a spoonful of cod liver oil, a dose of lime juice, a dab of Marmite. These do not improve the living and working conditions of people but rather make them fit for work (historically, as sailors or labourers) or bearing arms (notably in World War I). This has been carried forward: an ounce of education, a brief piece of advice, a mobile phone app. The legacy of this tradition is clear within DOHaD. Also clear is that certain views of bodies and food pervade the field: making women fit for childbearing and food as substrate for fetal growth.

What this approach neglects is the gendered, sociocultural, economic, and political contexts of food and food systems, and the everyday lives of women and their emotional wellbeing, that shape the many practices of how eating, care, and nourishment are done.

We acknowledge that some DOHaD efforts have been directed to these broader contexts [28, 29], and we would encourage much more of this. We know it remains important to address micronutrient deficiencies in pregnant women in many parts of the world [30], and folic acid supplementation is important to prevent neural tube defects [31]. However, different approaches are needed for obesity.

5.6 The Overweening Shadow of Historical Nutritional Research

The history of nutrition research and its emergence as a science, as represented in imperial and colonial accounts, emphasises advances made in the UK and the USA from the 1900s [32]. These advances prioritised the discovery of nutrients, descriptions of nutritional deficiencies, and factors affecting nutrient availability. In the UK, this history is marked by concerted government efforts to research specific public health problems and then mobilise a response on a large scale. Unparalleled elsewhere, this reflects the much greater involvement of the UK than the USA in the two world wars. Nutrition was an 'instrument of state' [33, p. 702], as outlined below, pressed into service to ensure the food security of troops as well as that of the home population, with the UK vulnerable to blockade and experiencing a shortage of agricultural labour (see [33, 34]).

As recounted by Acheson (who preceded Barker as the director of the MRC Environmental Epidemiology Unit and then became Chief Medical Officer 1983–1991), 'The story of the Government's triumphantly successful food policy in World War II has often been told …' [35, p. 210]. To ensure the food supply, there was rationing underpinned by nutrition science. Thus, staples of bread and potatoes were not restricted, while meat, fat, and sugar were; vitamins were distributed; expectant and nursing mothers had an extra allowance of milk. The physical health of the population, notably children, measurably improved [35].

Less well known is an older history of endeavours, for example, to avoid scurvy in troops in World War I. An appeal by the War Office led to Harriette Chick at the Lister Institute recommending the consumption of beans and lentils that had been germinated or sprouted [34]. The political situation (war) made the study of vitamins (then known as accessory food factors) an imperative, and the functional properties of certain foods were used to solve the problem of maintaining the health of troops within the constraints of army food supplies; pulses for germination were much easier to store and distribute than fresh fruits and vegetables.

Also noteworthy is the history of rickets [32], which manifests in children as bowed legs and other skeletal deformities. Rickets was perplexing in research, long the subject of apparently contradictory findings and debate. In retrospect, we know that this confusion was because rickets is due to a deficiency of vitamin D (needed to absorb calcium), which can be sourced from sunlight or from diet (while some cereals can reduce absorption of calcium). In 1914, the (then) Medical Research Committee funded Edward Mellanby to undertake research that included his famous experiments with dogs; he fed puppies different diets to see which resulted in rickets, systematically identifying a deficiency of a fat-soluble accessory food factor that must be responsible and testing 'anti-rachitic' diets. Mellanby concluded that rickets was a deficiency disease that could be cured by providing animal fats or cod liver oil. After World War I, clinical trials with children in Vienna (led by Harriette Chick) demonstrated that rickets could be treated and prevented by these means (or sunlight) [36].

Mellanby went on to have a long career providing advice to the Ministry of Health and to the War Cabinet in World War II. His early work set a pattern for the interaction of clinical and experimental work that he advocated in a book with that title and as Secretary for the MRC from 1933 to 1949. Mellanby was hugely influential through the positions he held, and biomedical and nutrition science was shaped by his historically resonant presence. (See, for example, the celebration of this research tradition in the 'Timeline of MRC research and discoveries' on the website of UK Research and Innovation.) This pattern of clinical and experimental work was carried forward by McCance and Widdowson in their work on fetal and infant growth after World War II [37] and was advocated and upheld in the DOHaD field as the biomedical model par excellence.

Thus, after the initial findings from observational epidemiological studies, animal experiments that are the hallmarks of 'proper' scientific nutritional research were soon undertaken. This was vital to prove the principle that dietary manipulations in pregnant animals can alter long-term metabolic function in offspring. Most of the research was undertaken in rats, with consequences for offspring of maternal low-protein diets, in particular, described in detail: altered fetal growth; reduced size of truncal organs (but brain sparing); hypertension; abnormal glucose and insulin responses; impaired inflammatory responses; and shortened lifespan (e.g. [38]).

But these experiments should not be interpreted as demonstrations of what should happen in humans, in the way the older experiments on deficiencies provided direct guidance on what to insert into the diet. Even research with laboratory animals induced to have large amounts of body fat (e.g. [39]) only proves that this condition can affect the morphology and physiology of offspring; it does not indicate when or how obesity in women forming families should be addressed. Kelly and Russo [40] have identified this mistake in reasoning: the mechanisms of aetiology for non-communicable diseases are not the mechanisms of prevention. Thus, identifying obesity as a cause of poor health is not enough; it is not a pathogen or isolated behaviour to be eliminated; it has complex social origins that need to be understood for prevention to be possible.

We do not question a role of basic nutrition science, but we question it being viewed as almost all that is necessary, as providing a guide for clinical trials and related actions. The reductionism apparent in nutrition and in biomedicine more broadly was as strong as ever in DOHaD research, perhaps firmly embraced in the effort to gain legitimacy. The early findings from cohort studies had received the standard criticisms of observational epidemiology (see [41]): findings might reflect bias or confounding, correlation is not causation, and what was the mechanism? So the response was to undertake experiments in which nutrition was manipulated and to pursue biological mechanisms (eventually epigenetics). But more than this type of knowledge is required, and Penkler [15] notes that DOHaD researchers are beginning to recognise this.

Biomedicine and the basic sciences have profoundly shaped the field of nutrition and health, leading to well-trodden patterns of organisation across the scientific community. Thus, nourishment is seen in reductionist terms, food and the food–body relationship are standardised, and expert knowledge is seen as the corrective. This hegemonic nutrition is decontextualised: it does not attend to the exigencies of everyday lives; the roles of place, racism, gender and gender relations; or the politics of food systems. It dominates at the expense of other ways of thinking about food and health and possibilities for intervention. Valdez refers to this pervasive logic as an 'epistemic environment' [42, p. 9], as it highlights how scientific knowledge production is shaped and 'how science imagines, manages and apprehends future health' [42, pp. 9, 10]. This boundary work involves selective foreclosures [43], and in the case of DOHaD, this foreclosure consistently locates the 'problem' in maternal diets and in women's reproductive bodies, not in the broader conditions of daily lives.

5.7 Biopolitical Deployment of Nutrition Interventions

The DOHaD field clearly reflects a genealogy of hegemonic nutrition that can be further understood through Foucault's concept of biopolitics. Foucault argued that a new form of power emerged in the nineteenth century, with governments seeking to control and manage populations from a distance through expectations of collective conduct. Through shaping expectations about appropriate ways to live and behave, and having citizens monitor themselves and others, governments did not have to exert overt power (e.g. through threats of physical punishment or imprisonment). This form of power is known as biopolitics. Citizens learned about these expectations and how to conform through institutions such as schools and clinics (that had become widely accessible), as well as laws and regulations. Although the strategies and technologies of biopower (the ways expectations are created and maintained) have changed over time, one enduring focus has been reproduction and the role of mothers in serving the health of their children and in maintaining the population needed for labour and war [44, 45]. The biopolitics of reproduction is now extended to the health of their children before birth [46].

Biopower works subtly as it operates horizontally in everyday worlds rather than appearing to be imposed directives. People are asked to take responsibility for their health through self-care and to work on their own bodies according to normalised standards (see [47]). Autonomy is emphasised, and this resonates with a liberalism ideology. (But as the example of obesity makes clear, individuals are not free to reject expectations to do this work.) Expectations for collective conduct are set in conjunction with a range of networked agencies and professional organisations that authorise and legitimise norms. The medical profession and the basic sciences have long been sources of authority drawn upon in biopolitics (sometimes notoriously, as in the eugenics movement) [48, 49]. Biopower can be useful in organising communities and improving health, but it can also entail harm when problems are purely individualised.

There is a history of research in which pregnancy, childbirth, and caring for children are considered through the lenses of medicalisation and biopolitics [44, 50]. Mothers-to-be and mothers are subject to expert advice, medical monitoring, and public scrutiny, with discourses on appropriate self-care proliferating in popular media. Conforming is a personal responsibility and a moral imperative, regardless of a woman's life circumstances or constraints. In general, biopolitics identifies certain groups as needing more scrutiny and guidance to comply with bodily self-regulation. The 'problem' groups are those that fall outside the normalised parameters of health or civility, such as the poor, the unemployed, migrants, or people of colour. Such groups are often represented as ignorant and uneducated, requiring heightened surveillance and education. In relation to pregnancy, women whose body size is classified as obese are now seen as a 'problem' group. Here lies the potential to re-inscribe discrimination.

Antenatal lifestyle interventions for pregnant women, particularly those with large body size [51], are an exemplar of gendered biopolitics. Women are typically counselled by dieticians and provided individual advice. There are now apps to track nutritional intake and physical activity and to receive behaviour modification messages. Other educational supports in the service of improving lifestyles include any number of pamphlets, social media sites, and food marketing. While the use of digital technologies gives this a veneer of twenty-first-century self-help, these lifestyle interventions have not significantly changed since the 1950s [42].

Conceptually, biopolitics helps us see how medicine, nutrition science, and health promotion – now integrated in DOHaD – direct women to put more effort into managing their pregnant bodies and securing the future health of their children. For some women, this may be useful and provide a sense of control, but for others it is a source of unfair pressure. The individualisation of responsibility means that women are blamed, or feel blamed, when they do not act appropriately [52, 53], and the difficulties faced by women in disadvantaged circumstances and/or ethnic minorities are not taken into account. Furthermore, meaningful support and social change do not occur.

We are not trying to deny that improvements in antenatal care have reduced maternal and perinatal mortality and morbidity, notably over the first half of the twentieth century. We are not suggesting that women are not agents in biopolitical processes (especially middle-class, white women). However, we do criticise lifestyle interventions in antenatal care as the dominant response to DOHaD in Western countries. From within this paradigm, there have been questions about the efficacy of the approach because it probably occurs too late to benefit fetal development [54], so a shift in focus to pre-conception care has been proposed [55]. That would simply shift the problem of foreclosure we identify to an earlier point in women's lives.

Biopolitics constructs health as an individual responsibility. But as Wells has argued, society has created 'metabolic ghettos' in which people are susceptible to obesity, and there are many steps that governments could take to address the commercial and corporate determinants of obesity and to support people to have healthier lives [56]. These are social justice initiatives – not the portable, insertable solutions exemplified by cod liver oil.

5.7 Interdisciplinary Approaches Are Needed

The challenges of broadening and transforming disciplinary boundaries are multiple, even for those working from within. Tensions in the field of nutrition concerning its disciplinary emphasis have long been recognised (e.g. [57]). In 2005, Cannon and colleagues [27] set out the basis for a 'new nutrition science' that was social and environmental as well as biological. Within the American Society for Nutrition, the case for 'mode 2' research (another term for applied research) has been made [58]. Several European nutrition entities have jointly proposed embracing broader research domains and disciplines, including anthropology, sociology, and cultural studies [59].

But where are the funds to be found? For decades, nutrition science has received enormous funding from industries involved with agricultural production and food manufacturing. We note that the food industry has a vested interest in human nutrition being framed as food composition, with consumers needing better education, as this deflects attention from the corporate determinants of health (via multinational corporations making huge profits from processed food that is high in salt, fat, and sugar [60]). It is unclear how to fund the volume of research needed to provide depth and variety in the eco-social knowledge of nutrition, especially when health and medical research councils continue to see nutrition in biomedical terms. DOHaD could become a strong advocate for such research diversity.

It is not just through biomedicine and nutrition science that a repressive approach to diet and nutrition proliferates. This is reproduced across health and educational institutions as well as popular culture. DOHaD ideas have generated a great deal of wider interest [61], so there is an opportunity to engage with institutions and communities to ask questions about the traditional framing of nutritional problems and their solutions and to showcase alternatives [4, 43].

5.8 Conclusion

In conclusion, we would first like to acknowledge some limitations of this piece. There is also entangled colonialism and racism that we have not explored, nor have we been able to do justice to the biopolitics of the foundations of antenatal care (to avert population decline) (see [62]). We have focused on hegemonic nutrition as seen in the UK and Australia (which ignores Aboriginal and Torres Strait Islander knowledge). We had to be selective with the references provided, and we acknowledge there are many other scholars whose work is relevant.

The UK, Australia, and similar countries have favoured individualised responses to obesity prevention, despite being urged to take a societal or systems approach [63]. So far, this is also the dominant response within DOHaD, and DOHaD ideas have not changed social or structural factors that shape the health of women and their children. Indeed, the ideas might have found acceptance in an era that emphasises individual responsibility precisely because they follow a well-trodden path and are not disruptive. From our interdisciplinary standpoint, we recommend looking beyond biomedicine and nutrition science for answers to problems that encompass socio-economic-political-material-bio systems. Broadening attention to social environments includes appreciating and attending to the power relations of multiple knowledges, to differing disciplinary knowledges, and to the situated knowledges of the people and communities that are the focus of DOHaD. Without such interdisciplinary and co-constituted attention, DOHaD will not be able to address health inequalities.

References

1. Roberts D. *Killing the Black Body: Race, Reproduction and the Meaning of Liberty.* New York: Pantheon Books, 1997.

2. Ross L, Solinger R. *Reproductive Justice: An Introduction.* Berkeley: University of California Press, 2017.

3. Shrecker T, Bambra C. *How Politics Makes Us Sick: Neoliberal Epidemics.* Houndmills, Basingstoke, UK: Palgrave Macmillan, 2015.

4. Hayes Conroy A, Hayes Conroy J. *Doing Nutrition Differently: Critical Approaches to Diet and Dietary Interventions.* Ashgate: London, 2013.

5. Sanabria E, Yates-Doerr E. Alimentary uncertainties: From contested evidence to policy. *BioSocieties* 2015; 10: 117–124.

6. Martin A. Science as culture. In Brock M, Raby D, Thomas R. (eds) *Power and Everyday Practices.* Toronto: Nelson Education, 2011; 161–181.

7. Fisher M, Baum FE, MacDougall C, Newman L, McDermott D. To what extent do Australian health policy documents address social determinants of

health and health equity? *J Social Policy* 2016; 45: 545–564.

8. Gieryn T. *Cultural Boundaries of Science: Credibility on the Line*. Chicago, IL: University of Chicago Press, 1999.

9. Lennon K, Whitford M. Introduction. In Lennon K, Whitford M. (eds) *Knowing the Difference: Feminist Perspectives in Epistemology*. London: Routledge, 1994; 1–16,

10. Department of Health and Social Security. *Report of a Working Group on Inequalities in Health*. London: DHSS, 1980.

11. Barker DJP. The foetal and infant origins of inequalities in health in Britain. *J Public Health Med* 1991; 13: 64–68.

12. Acheson D. *Inequalities in Health: Report of an Independent Inquiry*. London: HMSO, 1998.

13. Stiglitz J, Fitoussi J-P, Durand M. *Beyond GDP: Measuring What Counts for Economic and Social Performance*. Paris: OECD, 2018.

14. Paremoer L, Nandi S, Serag H, Baum F. Covid-19 pandemic and the social determinants of health. *Br Med J* 2021; 372: n129.

15. Penkler M. Caring for biosocial complexity. Articulations of the environment in research on the Developmental Origins of Health and Disease. *Studies in History and Philosophy Science* 2022; 93: 1–10.

16. Barker DJP, Gluckman PD, Godfrey KM, Harding JE, Owens JA, Robinson JS. Fetal nutrition and cardiovascular disease in adult life. *Lancet* 1993; 341: 938–941.

17. Barker DJP. Geographical variations in disease in Britain. *Br Med J* 1981; 283: 398–400.

18. Davis JE. Holism against reductionism. In Davis JE, Gonzales AM. (eds) *To Fix or to Heal: Patient Care, Public Health, and the Limits of Biomedicine*. New York: New York University Press, 2016;1–29.

19. Barker DJP. *Mothers, Babies and Disease in Later Life*. London: BMJ Publishing, 1994.

20. Godfrey K, Barker DJP. Fetal nutrition and adult disease. *Am J Clin Nutr* 2000; 71 (suppl); 1344S–1355S.

21. Ounsted M, Ounsted C. *On Fetal Growth Rate: Its Variations and Their Consequences*. London: Heinemann Medical, 1973.

22. Oken E, Gillman MW. Fetal origins of obesity. *Obes Res* 2003; 11: 496–506.

23. Moore V, Warin M. The reproduction of shame: Pregnancy, nutrition and body weight in the translation of developmental origins of adult disease. *Science, Technology, & Human Values* 2022; 47: 1277–1301.

24. Scrinis, G. *Nutritionism: The Science and Politics of Dietary Advice*. New York: Columbia University Press, 2013.

25. Warin M, Turner K, Moore V, Davies M. Bodies, mothers and identities: Rethinking obesity and the BMI. *Sociol Health Illn* 2008; 30: 97–111.

26. Krieger N. Proximal, distal, and the politics of causation: What's level got to do with it? *Am J Public Health* 2006; 98: 221–230.

27. Cannon G, Leitzmann C. The new nutrition science project. *Public Health Nutr* 2005; 8: 673–694.

28. Penkler M, Hanson M, Biesma R, Muller R. DOHaD in science and society: Emergent opportunities and novel responsibilities. *J Dev Orig Health Dis* 2019; 10: 268–273.

29. Strommer SL, Lawrence W, Shaw S, Correia Simao S, Jenner S, Barrett M, et al. Behavior change interventions: Getting in touch with individual differences, values and emotions. *J Dev Orig Health Dis* 2020; 11: 589–598.

30. Keats EC, Haider BA, Tam E, Bhutta ZA. Multiple-micronutrient supplementation for women during pregnancy. *Cochrane Database Syst Rev* 2019, 3. Art. No.: CD004905.

31. De-Regil L, Peña-Rosas J, Fernández-Gaxiola AC, Rayco-Solon P. Effects and safety of periconceptional oral folate supplementation for preventing birth

defects. *Cochrane Database Syst Rev* 2015, 12. Art. No.: CD007950.

32. Carpenter KJ. A short history of nutritional science: Part 3 (1912–1944). *J Nutr* 2003; 133: 3023–3032.

33. Cannon G. The rise and fall of dietetics and of nutrition science, 4000 BCE–2000 CE. *Public Health Nutr* 2005; 8: 701–705.

34. Smith R. The emergence of vitamins as bio-political objects during World War I. *Stud Hist Philos Biol Biomed Sci* 2009; 40: 179–189.

35. Acheson D. Nutrition monitoring of the health of the nation. *J R Soc Health* 1987; 6: 209–214.

36. Carpenter KJ. Harriette Chick and the problem of rickets. *J Nutr* 2008; 138: 827–832.

37. Buklijas T. Food, growth and time: Elsie Widdowson's and Robert McCance's research into prenatal and early postnatal growth. *Stud Hist Philos Sci* 2014; 47: 267–277.

38. Langley-Evans S. Fetal programming of cardiovascular function through exposure to maternal undernutrition. *Proc Nutr Soc* 2001; 60: 505–513.

39. Samuelsson A, Matthews PA, Argenton M, Christie MR, McConnell JM, Jansen E, et al. Diet-induced obesity in female mice leads to offspring hyperphagie, adiposity, hypertension, and insulin resistance. *Hypertension* 2008; 41: 383–392.

40. Kelly MP, Russo F. Causal narratives in public health: The difference between mechanisms of aetiology and mechanisms of prevention in non-communicable diseases. *Sociol Health Illn* 2018; 40: 82–99.

41. Joseph KS, Kramer MS. Review of the evidence on fetal and early childhood antecedents of adult chronic disease. *Epidemiol Rev* 1996; 18: 158–174.

42. Valdez N. *Weighing the Future: Race, Science and Pregnancy Trials in the Postgenomic Era.* Oakland: University of California Press, 2021.

43. Guthman J. *Weighing In: Obesity, Food Justice and the Limits of Capitalism.* Berkeley: University of California Press, 2011.

44. Ginsburg F, Rapp R. The politics of reproduction. *Annu Rev Anthropol* 1991; 20: 311–343.

45. Clarke A. *Disciplining Reproduction.* Berkeley: University of California Press, 1998.

46. Lupton, D. 'Precious cargo': Foetal subjects, risk and reproductive citizenship. *Crit Public Health* 2012; 22: 329–340.

47. Coveney J. *Food, Morals and Meaning: The Pleasure and Anxiety of Eating.* New York: Routledge, 2006.

48. Lemke T. The birth of bio-politics: Michel Foucault's lecture at the College de France on neo-liberal governmentality. *Econ Soc* 2001; 30: 190–207.

49. Rose N. The politics of life itself. *Theory Culture Soc* 2001; 18: 1–30.

50. Oakley A. The sociology of childbirth: An autobiographical journey through four decades of research. *Sociol Health Illn* 2016; 38: 689–705.

51. Flynn AC, Dalrymple K, Barr S, Poston L, Goff L, Rogonzinska E, et al. Dietary interventions in overweight and obese pregnant women: A systematic review of the content, delivery, and outcomes of randomized controlled trials. *Nutr Rev* 2016; 74: 312–328.

52. Warin M, Zivkovic T, Moore V, Davies M. Mothers as smoking guns: Fetal overnutrition and the reproduction of obesity. *Feminism Psych* 2012; 22: 360–375.

53. Richardson SS, Daniels CR, Gillman MW, Golden J, Kukla R, Kuzawa C, Rich-Edwards J. Society: Don't blame the mothers. *Nature* 2014; 512: 131–132.

54. Catalano P, deMouzon SH. Maternal obesity and metabolic risk to the offspring: Why lifestyle interventions may not have achieved the desired outcomes. *Int J Obes* 2015; 39: 642–649.

55. Vogel C, Kriznik N, Stephenson J, Barker M. Preconception nutrition: Building advocacy and social movements to

stimulate action. *J Dev Orig Health Dis* 2021; 12: 141–146.

56. Wells J. *The Metabolic Ghetto: An Evolutionary Perspective on Nutrition, Power Relations and Chronic Disease.* Cambridge: Cambridge University Press, 2016.

57. Waterlow JC. Crisis for nutrition. *Proc Nutr Soc* 1981; 40: 195–207.

58. Pelletier DL, Porter CM, Aarons GA, Wuehler SE, Neufeld LM. Expanding the frontiers of population nutrition research: New questions, new methods, and new approaches. *Adv Nutr* 2013; 4: 92–114.

59. Tufford AR, Calder PC, Van't Veer P, Feskens EF, Ockhuizen T, Kraneveld AD, Sikkema J, de Vries J. Is nutrition science ready for the twenty-first century? Moving towards transdisciplinary impacts in a changing world. *Eur J Nur* 2020; 59 (Suppl 1): 1–10.

60. Nestle M. *Unsavory Truth: How Food Companies Skew the Science of What We Eat.* New York: Basic Books, 2018.

61. Budds K. Fit to conceive? Representations of preconception health in the UK press. *Feminism Psych* 2021; 31: 463–482.

62. Hanson C. *A Cultural History of Pregnancy: Pregnancy, Medicine, and Culture 1750–2000.* Houndmills, Basingstoke, UK: Palgrave Macmillan, 2004.

63. Ulijaszek SJ, McLennan AK. Framing obesity in UK policy from the Blair years, 1997–2015: The persistence of individualistic approaches despite overwhelming evidence of societal and economic factors, and the need for collective responsibility. *Obes Rev* 2016; 17: 397–411.

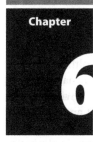

Gender, Racism, and DOHaD

Natali Valdez and Martine Lappé

6.1 Introduction

Contemporary scholars, many of whom are included in this edited volume, have highlighted the gendered dimensions of DOHaD research, noting its social and historical contours and consequences, particularly for women and mothers [1–4]. This chapter furthers these important discussions by highlighting how a gendered analysis of DOHaD must focus not only on how women's bodies and lives are taken up and affected by science but also on DOHaD's relationship to racism. By examining DOHaD through a feminist and critical race lens, we address how *both* gender and racism operate as relations of power in and through this science. Our analysis critically examines how gender has traditionally been studied as distinct from race and racism in DOHaD research, and the need to do otherwise.

This approach reflects our interest in transformational feminist interventions in the life sciences, and the need to centre reproductive justice and anti-racism in these efforts. Rather than seeing categories like gender, race, and class as discrete variables that merely need to be included or compared to one another in DOHaD and other areas of research, here we draw on Black feminist scholarship to highlight gender and racism as mutually constructed and reinforcing power relations that inform the history and contemporary contours of DOHaD and its ongoing effects. By analysing these dimensions of the science, this chapter reflects how gender and racism unequally survey and manage the living conditions and behaviours of Black, Brown, and Indigenous bodies, highlights the unequal impacts of DOHaD research, and reflects the need for a critical gender analysis of DOHaD and other postgenomic sciences [5]. Our analysis therefore focuses on how gender is always already bound up with racism and other forms of oppression, and how this shapes the practices and possible futures of DOHaD in critical ways.[1]

6.2 Gender, Reproduction, and Biopolitics

We begin this chapter with a review of feminist and critical race analyses of reproduction and an emphasis on biopolitics and processes of medicalisation that are central to the focus on pregnancy and early development in DOHaD research. Biopolitics refers to how the population emerged as a political problem to be managed by the state, and medicalisation focuses on how domains of social life become defined as medical problems [6, 7]. We discuss these concepts and their contributions to our analysis in relation to the

---

[1] For more on race in DOHaD research, see Meloni et al. in this volume.

'politics of reproduction', which Ginsburg and Rapp [8] developed to explore the vital role that reproduction plays in social and institutional organisations [9]. Engaging these approaches and their intersections is important, as DOHaD has increasingly become central to reproductive science, medicine, and conceptualisations of health and illness more broadly [10, 11]. Further, Lappé, Jeffries Hein, and Landecker have framed DOHaD and its sibling science environmental epigenetics as part of an 'environmental politics of reproduction' to address the intersections of the environment and reproduction in late capitalism [12].[2] This approach and others explicitly highlight the racialised politics of reproduction in contemporary DOHaD and environmental epigenetics research and how broader relations of power shape these sciences and their effects [13–15]. Drawing on this rich set of literature, this section positions gender and DOHaD as part of a larger feminist discussion on the biopolitics of reproduction and in relation to race/racism, a term that Valdez uses to intervene on references to race as if it were not always already embedded in racist logics [16]. While our own work is situated in the United States, Canada, and the United Kingdom, here we draw on scholarship across various locations to illustrate why a critical gender analysis is necessary anywhere DOHaD research is conducted and circulates.

Reproduction was and often still is conceived of only as a 'woman's issue' with the science and medicalisation of reproduction centred largely on cis-gendered women's bodies. Numerous scholars have analysed how DOHaD's focus on pregnancy reinforces this emphasis and positions cis-gender women as central objects of study and primary targets of intervention [17]. DOHaD researchers claim to study this period of the lifecourse because of the unique plasticity and programming of biological systems during 'critical windows' of fetal development. However, historians of maternal–fetal relations argue that this emphasis on pregnancy shapes and is shaped by gendered forms of social control and surveillance that have been central throughout the history of the reproductive sciences [1, 18].

Scholars of the contemporary also illustrate how a focus on the individual behaviours and exposures of pregnant people in DOHaD research overwhelmingly positions mothers as primarily responsible for the health of future generations. For example, Pentecost and Ross, Sharp and Richardson, Warin, Moore and Davies, Kenney and Müller, and others discuss how DOHaD emphasises pregnancy as an ideal time for research and intervention, despite the recognition that social environments shape health throughout the lifecourse [2, 4, 19, 20]. These authors and others show how the focus on early life and pregnant bodies within DOHaD studies relies on and reinforces self-surveillance and anticipatory care work for people with the capacity for pregnancy [11]. In their chapter in this volume, Chiapperino and colleagues also detail how DOHaD influences gendered responsibilities for health in ways that reinforce the gender binary and unequally impact women's bodies and lives. This occurs around food and nutrition, as Moore and Warin discuss in this volume, and in relation to pollutants, pesticides [21], and stress [22], in ways that disproportionately affect Black, Brown, and Indigenous lives [13, 23], as we discuss below.

---

[2] DOHaD often draws on epigenetic mechanisms to explain the links between gestational exposures and intergenerational health outcomes, and its focus on pregnancy and reproduction brings studies across DOHaD and epigenetics together, even while the fields also remain distinct.

Of course, as numerous scholars of gender, women's, and queer studies reflect, reproduction is not only the domain of cis-gender women. Recently, feminist science studies scholars in particular have brought attention to the missing science of men's reproductive contributions and paternal effects [24], providing a necessary intervention into discussions of gender and DOHaD [1]. Feminist science studies is a transdisciplinary area of scholarship that addresses how gender and other social categorisations shape and are shaped by science and technology. While these specific interventions are important to consider, our review of biopolitics, medicalisation, and the politics and environmental politics of reproduction in this section reflects that merely expanding scientific and medical surveillance to men deemed capable of reproduction will do little to address how power relations influence DOHaD science and its unequal impacts. Rather, we argue that a critical gender analysis must focus on the racial and gender politics of DOHaD and question the premise that individuals are the appropriate target for intervention at all. Doing so relies on well-established literature that actively positions reproduction as a topic crucial to social theory [25]. As we detail below, a continued focus on individual bodies as sites of intervention, rather than on broad social structures and power relations, reflects the convergence of biopolitics and reproductive politics within DOHaD and underscores the need to address the central logics that influence this science [6, 9].

Biopolitics and the politics of reproduction illuminate how social institutions like medical and population health programmes, as well as the military–industrial complex, provide the infrastructure that makes it possible to systematically collect health data and the unequal impacts of these efforts. This is important for our analysis because foundational observational studies that inform DOHaD's focus on the long-term health consequences of experiences and exposures during early development were originally based on the systematic collection of state and military health records [26]. The concept of biopolitics therefore allows us to address how power relations and social institutions have shaped DOHaD and its relationships to race/racism from its very beginnings and their ongoing effects today.

In his elaboration of the concept of biopolitics, Foucault argued that because of a fundamental shift in European nation-states during the seventeenth century, individual bodies became a key target for the maintenance of the nation. In that context, he argued that individual and aggregate bodies became important for protecting and defining the state, nation, or population, and keeping bodies healthy became crucial to produce labour and maintain the military. While Foucault focused on the management of 'families' as the fundamental units of the population [6], feminist scholars highlight that the 'family unit' Foucault imagined was primarily the bodies and behaviours of women [27]. Feminist scholars of colour have arbitrated further by emphasising that Black, Brown, and Indigenous reproduction is seen by the nation-state as a threat to the white supremacist imagination across multiple locations and time periods [23, 27].

The connection between individual bodies and the body of the nation has therefore justified the control and intervention of people's reproductive capacities in numerous ways. Public health campaigns from the nineteenth and twentieth centuries targeted poor women to reduce their fertility rates and prescribed a 'domestic science' of house cleaning for germ prevention [28]. Later approaches focused on behaviours related to alcohol and tobacco consumption [29] and breastfeeding [30]. In more contemporary examples, forced sterilisation of immigrant populations, family separation at the United States and other borders, expansive juvenile detention, and the overturning of Roe

v. Wade in the United States provide just a few of the state-endorsed reproductive and family policies that emerge from racist, nationalist, and xenophobic laws and policies [31–33].

The medicalisation of reproduction was also founded on the biopolitical aim of controlling and managing people's reproductive capacities and frames pregnancy as an illness that requires medical intervention and surveillance [34]. Riessman argues that the medicalisation of reproduction is a 'contradictory reality for women' [35, p. 16] as it provides certain women a way to gain some control and autonomy over aspects of reproduction while strengthening the control of biomedicine to define and survey reproductive experiences. We draw on this approach to emphasise that not all women and non-binary people experience 'reproductive freedoms'. Rather, as Black feminists argue, current notions of reproductive 'freedom' that focus on bodily autonomy and choice are based on systemic forms of control, exploitation, and oppression forced upon formerly enslaved people over the course of hundreds of years and continue to affect Black, Brown, and Indigenous lives today [27].

To study these dynamics of reproduction, feminist scholars have developed a varied repertoire of tools and frameworks important to a critical gender analysis of DOHaD. Central to these, and part of the politics of reproduction introduced at the beginning of this section, is Ginsberg and Rapp's notion of 'stratified reproduction'. This concept describes how political, economic, and social forces create the conditions under which people carry out reproductive labour [36]. Stratified reproduction emphasises the need to explore reproductive experiences based on social, racial, and gendered locations and reflects how the treatment of people's reproduction is not equally valued: certain people's reproduction is cherished, while the reproduction of others is denied and denigrated [13, 26, 35–37]. This is a critical lens through which to understand how gender has always been tied to race and racism within the sciences associated with reproduction, including DOHaD.

Another key concept for understanding the politics of reproduction, especially in a postgenomic era, is the Reproductive Justice (RJ) framework developed by the SisterSong collective [23, 38–40]. It focuses on how racism shapes reproductive experiences and prioritises the stories of women of colour as the foundation for new knowledge. Reproductive Justice also emphasises how social justice issues like mass incarceration, premature death, disinvestment in public services, and environmental justice are all reproductive issues. This approach highlights how the management of population health through the control of reproduction was operationalised at the level of the individual through ideas of responsibility that were always deeply connected to racist ideologies. Thus, the RJ framework aims to move beyond the individualistic and neoliberal dis-course of 'choice' to recognise that not everyone lives in an environment that provides them with the same options from which to choose [41].

Applying these feminist and critical race concepts allows us to explore how DOHaD theories *deepen* the stratification of reproduction. For example, in her book *Weighing the Future*, Valdez highlights how contemporary pregnancy trials that draw on DOHaD and epigenetic theories to study how maternal diet during pregnancy impacts children's health outcomes are akin to nineteenth- and twentieth-century biopolitical strategies that focus on controlling, managing, or surveying women's bodies and behaviours. Her analysis shows how, historically and presently, the surveillance and control of reproduc-tion are unevenly distributed across populations based on race and class. Through her ethnographic study, Valdez illustrates how this occurs through what she calls the 'politics of postgenomic reproduction', a framework that examines how new science and technology emergent in a postgenomic era, including the fields of epigenetics and DOHaD, create conditions that both enliven twentieth-century reproductive politics and stimulate novel iterations of surveillance, risk, and control in the twenty-first century [16].

This feminist lens critically attends to issues of race and gender in two main ways: its application is based on the premise that processes of racism are enacted in and through reproduction and that queering reproduction requires a reframing of the maternal environment that is not biologically and genetically essentialised or individualised to cis-gendered bodies deemed capable of reproduction. Queering reproduction reflects the need to rethink reproduction beyond heteronormative, cisgender, white supremacist, and biocentric ways of thinking and aligns with the ethic of recent feminist scholarship on the environmental politics of reproduction as well. Building on the politics of reproduction and the intellectual and advocacy movements of RJ and Environmental Reproductive Justice (ERJ), Lappé, Jeffries Hein, and Landecker's analysis of the environmental politics of reproduction critically addresses the intersections of lived experiences of oppression, environments of late capitalism, and postgenomic sciences to illustrate how human reproduction is increasingly bound up with environmental issues in ways that are always already connected to gender and racism [12]. Both the politics of postgenomic reproduction and environmental politics of reproduction therefore highlight how racism, white supremacy, and neocolonialism shape the unequal distribution of resources, lived experiences of reproduction, and the practices and ethics of emergent sciences [12, 41]. Alongside the concepts detailed above, this scholarship provides a critical entry point for addressing the intersections of gender and racism in DOHaD science today.

6.3 Don't Blame the Poor Black, Brown, and Indigenous Pregnant Person

Two examples from our own scholarship illustrate how the emphasis on the bodies and behaviours of cis-gendered pregnant women and a lack of attention to racism and stratification influence the practices and consequences of contemporary DOHaD science. Our findings and the work of others reflect that even when measures of race and socioeconomic status (SES) are incorporated into DOHaD studies, merely including these variables does little to address how *racism* shapes lived experiences or to dismantle the gendered and racial logics that inform many DOHaD studies [16, 45]. These examples show that inconsistent and superficial measures of race and class often stand in for the deeply embedded power relations that influence health outcomes of central interest in the studies we follow. Thus, both examples introduced in this section reinforce the need for critical gender analyses of DOHaD and other postgenomic sciences that attend to the ways that gender and race/racism shape research practices, knowledge claims, and the impacts they have on experiences of reproduction and the broader environments that influence health across the lifecourse.

The first example comes from Valdez's ethnographic study of contemporary postgenomic pregnancy trials in the United States and United Kingdom. Introduced briefly above, her influential project draws on critical race theory and Black feminist theory to address how race/racism is foregrounded at the recruitment phase of trials focused on maternal diet during pregnancy and children's future health and then disappears during the collection and analysis of the trials, only to return as significant in the comparison of outcomes in the publication of results [16, 42]. Her findings reflect how race is imbued with meaning, yet remains mercurial and mobilised in ways that distance it from the contexts and relations of power that shape the lives of trial participants.

Valdez's findings illuminate the need to shift the focus away from diversity and inclusion efforts in postgenomic research and instead theorise how *racist environments* impact maternal health outcomes across the lifecourse [16]. Her work shows that individual-level interventions, which are central to these trials, need to be read as symptomatic of systemic racism, rather than as a solution to multidimensional illnesses like diabetes and obesity that disproportionately impact communities of colour. This is because the 'underlying logics of individual lifestyle interventions are cut from the same ideological cloth that assumes poor, fat, and ethnically diverse individuals have risky bodies and are responsible for changing their bodies and behaviors' [16, p. 10].

While such individual lifestyle interventions are framed as if all bodies live in similar environments and have equal access to 'healthy' opportunities, choices, and material conditions, Valdez shows that the pregnant people classified as 'high risk' for diabetes and obesity that are targeted for these interventions live in racist and poorly resourced environments that make it nearly impossible for them to comply with the intervention during the trial or sustain the intervention changes after the trial is completed. These findings reflect a key aspect of our argument here, which is that gender analysis without a critical understanding of race/racism is not a comprehensive framework for understanding DOHaD science and its consequences. This is particularly so when numerous studies show that focusing solely on individual interventions in maternal nutrition or early care is ineffective in addressing health and disease inequities [43].

In our second example, Lappé's multi-sited ethnographic study of epigenetic research related to children's behavioural health finds a similar emphasis on cis-gender women and their individual care practices during pregnancy and early parenthood, rather than on the structural conditions that shape their lives. Lappé's project focuses on the production and circulation of epigenetic and DOHaD knowledge related to children's behavioural health across laboratories, clinics, and communities in the United States and Canada. By studying the material practices and epistemic cultures that inform this science and its translation, she shows how many studies and initiatives focus on early-life adversity (ELA) as central in their broader questions about children's behavioural health. She finds that scientists and others often use ELA to capture how myriad early-life experiences, including neglect, abuse, and poverty, shape health trajectories across the lifecourse [12, 44, 45].

Through her observations of behavioural epigenetic studies and their translation, Lappé describes how past and present DOHaD theories and findings critically inform the practices and impacts of these efforts [44, 45]. For example, even when epigenetic scientists, clinicians, and community members emphasised the health impacts of racism as primary motivations for their work, she finds that standardised measures of race and disadvantage used in many studies provide poor proxies for how racism and gender mutually shape lived experiences of pregnancy, parenting, and children's health. Often limited to self-reported race, maternal education, and SES, Lappé reflects how scientists themselves noted the limitations of these measures, which nevertheless became built into large-scale epigenetic studies of children's health. Her analysis shows how these measures and the primary focus on cis-gender women's behaviours do little to address how systemic oppression influences the outcomes of interest in the studies she follows [45].

Lappé also finds that epigenetic and DOHaD studies of early life often build on previous results from animal models to focus primarily on the effect that women's behaviours and experiences during pregnancy and early parenthood have on their children's future health. As a result, concerns about the health effects of racism become channelled through measures and analyses that emphasise the maternal–child dyad and women's care practices, rather than on how racist and sexist environments influence their lives. Even when studies aimed to improve children's health through supporting families, the focus on women's behaviours and experiences during pregnancy and postpartum had the effect of individualising responsibilities for children's health, rather than addressing the need for broader social and structural change [46].

The analyses provided in these two empirical examples reflect how narrow and persistently individualistic models in DOHaD and epigenetic research focus on binary notions of gender and do little to address how systemic racism shapes experiences of reproduction and health across the lifecourse. The absence of *racism* as a central factor in prominent DOHaD studies therefore helps perpetuate understandings of health and inequity that overemphasise comparisons across racial and ethnic groups while ignoring the role of systemic racism in shaping health inequities. Such understandings reflect how race and ethnicity continue to be used in DOHaD and postgenomics research despite the knowledge that it is *racism* that fundamentally shapes health inequities across all gradients of income [5, 47, 48].[3] Further, the focus on behaviours during pregnancy and early life in these and many other studies reinforces the individualised focus on cisgender pregnant women and mothers, rather than emphasising the unequal social environments that shape their lives.

These findings matter as new epigenetic and biopolitical strategies in the postgenomic era emphasise how present exposures and experiences may shape both intergenerational and transgenerational health. This extension of individualised responsibilities can further white supremacist and neoliberal notions of health by ignoring the connections between gender, racism, and reproduction. A feminist and critical race lens draws attention to these dimensions of DOHaD science and their unequal consequences, particularly when studies are overly dependent on individual-level interventions. The persistent focus on cisgender bodies and race, rather than racism, in DOHaD research also reflects how systemic racism and late liberalism shape science. The findings described in this section therefore reinforce the importance of addressing how gender and racism operate as mutually constituted power relations that shape DOHaD research and its effects in the world.

6.4 Conclusion

Over the past several decades, scholars have drawn more awareness to how systemic racism and other forms of oppression impact health, pointing to structural and institutional power relations, rather than individual actions, as critical sites for intervention. This work builds on a history of activism by Black, Brown, and Indigenous communities to address how racism, violence, and environmental injustice shape health inequities and

---

[3] See Meloni et al. in this volume on race and DOHaD research.

lived experiences of reproduction [49, 50]. As we have illustrated above, these agendas and those in critical gender studies offer opportunities for DOHaD researchers to examine their research, its history, and its current mobilisations to address how gender and racism shape this science.

Through the frameworks and empirical research introduced above, we have shown that merely including gender, race, ethnicity, and class as variables of interest in DOHaD research does little to address how the mutually constituted power relations of gender and *racism* shape science and its unequal impacts on people's lives. Addressing this is of utmost importance as Black, Brown, and Indigenous people have been and continue to be exploited through scientifically legitimised narratives that allow the state to remove their autonomy, force reproduction and sterilisation, and deny their reproductive rights [27, 51]. As reflected in rates of premature birth and maternal mortality among Black women in the United States regardless of SES, the relationships between gender and racism shape health inequities in clear and ongoing ways [48, 52]. These forms of 'obstetric racism' and the analysis we provide above reveal how gender is always already bound up with racism and other forms of oppression [34].

To address gender and racism in DOHaD, interdisciplinary engagements with this science must explicitly name how power relations shape research and its effects. In this chapter, we have highlighted how a feminist and critical race approach to gender and racism in DOHaD is necessary to accomplish this goal. In doing so, we advocate for critical gender analyses that push social and biological scientists alike to examine how systems of oppression inform research and its unequal impacts in the world. We end by highlighting the need to move beyond description and critique to create real change in the structures that affect people's lives. This requires not only rethinking how we analyse DOHaD science but also actively reshaping the racist environments that impact health [53, 54].

References

1. S. S. Richardson, The Maternal Imprint: The Contested Science of Maternal-Fetal Effects (Chicago, IL: University of Chicago Press, 2021).

2. G. C. Sharp, D. A. Lawlor, S. S. Richardson, It's the mother!: How assumptions about the causal primacy of maternal effects influence research on the developmental origins of health and disease. Social Science & Medicine. 213 (2018), 20–7.

3. B. Mansfield, J. Guthman, Epigenetic life: Biological plasticity, abnormality, and new configurations of race and reproduction. Cultural Geography. 22(1) (2015), 3–20.

4. M. Warin, T. Zivkovic, V. Moore, M. Davies, Mothers as smoking guns: Fetal overnutrition and the reproduction of obesity. Feminism & Psychology. 22(3) (2012), 360–75.

5. M. Meloni, T. Moll, A. Issaka, C. W. Kuzawa, A biosocial return to race? A cautionary view for the postgenomic era. American Journal of Human Biology. 34(7) (2022), 2–24.

6. M. Foucault, The Birth of Biopolitics: Lectures at the Collège de France, 1978–1979 (London: Palgrave Macmillan, 2010).

7. P. Conrad, Medicalization and social control. Annual Review of Sociology. 18 (1) (1992), 209–32.

8. F. Ginsburg, R. Rapp, The politics of reproduction. Annual Review of Anthropology. 20(1) (1991), 311–43.

9. E. Thacker, Necrologies: or, the death of the body politic. In: P. T. Clough, C. Willse, editors. Beyond Biopolitics. (New York: Duke University Press, 2011) pp. 139–62.

10. E. M. Armstrong, Reproduction, Health, and Medicine (United Kingdom: Emerald Publishing, 2019).

11. M. Waggoner, The Zero Trimester: Pre-Pregnancy Care and the Politics of Reproductive Risk (Oakland: University of California Press, 2017).

12. M. Lappé, R. J. Hein, Landecker, Environmental politics of reproduction. Annual Review of Anthropology. 48(1) (2019), 133–50.

13. N. Valdez, D. Deomampo, Centering race and racism in reproduction. Medical Anthropology. 38(7) (2019), 551–9.

14. A. Saldaña-Tejeda, P. Wade, Eugenics, epigenetics, and obesity predisposition among Mexican Mestizos. Medical Anthropology. 38(8) (2019), 664–79.

15. R. Rapp, Race & reproduction: An enduring conversation. Medical Anthropology Quarterly. 38(8) (2019), 725–32.

16. N. Valdez, Weighing the Future: Race, Science, and Pregnancy Trials in the Postgenomic Era (Oakland: University of California Press, 2021).

17. M. Pentecost, F. C. Ross, A. Macnab, Beyond the dyad: Making Developmental Origins of Health and Disease (DOHaD) interventions more inclusive. Journal of Developmental Origins of Health and Disease. 9(1) (2018), 10–14.

18. T. Buklijas, Transformations of the maternal-fetal relationship in the twentieth century: From maternal impressions to epigenetic states. In: B. Dohm, U. Helduser, editors. Imagination en des Ungeborenen/Imaginations of the Unborn (Heidelberg: Universitätsverlag Winter, 2018) pp. 213–33.

19. M. Pentecost, F. Ross. The first thousand days: Motherhood, scientific knowledge, and local histories. Medical Anthropology. 38(8) (2019), 747–61.

20. M. Kenney, R. Müller, Of rats and women: Narratives of motherhood in environmental epigenetics. BioSocieties. 12 (2016), 23–46.

21. N. Mackendrick, More work for mother: Chemical body burdens as a maternal responsibility. Gender & Society. 28(5) (2014), 705–28.

22. C. J. Mulligan, Early environments, stress, and the epigenetics of human health.

Annual Review of Anthropology. 45 (2016), 233–49.

23. L. J. Ross, R. Solinger, Reproductive Justice: An Introduction (Oakland: University of California Press, 2017).

24. R. Almeling, GUYnecology: The Missing Science of Men's Reproductive Health (Oakland: University of California Press, 2020).

25. F. D. Ginsburg, R. Rapp, Conceiving the New World Order: The Global Politics of Reproduction (Berkeley: University of California Press, 1995).

26. Z. Stein, M. Susser, G. Saenger, F. Marolla, Famine and Human Development: The Dutch Hunger Winter of 1944–1945 (New York: Oxford University Press, 1975).

27. D. E. Roberts, Killing the Black Body: Race, Reproduction, and the Meaning of Liberty (New York: Pantheon Books, 1997.

28. N. Tomes, The Gospel of Germs: Men, Women, and the Microbe in American Life (Cambridge, MA: Harvard University Press, 1999).

29. H. Graham, G. Der, Influences on women's smoking status. European Journal of Public Health. 9(2) (1999).

30. L. Schiebinger, Introduction: Feminism inside the sciences. Signs: Journal of Women in Culture and Society. 28(3) (2003), 859–66.

31. L. Briggs, Reproducing Empire: Race, Sex, Science, and U.S. Imperialism in Puerto Rico. 1st ed. (Berkeley: University of California Press, 2002).

32. R. P. Petchesky, Abortion and Woman's Choice: The State, Sexuality, and Reproductive Freedom (Boston, MA: Northeastern University Press, 1985.

33. D. P. Dixon, Feminist Geopolitics: Material States (London: Routledge, 2016).

34. D. A. Davis, Reproductive Injustice: Racism, Pregnancy, and Premature Birth (New York: New York University Press, 2019).

35. C. K. Riessman, Women and medicalization: A new perspective. Social Policy. 14(1) (1983), 3–18.

36. S. Colen 'Like a Mother to Them': Stratified reproduction and West Indian chilcare workers and employers in New York. In: F. Ginsburg, R. Rapp, editors. Conceiving the New World Order: The Global Politics of Reproduction (Berkeley: University of California Press, 1995) pp. 78–102.

37. D. A. Davis, The politics of reproduction: The troubling case of Nadya Suleman and assisted reproductive technology. Transforming Anthropology. 17(2) (2009), 105–16.

38. R. A. Kanaaneh, Birthing the Nation: Strategies of Palestinian Women in Israel (Berkeley: University of California Press, 2002).

39. L. Mullings, The necropolitics of reproduction: Racism, resistance, and the Sojourner Syndrome in the age of the Movement for Black Lives. In: S. Han, C. Tomori, editors. The Routledge Handbook of Anthropology and Reproduction (United Kingdom: Routledge, 2021) pp. 106–22.

40. J. M. Silliman, Undivided Rights: Women of Color Organize for Reproductive Justice (Cambridge, MA: South End Press, 2004).

41. E. Hoover, Environmental reproductive justice: Intersections in an American Indian community impacted by environmental contamination. Environmental Sociology. 4 (1) (2018), 8–21.

42. N. Valdez, The redistribution of reproductive responsibility: On the epigenetics of 'Environment' in prenatal interventions. Medical Anthropology Quarterly. 32(3) (2018), 1–18.

43. A. K. Conching, Z. Thayer, Biological pathways for historical trauma to affect health: A conceptual model focusing on epigenetic modifications. Social Science & Medicine. 230 (2019), 74–82.

44. M. Lappé, R. J. Hein, The temporal politics of placenta epigenetics: Bodies, environments and time. Body & Society (2022).

45. M. Lappé, F. F. Fahey, R. J. Hein, Epigenomic stories: Evidence of harm and the social justice promises and perils of environmental epigenetics. Science Technology & Human Values. (2022).

46. M. Lappé, R. J. Hein, You are what your mother endured: Intergenerational epigenetics, early caregiving, and the temporal embedding of adversity. Medical Anthropology Quarterly. 35(4) (2021), 458–75.

47. L. M. Hunt, M. S. Megyesi, The ambiguous meanings of the racial/ethnic categories routinely used in human genetics research. Social Science & Medicine. 66(2) (2008), 349–61.

48. S. Sullivan, Inheriting racist disparities in health: Epigenetics and the transgenerational effects of White racism. Critical Philosophy of Race. 1(20) (2013), 190–218.

49. A. Pollock, Sickening: Anti-Black Racism and Health Disparities in the United States (Minneapolis: University of Minnesota Press, 2021).

50. A. Nelson, Body and Soul (Minneapolis: University of Minnesota Press, 2011).

51. D. E. Roberts, Torn Apart: How the Child Welfare System Destroys Black Families– and How Abolition Can Build a Safer World (New York: Basic Books, 2022).

52. CDC, Racial/ethnic disparities in pregnancy-related deaths. 2022. www.cdc.gov/reproductivehealth/maternal-mortality/disparities-pregnancy-related-deaths/infographic.html (Accessed 12 July 2022.)

53. M. Penkler, Caring for biosocial complexity. Articulations of the environment in research on the Developmental Origins of Health and Disease. Studies in History and Philosophy of Science. 1(93) (2022), 1–10.

54. M. Penkler, C. M. Jacob, R. Müller, M. Kenney, S. A. Norris, et al. Developmental origins of health and disease, resilience and social justice in the COVID era. Journal of Developmental Origins of Health and Disease. (2021), 1–4.

DOHaD in Economics
Orthodox and Egalitarian Approaches

Jennifer Cohen

7.1 Introduction

The Developmental Origins of Health and Disease (DOHaD) is now an established area of inquiry in the economics discipline, cutting across subfields like health and demographic economics. Orthodox economists increasingly use econometric methods to make the case that individual-level epigenetic changes have measurable impacts on labour market outcomes. While some literature seeks to document disparities in health outcomes, most economic research considers the effects of health or economic shocks on educational attainment, employment, and wages. This focus on 'nonhealth endpoints' is guided by assumptions and definitions in orthodox economic thought that direct attention to concerns typically – or ultimately – related to market outcomes.

A wide range of *un*orthodox, egalitarian approaches within economics could contribute to DOHaD by integrating social forces, social structures, and social inequities. These approaches consider the origins and impacts of hierarchical power relations between groups. Compared to orthodox economists, egalitarian economists typically have a broader understanding of what an economy is and what an economy is for. Some view economics as the study of provisioning life or as the reproduction of society itself [1–3].

Differences between orthodox and egalitarian approaches are especially pronounced in analyses of the reproductive economy, an area of thought and policy relevant to DOHaD research. In orthodox economics, DOHaD research signals renewed interest in reproduction, but reproduction never fully disappeared from orthodox economic thought. Optimising economic outcomes through intervening in reproduction underlies eugenic research in economics, population control and 'family planning' in economic development, and DOHaD [4, 5]. The *work* and *function* of the reproductive economy, although essential for DOHaD, continue to attract little attention.

Some egalitarian economists highlight the critical roles of both. Reproductive labour includes the care work, housework, and other tasks associated with reproducing human life on a daily and intergenerational basis. Much of the work is unpaid. Functionally, production fundamentally depends on this unpaid labour, which reproduces the labour supply [2]. Despite its obvious economic importance, in the twentieth century, unpaid reproductive labour was defined outside of the boundaries of the mainstream economics discipline [6, 7]. This historical erasure of women and their economic contributions devalues women and the work they do, with material ramifications among other costs. Like the labour itself, economic research about it remains undervalued and marginalised in the discipline [6].

Hence, a resurgence of interest in reproduction by orthodox economists could be heartening. Yet when orthodox economists have been interested in reproduction historically, women have been instrumentalised in efforts to optimise economic outcomes such as gross domestic product (GDP) growth or income per capita by controlling reproduction. While women's 'maternal capital' [8] is sometimes recognised as playing a role in the creation of future value (e.g., offspring's wages), women themselves tend to be reduced to fetal environments, characterised as instruments of reproduction rather than as fully human people with valued lives.

Following a review of the literature, I demonstrate how egalitarian economic thought could usefully be brought to bear in DOHaD research, first by identifying weaknesses in the orthodox approach; second, by integrating social and historical context; and third, by suggesting areas for novel, socially grounded, collaborative DOHaD research. The egalitarian analysis indicates that richer understandings of social determinants of health could be a key contribution of DOHaD research. Egalitarians' sophisticated understanding of social structures and constructed categories can situate DOHaD in a real-world context. I conclude that egalitarian approaches can address a critique of DOHaD research both inside and outside economics: the failure to adequately integrate social structures. The analysis reveals the real-world risks of this failure for women and girls, linking DOHaD literature to political debates about 'fetal personhood', women's autonomy, and gender inequity.

7.2 DOHaD in Economic Research

To date, DOHaD-related empirical studies in economics take two main forms. One set attempt to document the effects of exposure to shocks, such as new access to medical technologies like antibiotics or adverse events like famines, epidemics, or recessions [9–12]. Many studies link women's bodies (as in utero environments) to offspring's childhood health or later-life outcomes. For studies in which health outcomes are dependent variables, health is a thing produced (an output) as a function of health investments (inputs) at different developmental stages of 'childhood' [13]. For example, some studies examine health outcomes such as adult height, a proxy for nutrition [14]. The second set of studies consider the efficacy of interventions to mitigate the detrimental effects of adverse events or social determinants of health, from public policy to micro-level service delivery [15]. This brief review of the literature focuses on the former studies as these are common in economics and can be foundational to the latter.

A distinguishing characteristic of economic research in DOHaD is the use of outcome variables aligned with most economic research: educational attainment, paid employment, and wages. According to Almond and Currie's original review of the DOHaD literature, the addition of 'nonhealth' endpoints is one of four major contributions from economics [16]. The other three contributions are (a) novel identification strategies for working around data availability issues, (b) the variety of exposures modelled, including infectious disease, pollution, and recessions, and (c) the argument that studies that focus on survivors are likely to find weaker relationships than they would if data accounted for those who did not survive. Conti et al. identify contributions from economics as 'rang[ing] from developing theoretical frameworks, to establishing causality, understanding mechanisms, and also computing costs and benefits of early interventions' [16].

The theoretical basis of nonhealth-endpoint studies is human capital theory [17]. Human capital is typically understood by orthodox economists to mean education. The definition in the literature is more expansive. Conti et al. describe human capital as '...the intangible stock of knowledge, skills, personality, and other attributes – including health – that produce economic value in the life of an individual' [15]. The economic model is an equation called a production function in which the thing produced, the output, is human capital. There are two periods of investment in the model discussed by Almond et al.: the in utero period of 'childhood' and the 'second period' of childhood [18]. In orthodox economic thought, human capital is the theoretical link between exposure to adverse events/shocks and wages: exposure impacts human capital that determines productivity, which in turn determines wages. Hence, for most economists, human capital is a key explanatory factor for labour market outcomes like wages – and wage inequality.

Empirically, the relationship between human capital and wages holds in general, but it does not hold for all people in all occupations. Where the relationship is present, its strength varies by demographic group because social inequities by race, gender, and disability status intervene. Racism, sexism, and ablism are oppressive systems of social relations that construct glass ceilings, glass elevators, and other impediments that constrain (or enable) advancement and mobility. For example, returns to human capital investment (education) have historically been lower for Black[1] people in the United States due to racial segregation [9]. Almond et al. note that long-run benefits of investment in human capital vary for Black men exposed to different degrees of segregation, '...suggesting that despite a strong economic climate (better early life conditions), institutional environment affects the rewards to investments in human capital' [18]. The institutional environment encompasses systems of social relations like racism, sexism, and ableism. Those systems can translate into inequitable 'returns to investment.' Institutional economics and related egalitarian approaches have much to offer such analyses.

Orthodox and egalitarian thoughts about labour markets and wages differ considerably. In orthodox economics, *occupational* segregation, or the concentration of certain demographics in certain occupations, is the result of individual investments in human capital. In other words, occupational segregation is interpreted as the result of freely made individual decisions. The orthodox explanation for occupational segregation by gender and women's lower earnings is that women choose to invest less in education or skills valued by employers and seek out jobs where experience plays little role in pay because they expect employment to be intermittent, due to their *reproductive responsibilities* [19, 20].

In some egalitarian approaches, gendered value systems and gender roles condition individual preferences, and gender discrimination crowds women into a subset of feminised occupations [21, 22]. Discrimination limits economic opportunities for the

---

[1] The term Black is often used interchangeably with 'African-American' in the United States. 'Black' primarily includes American descendants of slaves as well as other people who identify as Black such as Afro-Caribbean people and African immigrants. Racial segregation in the USA was implemented in the post-slavery period de facto and then through Jim Crow Laws formally passed in 1877. It was enforced in some US states up to the mid-1960s when the US Supreme Court ruled that racial segregation was unconstitutional. Polls (e.g., Gallup) indicate that Black adults have a slight preference for 'Black'. I follow the convention from the Associated Press by capitalising the term.

majority of the population – underrepresented men and women of all races – while restricting competition in occupations available to the minority [23]. Benefits for men include reduced competition for well-paid jobs and skilled employment in sectors that have historically been closed to women, such as economics and STEM fields [6, 24]. Directly related disadvantages for women include economic insecurity and a relatively weak ability to pursue divorce or to save for retirement.

Another explanation is that occupations become feminised *because* the people doing the work are themselves of low status [25]. Feminisation is a demographic process in which the proportion of women in an occupation rises, but it is also a process of devaluing those occupations as women enter them [6]. Evidence suggests that feminisation has a causal relationship with low pay and low status; hence, men have historically resisted women's entrance into higher education and male-dominated occupations [26]. Conti et al.'s definition of human capital as knowledge, skills, personality, health, and other attributes *'that produce economic value in the life of an individual'* offers some insight into the relationship between feminisation and value, economic and otherwise (emphasis added) [15]. In societies with gendered value systems in which women and men are valued inequitably, skills stereotypically associated with femininity and masculinity also tend to be valued inequitably [6]. Thus, some skills contribute far more than others to the economic value one's life may hold. Finally, the same skill may be valued in male workers and penalised in women workers.

In summary, orthodox economists brought later-life labour market outcomes into DOHaD research, which they connect to health through human capital theory: investments in human capital should have positive returns in the form of higher wages. However, as egalitarian economists point out, systems of social relations like racism and sexism generate inequitable 'returns to investment'.

This brief consideration of human capital theory reveals why social context matters in DOHaD literature. First, it is necessary for understanding existing economic analyses in which outcomes may be misinterpreted as the result of freely made individual-level choices. Egalitarian schools of thought, such as social economics, feminist economics, stratification economics, critical political economy, and institutional economics, draw insight from rich theoretical and practical understandings of the social context in which individuals make decisions. Egalitarian research offers historically grounded analyses of the origins and reinforcement of social structures. For example, feminist economists demonstrate how structural inequalities create gendered outcomes and explore how gender shapes understandings of economic activity [6, 7, 21, 22]. Some, especially women of colour, use intersectionality to describe how hierarchical social relations combine [27]. Institutional economists focus on evolving systems of power in which institutions coordinate economic behaviour, while social economists consider the ethical consequences of complex social interactions [28]. Stratification economics provides analyses of group-based inequality and is the product of research by Black economists [29].

Second, social context is also requisite for designing public policy to address the *causes* of inequitable *outcomes*. Egalitarianism contains justice-oriented guidance for policy and interventions because integrating power relations into analyses widens the scope for seeking social solutions to social challenges. Lastly, placing analyses in a social context may prevent the misinterpretation or misuse of DOHaD research for racist or sexist purposes.

In the remainder of the chapter, I demonstrate the usefulness of egalitarian thought in DOHaD. In Section 7.3, I make visible how the marginalisation of women's labour and, historically, of women's economic research contributes to the dehumanising instrumentalisation of women in orthodox economic research in DOHaD. The following section suggests that DOHaD could contribute to research on determinants of health, but its current contribution is limited by a narrow focus on molecular factors and uncritical use of demographic variables. I bring these points together in a short exploration of some real-world risks of dehumanising instrumentalisation for women and girls, linking DOHaD literature to political debates about 'fetal personhood', women's autonomy, and gender inequity.

7.3   Economic Orthodoxy and Reproduction

Most economists exhibit little concern about the unpaid reproductive labour typically done by women, like cleaning, cooking, and raising children, among other tasks [2, 22, 30]. Still, it is women's perceived responsibility for reproductive labour that links gender roles/norms to economic outcomes. The social expectation that women are responsible for the unpaid reproduction of life has economic consequences for women and men:

> [W]omen are less likely to [do paid] work, they earn less than men for similar [paid] work, and are more likely to be in poverty even when they work [for pay]. Women spend almost twice as much time on housework, almost five times as much time on childcare, and about half as much time on [paid] market work as men do [30].

Women's unpaid work has been defined out of the economics discipline theoretically, professionally, and empirically through decisions made by powerful actors in the field. In economic theory, disciplinary boundaries are established and enforced through gendered interpretations of value that treat unpaid work as a 'non-economic' activity [6]. Activities that are monetised are included on one side of this 'arbitrary line', while those 'services gratuitously rendered by women' are not [31]. Professionally, a process of 'defeminization' of the discipline took place in the early twentieth century, excising the study of the household by women economists [32]. Empirically, official state-based recordkeeping, such as the United States Census, excludes unpaid labour [7, 33]. The decision to exclude unpaid work from GDP was made by Richard Stone in pursuit of a 'universal method' against the advice of Phyllis Deane, a woman economist Stone hired to study the method's accuracy in colonial territories [33]. Despite critiques by Deane and the only two women on international committees on national income statistics at the time, Hildegarde Kneeland (League of Nations, 1947) and Margaret Mód (United Nations, 1968), the method was promoted globally and widely adopted [33]. GDP is among the most commonly used pieces of economic information about a given country; 'economic growth' refers to a positive change in GDP.

The gendered method of calculating GDP and the gendered definition of value reinforce a hierarchical gender division of labour: monetised, valued labour associated with masculinity and the 'public sphere' termed 'production' is at the top, and non-monetised, devalued labour associated with femininity and the 'private sphere' is at the bottom. The division is informed by *productivism*, a bias that privileges monetised economic contributions, one aspect of reproducing life, over others. The gender division of labour and associated value judgements are so naturalised that they inflect the definition of what 'The Economy' *is*; what activities it includes, both popularly and according to most economists; and the ends of economic activities. It is deeply embedded in economic thought, with implications far beyond the discipline because of the influence economics and economists have on policy [6].

Women's unpaid labour is the foundation of the reproduction of society on a day-to-day basis and intergenerationally. The term 'labour', as in 'going into labour', connects biological/physiological reproduction and the uncompensated work of social reproduction. There can be no production without the reproduction of life itself, including that of those in the paid labour force. If production is understood to constitute '*The Economy*', then there is no 'The Economy' without women's reproductive labour. Given this history and its negative effects on women materially and in terms of social status, orthodox economists' newfound interest in reproduction could be welcome: it presents an opportunity to take the value of women's reproductive labour seriously.

Historically, however, economic research on reproduction has embraced optimisation strategies that instrumentalise women. Eugenic projects sought to improve 'the race' with policy interventions like forced sterilisation that primarily targeted women, especially women of colour, in developed and underdeveloped countries from the United States to Sweden to Bangladesh as recently as 2020 [34, 35]. Forced sterilisation was thought to 'improve the race' in part by controlling population growth and therefore raising economic output (measured as GDP per capita). In this dehumanising project, women are reduced to instruments for economic growth.

DOHaD research in economics has often in similar ways emphasised the optimisation of economic growth, mainly by proposing forms of intervention in women's lives. Critically, optimisation is framed in economistic terms with effects on knowledge production beyond the discipline: scholars point to the '"growing adoption of economics" "cognitive infrastructures" or "epistemic infrastructures" in global health governance' [8]. DOHaD studies often employ economic language, framing economic benefits as 'resource savings' in the form of reduced child deaths, reduced morbidity, and the savings from potential adult chronic disease [8, 36]. Authors also find *returns on investment* in the forms of increased worker productivity, school attendance and achievement, and better employment in the future [36]. The economic logic driving some epigenetic research finds its rationale in human capital and the future earnings of fetuses.

Economistic thought, in which economic ends dominate other possible commitments, such as equity and justice, is enormously consequential. Some DOHaD research constructs women as vessels that [should] act in the interest of potential future progeny, a normative position that violates basic premises of orthodox thought. In some studies, the 'future value' of fetuses appears to take precedence over the value of actually - existing women, whose preferences are unaddressed. Women's autonomy – especially that of women of colour – may carry relatively little weight in studies that prioritise economic growth over justice (see Section 7.4.2.1). As Chiapperino and colleagues discuss in this volume, this introduces a set of moral paradoxes for DOHaD.

7.4 Egalitarianism in Economics and DOHaD

The critiques of (a) the devalorisation of women's reproductive labour and (b) of the dehumanisation and instrumentalisation of women in Section 7.3, and the implications that I explore below, exhibit the kind of historically grounded, socially informed insight that egalitarian economists can bring to DOHaD research. The analysis here makes two main points: first, it demonstrates how DOHaD research could contribute to more complete understandings of social determinants of health. Egalitarians integrate social context and can steer DOHaD analyses away from biological and/or cultural essentialism. Second, it shows how reducing women and girls to instruments of reproduction reinforces gender inequities.

7.4.1 DOHaD and Social Determinants of Health

A key contribution of DOHaD research could be in providing better explanations of existing social inequities and informing policies to address their causes. In contrast to imagining 'utopian visions of where life can be remade and further harnessed for economic gains' through technological innovations, this information could help make unjust social forces the primary targets for policy [36]. However, a common critique is that DOHaD literature, and a great deal of published research in economics, fails to integrate social forces, social structures, and social inequities [37]. Additionally, and related, some scholars criticise DOHaD research for endorsing biological and/or cultural essentialism [38]. Socially oriented economic research helps address these critiques through the theoretical and practical recognition that social variables reflect systems of social relations, not individual characteristics.

Racism and sexism are critically important determinants of health, including maternal, infant, and child health [39–41]. Notably, it is *racism*, not race, and *sexism*, not gender, that are social and structural determinants of health (SDH). The SDH are the systems of social relations that reinforce hierarchies of constructed categories to the detriment of people at the bottom of those hierarchies – women, people of colour, LGBTQI people, and those with disabilities – and benefit those at the top.[2] Variations across groups, such as disparities in health and other domains, largely reflect social dynamics and relations of power. DOHaD research may find disparities in outcomes, but the *origins* of those disparities are social.

One review of how empirical epigenetic studies integrate SDH began with 337 studies of social exposures ranging from low socio-economic status (child and/or adult), early-life adversity, to workplace or neighbourhood exposures, and adult DNA methylation [37]. Of those, over 115 studies included race or gender as variables *without an explanation of the social exposures the variables represented*. In other words, one-third of the studies misrepresented social categories as biological traits. To contribute to research on SDH, researchers must recognise that demographic variables serve as proxies for hierarchical power relations. Some scholars argue that researchers must try to measure the social structures and processes that result in the inequitable group-level distribution of resources [37].

Social determinants of health are widely acknowledged as primary determinants of health that encompass inequities resulting from social structures [39]. By collaboratively theorising and documenting the impacts of SDH, DOHaD research has the potential to shed light on the persistence and costs of *inequities*. Inequity is conceptually distinct from inequality; inequities are recognised as 'unfair or stemming from some form of

---

[2] The corresponding power relations to those listed are patriarchy, white supremacy and anti-blackness, heteronormativity, and ableism; discrimination may be based on [perceived] gender/gender identity, [perceived] race/ethnicity and related identities, [perceived] sexuality/sexual orientation, and disability status. An intersectional approach requires consideration of multiple, interacting hierarchies [42].

injustice' [43]. Economistic logic that prioritises economic growth may preclude alternative logics like the pursuit of equity and justice. Orthodox scholarship in economics does not typically centre these pursuits due to the economism that guides research. Theory, methodology, and foci can be path dependent, meaning that existing literature defines the future trajectory of research because scholars use it as a foundation, making it easier to publish related work and build the literature. These are nonetheless decisions made by researchers who could opt for alternative, egalitarian approaches.

There are substantial risks to the limited exploration of social structures. First, scholars may overemphasise findings that add little explanatory power beyond that of existing social systems. For example, based on animal models, Almond et al. conclude that 'it is highly likely that changes in the foetus or young child could be passed on to the next generation. This type of mechanism could offer *an additional reason* for the intergenerational persistence of poverty, and for the existence of poverty traps…' (emphasis added) [18]. The authors do not identify the *other* reasons for the persistence of poverty, but presumably they include the myriad social factors that reproduce poverty. In comparative terms, the impact of an additional, potentially epigenetic effect in an explanation of the intergenerational persistence of poverty is probably marginal. As articulated in Almond et al. and elsewhere in published DOHaD research, this type of conjecture overstates the likely impact. Such emphases can give the misguided impression that there may be individual-level solutions to social inequities.

Second, a small impact may still be worth investigating, but scholars often combine potential epigenetic mechanisms with social variables like race and gender. Without acknowledging that those variables are proxies for racism and sexism, analyses are open to misinterpretation – scholarly and popular – as identifying biological or cultural 'deficiencies' in certain gendered and/or racialised groups.

Instead of contributing better explanations of existing social inequities, a narrow focus on molecular factors combined with an uncritical use of social variables risks making inequity-generating social structures and their unjust consequences *less* visible. The gender division of labour is a core element of the social structure that reinforces gender inequities. The next part of Section 7.4 explores some real-world risks of the failure to integrate social structures into analyses. More specifically, it describes how reducing women and girls to instruments of reproduction reinforces gender inequities.

7.4.2 Instrumentalisation of Women and Girls: Gender Inequities

Egalitarian approaches reveal the ways that policies, interventions, and language can reinforce inequities. Egalitarian economists offer socially aware insight and may identify alternatives. In this analysis, by locating policies/interventions/language in a real-world social context, feminist political economy elucidates some stakes of DOHaD research for women and girls. I describe two ways that the dehumanisation and instrumentalisation of women and girls contribute to gender inequity: (a) limitations on women's autonomy and (b) the high costs of emphasising women-as-mothers vis-à-vis the low value of reproductive labour covered in Section 7.3.

7.4.2.1 Restrictions on Women's Autonomy

Women's dehumanisation is not an abstract danger. Some DOHaD literature is consistent with rhetorical and legislative strategies of pro-life political groups, which have 'transformed their framing of the abortion issue, from one that pits foetal rights against maternal rights to one that emphasises the unique and intimate bond between the woman and the "child"' [44]. In human capital models in the DOHaD literature, a zygote, embryo, and fetus – stages of in utero development – are described as part of 'childhood' (e.g., [18]). Thus the DOHaD literature overlaps with political debates about 'fetal personhood' and women's autonomy.

For example, personhood laws in the United States have sought to establish fertilised eggs, embryos, and fetuses as entities with rights independent of those of a pregnant person [45]. The 1973 Supreme Court decision in Roe v. Wade 'explicitly rejected the claim that foetuses, even after attaining viability, are separate legal persons with rights independent of the pregnant women who carry, nurture, and sustain them' [45].

Hundreds, perhaps thousands, of women have nonetheless been arrested and prosecuted for 'crimes' against fetuses in the period between 1973 and 2022. Between 1973 and 2005, there were 413 such cases in which women were deprived of freedom through arrests or forced medical interventions [45]. Almost three-quarters of those women were African American [45]. Judges, juries, prosecutors, healthcare practitioners, and social workers have all represented the purported interests of fetuses at the expense of women's physical freedom. For orthodox economists, gender-specific constraints on women, and the treatment of women's preferences more generally, present theoretical, methodological, and practical challenges. Of further concern for DOHaD scholars should be the fact that criminal charges were typically based on the *risk of harm* without evidence of harm. The 2022 Supreme Court judgement overturning the 1973 Roe v. Wade decision brings these issues to the fore.

7.4.2.2 Women-as-Mothers and the Low Perceived Value of Reproductive Labour

Feminists in economics have long been deeply concerned about economic research that simultaneously reduces women and girls to instruments for productivity and economic growth and assigns them responsibility for the same. For example, microcredit schemes target women as sources of social capital based on gender stereotypes (i.e., cooperation) [46]. Reducing women and girls to their reproductive capacities similarly instrumentalises them as containers of 'maternal capital'. DOHaD research inside and outside economics adopts the language of 'capital': health capital, human capital, maternal capital, somatic capital, cognitive capital, resource capital, and offspring capital all appear in the literature [4, 8, 16, 47]. The language places responsibility on individual women for accruing and maintaining their 'maternal capital' during potential childbearing years. For most women, this accounts for half of their lifetimes, starting prior to adulthood, sometimes as early as six or seven years old [48]. As Currie recognises in an interview, this implies a shift in the logic of intervention:

> It really means you should be targeting a whole different population than, say, 15 years ago, when we thought, Oh, we need to be targeting preschool kids instead of kids once they reach school age. Now we're kind of pushing it back . . . *Now the implication is that we've got to reach these mothers before they even get pregnant if we really want to improve conditions.*
>
> (emphasis added) [8]

Any such effort to reach 'potential mothers' would likely need to cover half of the general population over time. Yet most DOHaD literature does not target that half of the population *as* women or girls; it targets them as potential fetal environments. Imagining all women and girls as 'mothers' reduces them to their reproductive role, overvaluing the fetal environment and undervaluing the people embodying it.

The emphasis on women-as-mothers has ramifications in other domains. Gender roles in reproductive labour link framing women-as-mothers and material and social impacts. I argue elsewhere that constructing women-as-mothers contributes to gender disparities in pay [6]. That is, gender inequity contributes to gender pay gaps, including those related to occupational segregation. In turn, pay gaps contribute to women's economic dependence on men and penalise single women by making it more difficult to save for a down payment for a home or to save adequately for retirement.

The reduction of women to instruments of reproduction is a disciplinary mechanism with material consequences. It imagines dependent children and responsibility *even where none exists* to a punitive effect in the labour market. Critically, DOHaD's concern with maternity is not likely to do women any favours materially without a dramatic shift in the perceived value of reproductive labour.

7.5 Conclusion

Orthodox economists brought later-life labour market outcomes into DOHaD research, which they connect to health through human capital theory: investments in human capital, including health, should have positive returns in the form of higher wages. However, systems of social relations like racism and sexism are sources of inequitable 'returns on investment'. Further, inequity-generating social structures and their unjust consequences are made *less* visible by research that uncritically uses social variables. The gender division of labour is part of the social structures that reinforce gender inequities.

Reproductive labour, and who is believed to be responsible for this low-status, poorly paid, and unpaid work, is key to understanding persistently gendered and racialised inequity. Social structures that devalue women and 'women's work' are institutionalised in practices like gender-based discrimination in the labour market. Women are discriminated against in the labour market *because* of their perceived responsibility for reproductive labour (i.e. because of gender roles). Women are obviously more than instruments of reproduction but have been instrumentalised in the interest of optimising economic outcomes. DOHaD research continues this tradition, but it does not need to.

Many opportunities remain in the field for 'exploring structural factors that capture intersectional and interlocking systems of oppression' [37]. Egalitarian economists are well equipped theoretically and methodologically for analyses of social structures and oppressions. Many of the people conducting equity-oriented research in economics are members of underrepresented groups and have related experiences that inform their research. Those experiences can be sources of insight from which a diverse group of economists develop economic theories that better reflect power dynamics in the social world.

References

1. M. Power. Social Provisioning as a Starting Point for Feminist Economics. Fem Econ 10 (2004), 3–19.

2. B. Laslett, J. Brenner. Gender and Social Reproduction: Historical Perspectives. Annu Rev Sociol 15 (1989), 381–404.

3. J. Cohen. What's 'Radical' about [Feminist] Radical Political Economy? Rev Radic Polit Econ 50 (2018), 716–726.

4. M. Murphy. The Economization of Life (Durham, NC; London: Duke University Press, 2017).

5. G. N. Price, W. Darrity Jr, R. V. Sharpe. Did North Carolina Economically Breed-

Out Blacks During Its Historical Eugenic Sterilization Campaign? Am Rev Polit Econ **15** (2020), 1–22. https://doi.org/10.38024/arpe.pds.6.28.20

6. J. Cohen. The Queen of the Social Sciences: The Reproduction of a [White] 'Man's Field.' Hist Polit Econ **54** (2022), 259–282.

7. N. Folbre. The Unproductive Housewife: Her Evolution in Nineteenth-Century Economic Thought. Signs **16** (1991), 463–484.

8. T. Moll, M. Meloni, A. Issaka. Foetal Programming meets Human Capital: Biological Plasticity, Development, and the Limits to 'the Economization of Life' (unpublished).

9. S. Bhalotra, A. S. Venkataramani. Shadows of the Captain of the Men of Death: Health Innovation, Human Capital Investment, and Institutions (United Kingdom: University of Essex, 2015).

10. G. Conti, S. Poupakis, P. Ekamper, et al. Severe Prenatal Shocks and Adolescent Health: Evidence from the Dutch Hunger Winter. Working Paper 2021-056. (HCEO Working Paper Series, 2021).

11. D. Almond, B. Mazumder. The 1918 Influenza Pandemic and Subsequent Health Outcomes: An Analysis of SIPP Data. Am Econ Rev **95** (2005), 258–262.

12. G. J. van den Berg, M. Lindeboom, F. Portrait. Economic Conditions Early in Life and Individual Mortality. Am Econ Rev **96** (2006), 290–302.

13. F. Cunha, J. Heckman. The Technology of Skill Formation. Am Econ Rev **97** (2007), 31–47.

14. C. Bozzoli, A. Deaton, C. Quintana-Domeque. Adult Height and Childhood Disease. Demography **46** (2009), 647–669.

15. G. Conti, G. Mason, S. Poupakis. Developmental Origins of Health Inequality: Oxford Research Encyclopedia of Economics and Finance. (Oxford: Oxford University Press, 2019). www.iza.org/publications/dp/12448/developmental-origins-of-health-inequality.

16. D. Almond, J. Currie. Killing Me Softly: The Fetal Origins Hypothesis. J Econ Perspect **25** (2011), 153–172.

17. J. Yi, J. J. Heckman, J. Zhang, et al. Early Health Shocks, Intra-Household Resource Allocation and Child Outcomes. Econ J **125** (2015), F347–F371.

18. D. Almond, J. Currie, V. Duque. Childhood Circumstances and Adult Outcomes: Act II. J Econ Lit **56** (2018), 1360–1446.

19. S. W. Polachek. Occupational Self-Selection: A Human Capital Approach to Sex Differences in Occupational Structure. Rev Econ Stat **63** (1981), 60–69.

20. P. England, I. Browne. Trends in Women's Economic Status. Sociol Perspect **35** (1992), 17–51.

21. B. Bergmann. Occupational Segregation, Wages and Profits When Employers Discriminate by Race or Sex. East Econ J **1** (1974), 103–110.

22. J. Cohen. Precarity of Subsistence: Social Reproduction among South African Nurses. Fem Econ **29** (2023), 236–265.

23. C. D. Goldin. The Role of World War II in the Rise of Women's Employment. The Am Econ Rev **81** (1991), 741–756.

24. E. A. Cech. The Intersectional Privilege of White Able-bodied Heterosexual Men in STEM. Sci Adv **8** (2022), eabo1558.

25. P. England. The Failure of Human Capital Theory to Explain Occupational Sex Segregation. J Hum Resour **17** (1982), 358–370.

26. A. Levanon, P. England, P. Allison. Occupational Feminization and Pay: Assessing Causal Dynamics Using 1950–2000 U.S. Census Data. Social Forces **88** (2009), 865–891.

27. N. Banks. Black Women in the United States and Unpaid Collective Work: Theorizing the Community as a Site of Production. Rev Black Polit Econ **47** (2020), 343–362. https://doi.org/10.1177%2F0034644620962811

28. I. van Staveren, P. Knorringa. Unpacking Social Capital in Economic Development: How Social Relations Matter. Rev Soc Econ **65** (2007), 107–135.

29. G. Chelwa, D. Hamilton, J. Stewart. Stratification Economics: Core Constructs and Policy Implications. J Econ Lit **60** (2022), 377–399.

30. E. Duflo. Women Empowerment and Economic Development. J Econ Lit **50** (2012), 1051–1079.

31. M. A. Pujol. Feminism and Anti-feminism in Early Economic Thought (Aldershot, Hants, England; Brookfield, VT, USA: E. Elgar, 1992).

32. D. Philippy. Ellen Richard's Home Economics Movement and the Birth of the Economics of Consumption. J Hist Econ Thought **43** (2021), 378–400.

33. L. Messac. Outside the Economy: Women's Work and Feminist Economics in the Construction and Critique of National Income Accounting. J Imp Commonw Hist **46** (2018), 552–578.

34. P. Patel. Forced Sterilization of Women as Discrimination. Public Health Rev **38** (2017), 15.

35. National Women's Law Center. Forced Sterilization of Disabled People in the United States. (2021). https://nwlc.org/wp-content/uploads/2022/01/%C6%92.NWLC_SterilizationReport_2021.pdf (Accessed 2 August 2022)

36. M. Pentecost. The First Thousand Days: Epigenetics in the age of Global Health. In M. Meloni, J. Cromby, D. Fitzgerald, S. Lloyd, eds., The Handbook of Biology and Society (London: Palgrave Macmillan, 2018), pp. 269–294.

37. L. Evans, M. Engelman, A. Mikulas A, et al. How Are Social Determinants of Health Integrated into Epigenetic Research? A Systematic Review. Soc Sci Med **273** (2021), 113738.

38. T. Zuberi, E. Patterson, Q. Stewart. Race, Methodology, and Social Construction in the Genomic Era. Ann Am Acad of Polit SS **661** (2015), 109–127.

39. World Health Organization. Social Determinants of Health. Social Determinants of Health. n.d. www.who.int/westernpacific/health-topics/social-determinants-of-health (Accessed 1 August 2022).

40. Z. D. Bailey, J. M. Feldman, M. T. Bassett. How Structural Racism Works – Racist Policies as a Root Cause of U.S. Racial Health Inequities. New Engl J Med **384** (2021), 768–773.

41. P. A. Homan. Structural Sexism and Health in the United States: A New Perspective on Health Inequality and the Gender System. *Am Sociol Rev* (2019), Epub ahead of print.

42. K. Crenshaw. Demarginalizing the Intersection of Race and Sex: A Black Feminist Critique of Antidiscrimination Doctrine, Feminist Theory and Antiracist Politics. Univ Chic Leg Forum **1989** (1989), 139–167.

43. I. Kawachi, S. V. Subramanian, N. Almeida-Filho. A glossary for Health Inequalities. J Epidemiol Community Health **56** (2002), 647–652.

44. G. Halva-Neubauer, S. Zeigler. Promoting Fetal Personhood: The Rhetorical and Legislative Strategies of the Pro-Life Movement after Planned Parenthood v. Casey. Feminist Formations **22** (2010), 101–123.

45. L. M. Paltrow, J. Flavin. Arrests of and Forced Interventions on Pregnant Women in the United States, 1973–2005: Implications for Women's Legal Status and Public Health. J Health Polit Policy Law **38** (2013), 299–343.

46. S. Bergeron. The Post-Washington Consensus and Economic Representations of Women in Development at the World Bank. Int Fem J Polit **5** (2003), 397–419.

47. S. S. Richardson. The Maternal Imprint: The Contested Science of Maternal-fetal Effects (Chicago: University of Chicago Press, 2021).

48. A. Ghorayshi. Puberty Starts Earlier Than It Used To. No One Knows Why. The New York Times. (2022). www.nytimes.com/2022/05/19/science/early-puberty-medical-reason.html (Accessed 4 August 2022).

Chapter

The 'Moral Paradox' of DOHaD

Luca Chiapperino, Cindy Gerber,
Francesco Panese, and Umberto Simeoni

8.1 Introduction

Knowledge of the molecular and physiological mechanisms of the Developmental Origins of Health and Disease (DOHaD) is no longer confined to the lab and/or to research. Rather, the idiom of DOHaD is part and parcel of a scattered landscape of policy initiatives; that is, endeavours directed at translating DOHaD's central tenets into political discourses, programmatic statements, as well as implemented public health measures. Policy initiatives around DOHaD both inspire new policy approaches in public health [1, 2] and cast a new outlook on several policy domains in our societies – crafting, in some cases, previously overlooked links between existing policies and novel opportunities for intergenerational health promotion [3].

Yet, the central policy messages of DOHaD research are not devoid of criticism, especially on the side of the social sciences and/or ethical, legal, and social aspects (ELSA) analyses. The reason is that translating DOHaD messages into policy means walking a difficult tightrope. On the one hand, the field has the political potential to illuminate the temporal extension and far-reaching implications of the social determinants of health [4]. What happens during the developmental period has ramifications that extend to the lifecourse of parents (not just the pregnant mother-to-be), much like to the relational, social, and material environment of gestating bodies, or the structural patterning of health inequalities in our societies. If anything, DOHaD is – to this reading – only a demonstration that social inequalities hit harder in developmental times. As such, DOHaD policies would be expected to lean towards a syndemic approach to health; that is, to affirm a holistic conception of health, which considers risks as biosocial complexes emerging at the intersection of biological predispositions as well as social and environmental modulators of disease [5]. On the other hand, scientific literature and circulating evidence often provide a rather different take-home message from DOHaD research. This message affirms the importance of maternal–offspring dynamics for the programming of adult health and only recently has expanded into a broader focus on periconceptional and family-related dynamics, including effects following the paternal line [6]. Key to the enactment of DOHaD findings is – to this alternative reading – behaviour change, parental (and especially maternal) lifestyles, and more generally responsible actions based on literacy of developmental effects. In a nutshell, the key policy objectives of DOHaD research are highly idiosyncratic and taken in a tension. What could be called the 'moral paradox' of DOHaD is the idea that, while the scope, foundations, and

This work is part of the Swiss National Science Foundation (SNSF) Ambizione project 'Constructing the Biosocial: An Engaged Inquiry into Epigenetics and Post-genomic Biosciences' (PZ00P1_185822).

practical implications of DOHaD research call for structural interventions addressing social determinants of health over the lifecourse, DOHaD messages can at times boil down to simplistic claims of individual responsibility [7, 8].

In what follows, we attempt an explanation of these paradoxical implications of DOHaD research. We do so by offering a comprehensive analysis of claims towards *individual responsibilities* in the DOHaD literature. The chapter draws from a systematic literature review documenting the whole spectrum of policy and normative discourses in DOHaD research. Within this diverse set of policy interventions, the chapter unpacks the often-underlying normative claims pointing to the responsibilities of individuals (e.g. parents, parents-to-be, etc.). Complementing previous publications from our group [9–11], the literature review highlights the complexities of scientists' engagements with the moral and societal aspects of DOHaD research. Systematically analysing scientific publications allows us to unpack the intricate processes that bring about an economy of individual-oriented norms, responsibilities, and obligations [12] to the detriment of other ethical orientations of the field. DOHaD scientists, we argue, hardly make any straightforward argument in favour of individual responsibilities for health. The 'moral paradox' of DOHaD rather arises from an ambiguous stance on the possibilities of health promotion strategies inspired by DOHaD. This stance mixes up the current practical possibilities of the field with its policy framing, opportunities, and political ambitions.

By clarifying the normative scope and limitations of policy debates around individual responsibility in DOHaD research, we hope to prompt a deeper appreciation of the political ramifications of DOHaD knowledge and concepts. A higher awareness of the normative ambiguities and moral idiosyncrasies that raise critique of DOHaD research may help redefine the boundaries, priorities, objects, and representations of this research. In the discussion, we elaborate on how knowing the modalities and emergence of the 'moral paradox' of DOHaD calls into question the policy advocacies currently animating the field and points to the need for finally embracing the social justice framing of the field David Barker had hypothesised [2].

8.2 The Hyper-responsibilisation Critique of DOHaD Research

Several critiques have addressed normative and policy discourses in DOHaD research or the way its concepts and evidence circulate in the wider society. Anthropologist Megan Warin and colleagues have followed the genealogy of obesity discourses in Australia and highlighted the gender inequalities 'squeezed out' of Barker's hypothesis. How did his research programme – inaugurated with the discovery of a gendered socio-economic patterning of undernutrition and its effects on adult health – end up paradoxically reinforcing the social acceptability of a gendered stigma for obesity [13]? Along the same lines are those critiques that underline the reduction of the maternal body in DOHaD research to a 'vector' [14], or a 'capital' holder [15] for the healthy development of the child. According to these scholars, there is a risk that DOHaD research inspires a hyper-responsibilisation of women in contemporary societies [16]. Not only does DOHaD evidence replicate narratives of responsibilisation for women [17], but it also adds an ethics of stewardship and responsibility for future generations, which virtually extends over multiple generations [8, 18] (see also the chapters by Valdez and Lappé as well as Warin and Moore).

Others have shifted the focus of normative critique of DOHaD to studies of the epigenetic mechanisms of inheritance via the gametes – hence potentially *both* from the paternal and the maternal lines [10]. This line of research reaches beyond the intrauterine environment to include epigenetic predispositions via both parental gametes. While the increasing role assigned to paternal influences partly counterbalances 'the tendency to pin poor outcomes on maternal behaviour' [19], these attempts are not devoid of criticism. Besides raising questions as to their stereotypical treatment of paternal roles and responsibilities,[1] studies of *parental* effects still tend to support over-simplistic attributions of individual responsibilities. In fact, they only mark a switch to an extended version of gendered claims of individual responsibilities for health, which includes the environments, behaviours, life trajectories, and actions of the father (and fathers-to-be). In other words, the 'moral paradox' of DOHaD holds even without an exclusive gendered emphasis on women's bodies. We could in fact reformulate it as follows, by including also the injunction to protect one's gametes that virtually applies to *all* individuals of reproductive age: how did a research field founded on the socio-economic patterning of parental influences over development end up promoting discourses of individual behaviour change, *parental* responsibilities, and health literacy to promote the health of future generations? Let us turn to a tentative answer drawn from scientists' treatment of these normative matters in the DOHaD literature.

8.3 Methods and Materials

The literature review draws from peer-reviewed publications indexed on Web of Knowledge and follows the PRISMA guidelines for systematic literature reviews and meta-analyses [20]. Data collection took place between October 2020 and January 2021; source consultation and analysis were led by Luca Chiapperino (LC) and Cindy Gerber (CG) between March 2021 and December 2021. Francesco Panese (FP) and Umberto Simeoni (US) intervened later in data analysis. We searched Web of Knowledge for papers including the phrases '1000 days', 'developmental origin*', 'DOHaD', and 'fetal origin*', each accompanied by the specific search term 'polic*'. The star at the end of search terms allowed us to include papers using any derivative of these terms (e.g. in plural and singular forms). This database query returned different kinds of articles: reviews, editorial papers, perspective articles, commentaries, and theoretical discussions, much like empirical studies (n = 287). The substantive number of duplicate records across the different combinations of search terms (n = 93) hints at the evidence that '1000 days', 'DOHaD', or 'fetal origins' are often used interchangeably within the literature. After these duplicate items were removed from the database, CG and LC proceeded independently with the screening of records through abstract reading. This excluded a set of articles as out-of-topic items (n = 33). Either these articles did not inscribe themselves within DOHaD literature (e.g. they mentioned DOHaD for comparison, or in opposition to their subject matter) or they mentioned policy/policies in ways unrelated to translations of DOHaD in society (e.g. the manuscript mentioned policies on animal research or, more broadly, ethics policies governing research). The remaining records retrieved (n = 161) were grouped and imported into Nvivo for coding and analysis.

---

[1] Paternal influence is often confined to sperm-mediated effects, which calls into question how these studies may reconfigure gendered figurations of parental influences in DOHaD. We called this experimental and social construct the 'father-as-sperm' (10).

A preliminary screening of sample records (n = 20) conducted by LC and CG revealed that some papers included a mention of policies that was rather abstract or rhetorical. With this, we mean papers that offered only a generic appeal to the 'need to bring DOHaD evidence closer to policy-making' without really expanding on the reasons, motives, nor the strategies and objectives to be achieved through these translations. We excluded these papers (n = 50) due to their poor informational value for the present analysis. This iterative screening, selection, and analysis retained a total of 111 articles, which were coded through Nvivo. Within this set of papers, 50 offered at least one reference for coding to potential policies and interventions addressed at individuals (e.g. behaviour change, lifestyle change, ensuring breastfeeding, and health responsibilities) or made an explicit mention of 'mothers, fathers and families' as 'critical agents for change in setting up healthier trajectories for their children' (e.g. [21]).

8.4 The 'Paradox' Explained: Ambiguities and Difficulties of Translating DOHaD into Policy

All papers included in the analysis argue – through different formulations and to different degrees – for 'a process of broad societal engagement' ensuring that individuals adopt 'DOHaD-informed practices as feasible, positive and lifelong options' [21]. Of note, even the articles offering a substantively individual-centred rhetoric (e.g. putting a strong emphasis on the need to inform/educate mothers-to-be about healthy lifestyles) still acknowledge that choices and lifestyles of individuals are tied to broader 'political or financial incentives' that could motivate people to 'change modifiable risk factors for adverse health outcomes' [22]. In simpler terms, the main result of our review is that *DOHaD researchers do not make straightforward arguments in favour of individual responsibilities for health.* We did not find a paper treating individual obligations to adopt a healthy lifestyle in the periconceptional period in isolation from the need to target institutional or collective factors. Rather, individual and collective, public and private actors eminently mix and overlap as those responsible for a societal implementation of DOHaD research. Some, for instance, plead for the 'establishment of properly functioning economic and financial structures which supports children from underprivileged households' [23]. Others argue for the reduction of exposures to environmental chemicals found in the air, water, and soil [24]. Researchers from the Global South argue that 'nutrition-sensitive agricultural investments' are required to achieve 'income generation and nutrition outcomes' [25]. Finally, even marketing regulation is a widely recommended measure by DOHaD researchers [22, 26].

Thus, the 'moral paradox' of DOHaD is partly explained at least by the ambiguities and challenges scientists face in elaborating these normative claims. DOHaD authors do recognise that the developmental patterning of health inequalities largely depends on structural configurations of our societies. However, when turning these considerations into values, norms, and expectations, they still reproduce figurations, claims, and expectations that situate action at the individual level. None of the articles we analysed dwells in fact on a simplistic injunction towards behaviour or lifestyle change to be promoted with policies that, for instance, 'simply [recommend] a "good diet" to optimizing nutrient delivery for the developing child' [27]. Rather, scientists' policy thinking often acknowledges the need to consider 'direct education, social marketing, and policy, systems, and environmental changes' that could accompany the promotion of 'healthy diets for mothers, infants, and young children in the first 1000 days' [27]. What seems to be missing from these different policy articulations of DOHaD is a recognition one could easily draw from the fairly developed body of social sciences and/or ELSA scholarship on these matters [8, 9, 28]. Healthy eating, lifestyle changes, and healthy behaviours during this crucial time – or, in normative terms, individual responsibilities to act on DOHaD knowledge – cannot really be separated from social, economic, and political structural conditions of agency – much like, it should be added, from other material determinants of programming such as genetic variation and stochasticity [11]. The responsibilities for epigenetic and developmental predispositions to disease can therefore hardly be handled individually, or 'easily' translated into practice through 'modifiable behaviours that can be targeted during pregnancy' such as 'diet and exercise' [29].

Of interest is how DOHaD authors guard their work against simplistic responsibility claims [1]. The publications we analysed often situate the objective of acting on the determinants of developmental programming, such as, for instance, maternal nutrition, within 'multisectoral and broad double-duty actions by policymakers' [26]. Yet, in most cases, these articles fail to advocate straightforwardly in favour of addressing these responsibilities as a collective matter. The 'moral paradox' of DOHaD thrives therefore in the following ambiguity: failing to underline and prioritise social and political interventions – instead of individual behaviour change – as critical instruments of health promotion policies. This is the reason, we argue, policy translations of DOHaD research lend themselves to critiques alleging them to reinforce the idea we are morally accountable for these predispositions as individuals. In what follows, we draw from our literature review to offer several illustrations of this ambiguous stance as it touches upon a) reflections on the actors in charge of enacting DOHaD knowledge; b) the concrete policy proposals DOHaD should inspire; and c) the kind of health promotion interventions derived from DOHaD knowledge.

8.4.1 Mothers, Fathers, Families, and Society: Who Are the Actors of Change?

A first striking ambiguity in DOHaD researchers' writing on public health policy and intervention relates to the actors they designate for social change and for producing the public health benefits of this knowledge. Reflections on the scale and distribution of agency inspired by DOHaD research are fundamentally blurred, and the discourses of scientists often waver on *who should be the bearer of responsible action* over evidence of developmental programming of health.

For instance, a recent review by clinical scientists Birgit Arabin and Ahmet Alexander Baschat [30] draws insights from research on the 'Barker hypothesis' and 'reverse Barker hypothesis' into reflections on intervention and public health policy. The former is the typical knowledge claim of DOHaD research: that is, the recognition that poor maternal health conditions accelerate the risks and susceptibility to chronic diseases in the offspring. The latter is instead the idea that evidence of health issues in pregnancy predicts also the mother's future health or even the grandparents' risk for chronic diseases. This knowledge base, the authors argue, positions pregnancy as a unique window of opportunity to protect the future health of the mother and the child, revealing that the 'disease risks' of 'today and tomorrow' are fundamentally linked [30].

If anything, one could read the evidence Arabin and Baschat mobilise as a demonstration that the *origins* of intergenerational health inequalities largely extend beyond pregnancy. These rather stem from the multi-generational reproduction of patterns of inequality that affect family units – see [31] for an example of DOHaD researchers developing this perspective. And, in fact, Arabin and Baschat do recognise that DOHaD and epigenetic 'findings relate to questions of social and environmental justice and not only to individual responsibility' [30]. However, at the same time, their article forecloses this normative and political reflexivity by putting forward suggestions for primary prevention that can be resumed into 'personalized care paths for mothers and infants' (p. 13). The social and historical processes patterning health inequalities through the developmental period get here evacuated to give way to an implementation of DOHaD as 'sentinel risk profiles', 'lifestyle interventions', and maternal health 'passports' – if they do not consist in explicitly leveraging the 'fact that pregnant women are more sensitive for healthcare advices' as 'a chance to intervene' during pregnancy (p. 13).

Reducing practical options for implementing DOHaD evidence to the actions and behaviours of pregnant women has consequences for the political potential of the field. We do not mean to suggest that we expect clinical scientists to formulate a coherent community-based or intergenerational social policy strategy for primary prevention of developmental susceptibilities to diseases. Nor are we focusing on Arabin and Baschat's paper because we consider it particularly problematic compared to others (see [6, 32]). Our point is a different one. As DOHaD gains relevance in policy settings, it becomes crucial that scientists adequately consider the complexity of the contextual and social dimensions of DOHaD effects. While we agree that pregnancy is an underestimated window of opportunity, we also warn DOHaD researchers against the conceptual slippage of mixing up those who are mostly *affected* (mothers and children) with those who *should act* upon the social, individual, and biological determinants of developmental programming. The risk is not simply of making advice inert and unspecific; that is, turning the complex temporal and socio-environmental ramifications of health into banal advice towards balanced lifestyles in preconception and pregnancy. Rather, this unwarranted conceptual move risks tanking the political implications of DOHaD for health promotion. Can the multi-generational effects of the social determinants of health be simply translated into an injunction towards responsible behaviours of parents-to-be? How are matters of families, communities, and the wider society, which have often also longer histories than the people affected, to be solved just through individual action?

8.4.2 Education, Education, and Education: How Effective Is It?

Education is the most frequent individual-level intervention discussed by DOHaD researchers. Although educational policies take many different forms, they often invite the translation of DOHaD-inspired health 'recommendations into simple messages provided through an attractive graphical format' [33]. This effective communication is the pivot of this kind of DOHaD translation, targeting 'specific consumer [and] groups' and inspiring behaviour change [33]. As a corollary, this also raises the question as to who should oversee this communication most effectively. For instance, nurses are at the centre of these debates, as arguments abound that claim that they are in a unique position 'to disseminate information and promote maternal and infant mental health at every level of policy advocacy, public education, primary prevention, screening and intervention' [34].

Health literacy and effective communication are also an issue DOHaD researchers problematise as part of scientific practices (e.g. making sure one's research reaches out to critical actors for change; [21]), or as crucial activities of scientific societies. This is, for instance, the case of the 'DOHaD Society of Australia and New Zealand' (DOHaD ANZ), which has established several working groups (WGs) – including one on 'Translation, Policy and Communication' – to promote the 'collective identity' of the field and advance its agenda in science and society. Educating at-risk individuals is one of the core strategies the society has given itself 'to decrease the incidence and severity of noncommunicable diseases in Australia and New Zealand' (p. 438). The WG 'Translation, Policy and Communication' reports on its activities in 'three broad areas: knowledge synthesis, communicating this knowledge and translating this knowledge' (p. 438). The point for its policy uptake, translation, and communication is just to keep the DOHaD message simple and present it consistently by taking into account 'the mindset of each user group' [35].

It could be questioned whether mass communications directed at individuals are an effective strategy of health promotion – and, incidentally, a good way to bring DOHaD closer to societal action, whether individual or collective. Although a body of work on 'right messages' in health communication is built on intuitive assumptions about the receptiveness of intended audiences, a whole social epidemiology literature exists on what some call 'communication inequalities' [36]. These inequalities result from social determinants (e.g. class, social networks, education access and quality, neighbourhood, and built environment) that act on health literacy – much like they do on the individual capacity to be an actor for change in one's health. Health literacy and its translation into responsible health-related behaviours go therefore *beyond the process of tailoring the right message to the right individual*: rather, literacy demands the empowerment of the individuals concerned and entails an interactional process between them and their social environments [37–39].

The issue of DOHaD-related education requires therefore that language, metaphors, and arguments adequately consider such multi-level and integrated views of literacy and behaviour change for health. A nuanced critique of the centrality of behaviour change for DOHaD-related policymaking can be found in a paper by DOHaD researchers Luseadra McKerracher and colleagues [40]. They show that DOHaD knowledge translation (KT) can be made compatible to different degrees with an emphasis towards social, community, and institutional change. First, they put forward the 'pragmatic and moral reasons' against DOHaD KT. Educational interventions, they argue, could be detrimental to mothers-to-be by placing 'yet another layer of psychological responsibility (essentially blame) on the[ir] shoulders' (p. 424). To prevent this outcome, DOHaD KT should take into consideration that individuals or communities 'of lower socioeconomic status' are often simply 'unable to prevent nutritional shortfalls, to avoid environmental contaminants, or to avoid (or reduce) psychological and/or physiological stress in the environments' (p. 424). It is thus 'morally arbitrary' to expect that improving the health literacy of parents-to-be suffices as a policy translation of this field.

Second, the authors plead for the centrality of DOHaD KT to individuals in the policy agenda of the field and consider it a duty 'to actively disseminate crucial information regarding pregnancy nutrition' (p. 424). There are, they maintain, a few 'teachable moments' (p. 423) at different life stages (e.g. adolescence and pregnancy) where the dissemination of health-related information may be effective. This is due to a combination of higher individual information-seeking and higher receptiveness and will to engage in behavioural change. The fact, the authors conclude, that 'expecting mothers/ couples, or people planning pregnancies are not being targeted' represents 'a surprising gap' in current programmes. As problematic as DOHaD KT may be, the authors recommend to multiply and reinforce KT strategies in more receptive populations: access to information is a pillar of the policy translation of DOHaD [40].

McKerracher and colleagues attempt to formulate a balanced view concerning the importance of sustaining direct-to-public KT efforts. They underline the importance of KT all while ensuring 'that public institutions hold the lion's share of moral responsibility for ensuring environmental nutrition/health equity' (p. 425). Their strategy starts from the recognition that DOHaD researchers, much like the concerned individuals, cannot change the structural factors that shape 'developmental environments, developmental trajectories, disease risks over the lifecourse and long-term health outcomes' (p. 425). It also puts at the centre the importance of KT initiatives: parents-to-be, especially prospective mothers, ought to be informed while also being reassured about the fact that their 'capacity to improve their children's developmental environments, their bodies and behaviours' is just 'a small piece of a large and complex environmental puzzle' [40]. In the words of another DOHaD author critically addressing the field's emphasis on literacy and education, this issue should be treated with a nuanced view of what actions are really available to a given person in a given context: 'having information about healthier diets and some of the skills does not necessarily mean that choosing the healthier options is easy in today's society' [41].

8.4.3 Behaviour Change for the Sake of Pragmatism

Another conspicuous source of ambiguity in the policy discourses of DOHaD scientists stems from a mismatch between tools, ways of knowledge-making, and the scope of a clinical and/or public health science like DOHaD. While some pursue the line of research inaugurated by Barker's hypothesis (focusing on the populational effects of geographical and socio-economic conditions), current epigenetic studies of developmental programming in, for instance, a mother–child cohort often cast a far narrower outlook on these issues. This understanding of aberrant developmental effects during pregnancy is located in women's bodies, and the corresponding interventions are putatively supported by this evidence within the sphere of individual action and/or behaviour change. Thus, when presenting their results and their relevance for public health, DOHaD researchers often need to make multiple conceptual leaps: from the evidence produced at the individual level to a concept developed at the populational level; from the molecular mechanisms of developmental processes to the social and epidemiological factors that influence them; or even from the animal models providing mechanistic knowledge of developmental programming to the humans at the centre of clinical/primary prevention practice. Holding these multiple layers of evidence – and potential policy interventions – together is a difficult task. While awareness of the need to consider how all these factors interact is not lacking in the literature, a whole different task is to produce compelling evidence to intervene in these complex biosocial processes [42].

The challenge of holding together the individual and the collective, the clinical and the populational, the behavioural and the structural constitutes a third (and last) way DOHaD researchers end up legitimising – perhaps unwillingly – individual responsibilities for health. Take, for instance, a series of papers by influential DOHaD researchers – and contributors to this handbook – Mark Hanson, Peter Gluckman, and Lucilla Poston [1, 42, 43]. The complex social ramifications of DOHaD could not be stated in a clearer way in their work: 'if the result is a culture of blame or shame, the resistance to change induced [by DOHaD] will make the battle against NCD[s] even harder' [43]. And yet, these authors also affirm that there are 'pragmatic' reasons to support and promote lifestyle improvements in 'women and young girls', much like in 'men' and 'adolescents' [43].

With pragmatism, Hanson, Gluckman, and Poston have in mind an argument we partly encountered already above: there exist 'teachable moments' during anyone's lifetime that are a promising opportunity for an investment into health literacy with long-term consequences. Educating adolescents could have a dramatic impact on individual 'self-efficacy' and capacity 'to make decisions about lifestyle themselves' [43]. Therefore, although 'sensitivity' and a 'focus on empowerment' are paramount [43], translations of DOHaD knowledge into policy cannot afford to give up on the promotion of behaviour change and healthy lifestyles in vulnerable populations. The challenge for DOHaD scientists is striking the right balance between the need to offer 'evidence-informed strategies and where possible [also] pragmatic solutions' [1]. More than formulating a theory of DOHaD-inspired health justice, the challenge of DOHaD researchers is what can be 'back [ed] with impunity' [1], or what 'policy interventions may be most efficacious' [44].

While tapping into the political potential of DOHaD would encompass 'population-based complex interventions', the efforts of DOHaD researchers are limited by available evidence and the affordances of the science they practice. Policy translations that support lifestyle changes for women and their partners are often simply 'a more immediate message' [1], which they can offer with assurance and factual support. This raises the question of what DOHaD scientists can do from where they stand. In the absence of a complex, systems-based approach to the multi-generational mechanisms of developmental programming and the social determinants of health, the promotion of individual responsibilities for health – although tempered by DOHaD scientists' own critical reflexivities – appears to be a policy option with strong practical hold.

8.5 Discussion

Our systematic and critical review reveals that DOHaD scientists are no less concerned than public health advocates or ELSA scholars with the pathogenic environments and the social determinants of health that modulate developmental predispositions to adult disease. While they do not lack awareness of the relevance of these complex and multi-level processes for DOHaD thinking, they also know too well that reordering those socio-material circumstances is beyond their reach. As one gets closer to the ways DOHaD scientists write about individual agencies, parental behaviours, maternal/paternal lifestyles, and periconceptional health promotion, one cannot but notice their difficult position. On the one hand, they deplore the social, environmental, and multi-generational inequalities that pattern developmental exposures and reproduce health inequities in our societies. On the other hand, they lack the evidence (validated knowledge), tools, and influence to fully take issue with the complex biosocial origins of developmental programming and act upon the structural problems that interfere with periconceptional health behaviours, gestational lifestyles, or infant health. In the face of this situation, what remains open to these practitioners is the possibility to address DOHaD knowledge and advice to parents-to-be, pregnant women, prospective fathers, or couples in a reproductive project. Hence, the primary finding of our critical review is that the 'moral paradox' of DOHaD gets in part explained by *the challenges scientists face when elaborating upon the policy options backed up by their research and practice.* A thorough appreciation of their situatedness reveals that appeals towards individual responsibility in DOHaD are far from being (yet) another neoliberal disciplining strategy for health promotion. Quite the contrary, they are a suboptimal compromise. It is the necessity of tailoring the complex policy messages of DOHaD to the concrete opportunities for action and change available to most periconceptional health practitioners. To them, what is better, rather than worse, in the absence of an opportunity for structural change, is to encourage and educate prospective parents to become the actors for change and protect the health of their future children.

This does not mean that the hyper-responsibilisation critique we highlighted above is misplaced or unfounded. The truth is that, although grounded on pragmatic reasons, the public policy strategies of DOHaD researchers often boil down to providing mothers, fathers, and families with the 'right' information and to warning them about the long-term health consequences of their lifestyles and behaviours. In this respect, social scientists and ELSA scholars hit the right note when writing about (what we call) the 'moral paradox' of DOHaD. By foreclosing the reflexivity on the syndemic and multi-level implications of their knowledge, DOHaD scientists offer an ambiguous societal uptake of this evidence. This paradoxically ends up reinforcing problematic discourses of individual responsibility for health, especially in their uneven, gendered version that overburdens pregnant women and mothers-to-be. By targeting health behaviours as a main interventional strategy within their reach, DOHaD authors hamper the production of more elaborate policy imaginaries flowing out of their field. Thus, the hypothesis by David Barker that gestational socio-economic hardship translates into an unequal distribution of non-communicable adult disease turns into an admonishment to individuals on how to behave 'best', urging them to take the kind of control over their health that may simply be unaffordable to them from their own social and environmental positionality. Here lies our second conclusion: the 'moral paradox' of DOHaD represents an ambiguous normative stance that mixes up the pragmatic possibilities of clinical and public health sciences with the policy discourses, practical ambitions, and political potential of a scientific field.

So, what can scientists do to avoid this situation? Taking scientists' situatedness seriously, no ready-made solution exists to complexify DOHaD knowledge and its policy translations. This notwithstanding, scientists could at least embark upon two kinds of concrete actions that might defuse the 'moral paradox' of DOHaD. *First,* they could make explicit the tensions highlighted above at the core of their research: between the individual intervention and the social aetiology of a condition, between the behavioural recommendation and the need for political/structural change, between the tools and knowledge of biomedical sciences and the possibilities of populational health research, or, finally, between mechanistic knowledge and the need to remove the so-called 'causes of the causes' of diseases [4]. When discussing their data, presenting their results, and, especially, when positioning their science's implications for policy and society, they could explicitly acknowledge that what can be proven in the context of their research does not capture the complex biosocial dynamics that bring about these phenomena in the real world. DOHaD scientists could – as some of the authors we studied have already done – clearly state in their writing that the individual 'capacity to improve . . . children's developmental environments, their bodies and behaviours' is just 'a small piece of a large and complex environmental puzzle' [40]. While the knowledge they produce is of immense value to shed light on bits and pieces of this puzzle, they can advocate caution in extrapolating general solutions from partial knowledge. If such a provision were systematically part of the discussion sections of DOHaD papers investigating any of the biological, behavioural, relational, social, structural, and environmental dimensions of early-life programming (studied in conjunction, as much as in isolation – as they often are), there would be little doubt about the policy framings of DOHaD research. The 'moral paradox' of DOHaD would simply be dispelled.

Second, another opportunity to counter the 'paradox' is to ensure that explanations, interventions, and policy discourses support or initiate social interventions in relevant developmental windows and biosocial pathways of disease. This is, of course, easier said than done, as detailed by sociologist Michael Penkler in the context of DOHaD studies of social-biological transitions [45] leading to diseases [46]. The challenge is not simply identifying early-life predictive (epigenetic) biomarkers of relevance to adult disease [47]. Rather, it resides also in the identification of the structural 'windows of plasticity' and intervention in body–environment interactions [48]. Resilience and reversibility of programming processes at different life stages are also largely unexplored corollaries of DOHaD evidence; a far more complex biopsychosocial approach to early life in research settings is in order for the proliferation of different DOHaD policy discourses.

The present work has tried to sketch a few points of normative ambiguity in scientific writing as potential paths of improvements for the social and political circulation of DOHaD research. In the wish to make social science critique instructive of novel avenues of biosocial research, these suggestions should be read as no more than an analytical contribution to finally dispel the 'moral paradox' of DOHaD. And, perhaps, also as a contribution to a collaborative push to unleash DOHaD's full political potential for social reform, development, and change.

References

1. Hanson MA, Poston L, Gluckman PD. DOHaD – The challenge of translating the science to policy. Vol. 10, Journal of Developmental Origins of Health and Disease. Cambridge: Cambridge University Press; 2019. pp. 263–7.

2. Jacob CM, Hanson M. Implications of the Developmental Origins of Health and Disease concept for policy-making. Current Opinion in Endocrine and Metabolic Research. 2020 1 Aug;13:20–7.

3. Goodman JM, Boone-Heinonen J, Richardson DM, Andrea SB, Messer LC. Analyzing Policies Through a DOHaD Lens: What Can We Learn? Vol. 15, International Journal of Environmental Research and Public Health. Basel: MDPI; 2018: Article 2906.

4. Marmot M. Inclusion health: Addressing the causes of the causes. The Lancet. 2018 20 Jan;391(10117):186–8.

5. Singer M, Bulled N, Ostrach B, Mendenhall E. Syndemics and the biosocial conception of health. The Lancet. 2017 Mar;389(10072):941–50.

6. Soubry A. POHaD: Why we should study future fathers. Vol. 4, Environmental Epigenetics. Oxford: Oxford University Press; 2018. https://academic.oup.com/eep/article/4/2/dvy007/4987171

7. Meloni M, Testa G. Scrutinizing the epigenetics revolution. BioSocieties. 2014;9(4):431–56.

8. Penkler M, Hanson M, Biesma R, Müller R. DOHaD in science and society: Emergent opportunities and novel responsibilities. Journal of Developmental Origins of Health and Disease. 2018;10:268–73. www.cambridge.org/core/

journals/journal-of-developmental-origins-of-health-and-disease/article/dohad-in-science-and-society-emergent-opportunities-and-novel-responsibilities/A8395958BF322CE66429E1D2728AA6E6

9. Chiapperino L. Epigenetics: Ethics, politics, biosociality. British Medical Bulletin. 2018 1 Dec;128(1):49–60.

10. Chiapperino L, Panese F. Gendered imaginaries: Situating knowledge of epigenetic programming of health. Sociology of Health & Illness. 2018 1 Sep;40(7):1233–49.

11. Chiapperino L. Luck and the responsibilities to protect one's epigenome. Journal of Responsible Innovation. 2020;7(2):S86–S106. www.tandfonline.com/doi/full/10.1080/23299460.2020.1842658.

12. Fassin D. Moral economies revisited. Annales Histoire, Sciences Sociales. 2009 1 Dec;64th Year(6):1237–66.

13. Warin M, Moore V, Zivkovic T, Davies M. Telescoping the origins of obesity to women's bodies: How gender inequalities are being squeezed out of Barker's hypothesis. Annals of Human Biology. 2011 Jul;38(4):453–60.

14. Richardson SS, Stevens H, editors. Postgenomics: Perspectives on Biology after the Genome. Durham, NC: Duke University Press; 2015. 294 p.

15. Wells JCK. Maternal capital and the metabolic ghetto: An evolutionary perspective on the transgenerational basis of health inequalities. American Journal of Human Biology. 2010 Jan;22(1):1–17.

16. Richardson SS. The Maternal Imprint: The Contested Science of Maternal–Fetal Effects. Chicago: University of Chicago Press; 2021. 318 p.

17. Pentecost M, Ross F. The first thousand days: Motherhood, scientific knowledge, and local histories. Medical Anthropology. 2019 4 Apr;0(0):1–15.

18. Pentecost M, Meloni M. The epigenetic imperative: Responsibility for early intervention at the time of biological plasticity. The American Journal of Bioethics. 2018 2 Nov;18(11):60–2.

19. Richardson SS, Daniels CR, Gillman MW, Golden J, Kukla R, Kuzawa C, et al. Society: Don't blame the mothers : Nature News & Comment. Nature. 2014 14 Aug;512:131–2.

20. Page MJ, McKenzie JE, Bossuyt PM, Boutron I, Hoffmann TC, Mulrow CD, et al. The PRISMA 2020 statement: An updated guideline for reporting systematic reviews. BMJ. 2021 29 Mar;372:n71.

21. Norris SA, Daar A, Balasubramanian D, Byass P, Kimani-Murage E, Macnab A, et al. Understanding and Acting on the Developmental Origins of Health and Disease in Africa Would Improve Health across Generations. Vol. 10, Global Health Action. Abingdon: Taylor & Francis Ltd; 2017.

22. Arabin B, Timmesfeld N, Noever K, Behnam S, Ellermann C, Jenny MA. How to improve health literacy to reduce short- and long-term consequences of maternal obesity? Vol. 32, Journal of Maternal-Fetal & Neonatal Medicine. Abingdon: Taylor & Francis Ltd; 2019. pp. 2935–42.

23. Akombi BJ, Agho KE, Hall JJ, Merom D, Astell-Burt T, Renzaho AMN. Stunting and severe stunting among children under-5 years in Nigeria: A multilevel analysis. BMC Pediatrics. 2017 13 Jan;17:1–16.

24. Barouki R, Gluckman PD, Grandjean P, Hanson M, Heindel JJ. Developmental origins of non-communicable disease: Implications for research and public health. Environmental Health. 2012 20 Jun;11: Article number 42. https://ehjournal.biomedcentral.com/articles/10.1186/1476-069X-11-42#citeas.

25. Albert J, Bogard J, Siota F, McCarter J, Diatalau S, Maelaua J, et al. Malnutrition in rural Solomon Islands: An analysis of the problem and its drivers. Maternal and Child Nutrition. 2020 Apr;16(2):1–12.

26. Schott W, Aurino E, Penny ME, Behrman JR. The double burden of malnutrition

among youth: Trajectories and inequalities in four emerging economies. Economics & Human Biology. 2019 Aug;34(SI):80–91.

27. Schwarzenberg SJ, Georgieff MK, Nutr C. Advocacy for improving nutrition in the first 1000 days to support childhood development and adult health. Pediatrics. 2018 Feb;141(2):e20173716. https://doi .org/10.1542/peds.2017-3716

28. Dupras C, Saulnier KM, Joly Y. Epigenetics, ethics, law and society: A multidisciplinary review of descriptive, instrumental, dialectical and reflexive analyses. Soc Stud Sci. 2019 Oct 1;49 (5):785–810.

29. Bansal A, Simmons RA. Epigenetics and developmental origins of diabetes: Correlation or causation? American Journal of Physiology-Endocrinology and Metabolism. 2018 Jul;315(1):E15–28.

30. Arabin B, Baschat AA. Pregnancy: An Underutilized Window of Opportunity to Improve Long-term Maternal and Infant Health-An Appeal for Continuous Family Care and Interdisciplinary Communication. Vol. 5, Frontiers in Pediatrics. Lausanne: Frontiers Media SA; 2017.

31. Lewis AJ, Galbally M, Gannon T, Symeonides C. Early life programming as a target for prevention of child and adolescent mental disorders. Vol. 12, BMC Medicine. London: BMC; 2014.

32. Barnes MD, Heaton TL, Goates MC, Packer JM. Intersystem implications of the developmental origins of health and disease: Advancing health promotion in the Twenty-first century. Healthcare. 2016 Sept;4(3).

33. Koletzko B, Brands B, Grote V, Kirchberg FF, Prell C, Rzehak P, et al. Long-term health impact of early nutrition: The power of programming. Annals of Nutrition and Metabolism. 2017;70 (3):161–9.

34. DeSocio JE. Epigenetics, maternal prenatal psychosocial stress, and infant mental health. Vol. 32, Archives of Psychiatric Nursing. Philadelphia, PA:

W B Saunders CO-Elsevier INC; 2018. pp. 901–6.

35. Prescott SL, Allen K, Armstrong K, Collins C, Dickinson H, Gardiner K, et al. The establishment of DOHaD working groups in Australia and New Zealand. Vol. 7, Journal of Developmental Origins of Health and Disease. Cambridge: Cambridge University Press; 2016. pp. 433–9.

36. Viswanath K, Emmons KM. Message effects and social determinants of health: Its application to cancer disparities. Journal of Communication. 2006 1 Aug;56(suppl_1):S238–64.

37. Tengland PA. Empowerment: A goal or a means for health promotion? Medicine, Health Care and Philosophy. 2007 Jun;10 (2):197–207.

38. Tengland PA. Empowerment: A conceptual discussion. Health Care Analysis. 2008 Jun;16(2):77–96.

39. Ishikawa H, Kiuchi T. Health literacy and health communication. Biopsychosoc Med. 2010 Nov 5;4:18.

40. McKerracher L, Moffat T, Barker M, Williams D, Sloboda DM. Translating the Developmental Origins of Health and Disease concept to improve the nutritional environment for our next generations: A call for a reflexive, positive, multi-level approach. Vol. 10, Journal of Developmental Origins of Health and Disease. Cambridge: Cambridge University Press; 2019. pp. 420–8.

41. Levy LB. Food policy and dietary change. Proceedings of the Nutrition Society. 2009 May;68(2):216–20.

42. Gluckman PD, Hanson MA. Developmental plasticity and human disease: Research directions. Vol. 261, Journal of Internal Medicine. Malden, MA: Wiley-Blackwell; 2007. pp. 461–71.

43. Hanson MA, Gluckman PD. Developmental origins of health and disease: Moving from biological concepts to interventions and policy. International Journal of Gynaecology and Obstetrics. 2011 Nov;115 Suppl 1:S3–5.

44. Gluckman PD, Hanson MA, Low FM. Evolutionary and developmental mismatches are consequences of adaptive developmental plasticity in humans and have implications for later disease risk. Vol. 374, Philosophical Transactions of the Royal Society B-Biological Sciences. London: Royal Soc; 2019: Article number: 20180109. https://royalsocietypublishing.org/doi/10.1098/rstb.2018.0109.

45. Blane D, Kelly-Irving M, D'Errico A, Bartley M, Montgomery S. Social-biological transitions: How does the social become biological? Longitudinal and Life Course Studies. 2013;4(2):136–46.

46. Penkler M. Caring for biosocial complexity. Articulations of the environment in research on the Developmental Origins of Health and Disease. Studies in History and Philosophy of Science. 2022 Jun;93:1–10.

47. Shanthikumar S, Neeland MR, Maksimovic J, Ranganathan SC, Saffery R. DNA methylation biomarkers of future health outcomes in children. Molecular and Cellular Pediatrics. 2020 9 Jul;7(1):7: Article number 7. https://molcellped.springeropen.com/articles/10.1186/s40348-020-00099-0.

48. McEwen BS. Allostasis and the epigenetics of brain and body health over the life course: The brain on stress. JAMA Psychiatry. 2017 Jun 1;74(6):551–2.

Intra- and Intergenerational Justice, Law, and DOHaD

Isabel Karpin

9.1 What's Law Got to Do with It?

9.1.1 Introduction

Developmental Origins of Health and Disease (DOHaD) research focuses on the environmental causes of disease in the preconception, prenatal, and early-life periods of human development. Epigenetics is a key mechanism that underlies this research and refers to non-genetic inheritable changes that impact gene expression. DOHaD and epigenetics research can provide a critical resource for legal thinkers determining the lines of responsibility for environmental harms (both physical and psychosocial) that affect a child's growth and development. The epigenetic research that makes these claims is both contested and controversial; nevertheless, some DOHaD scholars argue it provides evidence of the origin of early-life health harms in events that occurred during pregnancy [1–3].[1] Additionally, some researchers argue that it is possible for disadvantageous epigenetic changes to occur in future children who were not even conceived at the time of the harm to their putative parents and thus were never directly exposed. Moreover, there is a body of scientific research that provides evidence that those suffering disadvantage throughout their lifecourse in conditions of systemic oppression, such as that arising from racism, sexism, or poverty, for example, may be disproportionately subject to epigenetic molecular changes creating harmed subgroups that are then intergenerationally reproduced as socially disadvantaged communities [4–10]. This chapter argues that, despite the tendency in Western common law systems to individualise responsibility, epigenetics may provide the key to an alternative approach that highlights interconnectedness within and across generations. In this way, whole communities and State systems may be held responsible rather than individuals.

Using examples from Australian, US, and Canadian legal systems, this chapter asks what legal obligations, if any, should or can be imposed on contemporary society to ensure not just the future 'health' of existing children (as they grow into adults) but also the generations of people yet to be born? It examines the possibility of *legal* protections and remedies for early-life and pre-life harms (ultimately manifesting as epigenetic changes), including from psychosocial adversity stemming from systemic mistreatment.

When identifying a 'risk pathway' for the attribution of responsibility in DOHaD research, there is a significant body of literature focusing on maternal causes for poor

---

[1] For a sociological perspective considering the contestable nature of this scientific research see Richardson S, this volume.

health outcomes in children. At the same time a growing body of literature in the interrelated field of epigenetics, highlights multiple and intersecting transmission pathways of harm stemming from marginalisation and disadvantage, including via the paternal line [11–13]. Epigenetic and DOHaD research show that social harms emanating from both psychosocial and physical environments can have long-term intergenerational effects. This poses a challenge to the standard reflexive response in law that identifies maternal responsibility and reinforces individualised models of blame. Epigenetics as an explanatory discourse makes a case, I argue, for a legal duty owed by the State for the harms caused by environments of systemic disadvantage. This would be a duty owed *to* parental actors rather than *by* them – an approach that would demand laws and public policy distribute responsibility across the community and demand State action.

9.1.2 Legal Persons and the Rights of Future Generations

The attribution of interests and rights (and thereby a capacity to be harmed) to an imagined future person whose development and birth are highly contingent challenges liberal legal and feminist views that rights should only accrue to legal persons. This is because what constitutes a legal person in law is not settled. The environmental and animal law fields have already had some success in attaching personhood status to natural entities such as rivers and non-human animals [14, 15]. However, there is ongoing concern that a flexible idea of personhood will be, if it has not already been, co-opted to control women's reproductive autonomy through the attribution of personhood to fetuses. Feminist disability scholars such as Rosemarie Garland-Thomson have come up against this problem when trying to create a space for autonomous decision-making in the abortion context alongside a deeper understanding of people with disability [16]. The risk of harm to 'future persons', for example, is already a justification used for a range of policy and regulatory strategies in Australia and the UK in laws around assisted reproductive technology [17, 18].[2] In those laws, the welfare of the future child is paramount or must be considered carefully when making reproductive decisions. The attribution of welfare rights to future individuals imposes a duty on existing persons.[3] An alternative and arguably more just approach, in keeping with feminist accounts of the self, involves articulating a collective duty (moral, political, and legal) to future generations. Edith Brown Weiss, for instance, argues that 'each generation receives a natural and cultural legacy in trust from previous generations and holds it in trust for future generations' [19, p. 2]. Given that it is a certainty that there will be a

---

[2] Other signs include recent prosecutions in the US for stillbirth and miscarriage after drug use as reported in the media in: Aspinwall C, Bailey B, and Yurkanin, A. They lost pregnancies for unclear reasons. Then they were prosecuted. *Washington Post*, September 12, 2022 www.washingtonpost.com/national-security/2022/09/01/prosecutions-drugs-miscarriages-meth-stillbirths/ accessed 28/11/2022 and Dwyer D and See P, Prosecuting pregnancy loss: Why advocates fear a post-Roe surge of charges. *ABC News* 28 September, 2022. https://abcnews.go.com/Politics/prosecuting-pregnancy-loss-advocates-fear-post-roe-surge/story?id=89812204 accessed 28/11/2022.

[3] *Assisted Reproductive Treatment Act 2008* (VIC) s 5(a)'; *Human Reproductive Technology Act 1991* (WA) s 4(d)(iv); *Assisted Reproductive Treatment Act 1988* (SA) s 4A; *Human Fertilisation and Embryology Act 1990* (UK) s13(5)

next generation, arguably, we can and must articulate legal and ethical duties in relation to those future communities. Claims about the intergenerational transmission of harms via epigenetic changes, however, demand a more complex articulation of the call for intergenerational justice, one that incorporates or understands the impact of *intra-generational injustice* – the unequal distribution of harms and resources within a generation. Eisen et al. argue, for instance, that the

> [T]endency in the orthodox intergenerational justice literature to define the 'interests' of a given generation as an aggregate of all individual interests, is both misleading as description and perilous as prescription. It glosses over the significant disparities within generations, and thus cannot provide the analytical tools to think about how those disparities persist and transform over time. [20, p. 5]

Epigenetic effects manifest when the body responds at a molecular level to the external physical and psychosocial environment [21]. This may happen by activating biochemical changes to methyl groups that modify the histones that wind around DNA, for example. These epigenetic changes can alter the usual trajectory of a gene towards activation or deactivation. In such cases, the outcome may be a disease or deficit that would not have otherwise eventuated. The resulting harms can be significant and serious, including heart disease, cognitive impairment, diabetes, and neurological disorders among others [9, 22, 23]. DOHaD research evidences epigenetic changes that occur to an existing person or to a fetus during pregnancy. But, as foreshadowed above, there is also research showing that even before a person becomes pregnant, changes to their or their partner's epigenetic system brought on by environmental harms may be passed on to the not-yet-conceived [1–3]. While this research is still nascent and contested, it is significant that epigenetic research is increasingly claiming to evidence the physical impact of systemic psycho-social harms such as racism, colonisation, slavery, child abuse, gendered violence, and socio-economic disadvantage [4–10, 24].

It is critically important to the development of a legal response to examine how DOHaD scholars and those working in the field of epigenetics articulate these harmful effects, because this will influence the way those harms are understood in the legal context. Epigenetic understandings may fundamentally challenge the reliance on ideas of individual responsibility in common law Western legal systems. I have argued elsewhere that if law incorporated an epigenetic understanding, the response to cases of systemic mistreatment would need to acknowledge the impact of a cultural milieu of hostility to certain groups [25]. As epidemiologist Nancy Krieger states, 'We live embodied – and our bodies each and every day biologically integrate each and every type of unjust, and also beneficial, exposure encountered, at each and every level' [26, p. 45].

The attribution of an obligation of care towards future persons is problematic because, historically, the State's interest in promoting the well-being of future persons has been enacted on and through the presumptively recalcitrant bodies of reproductive women. This has occurred using disciplinary legislative, medical, and public health regimes that attribute culpability to individuals, and women in particular, for failure to avoid poor reproductive outcomes [27]. However, this individualised model of blame can only gain traction if we see the future child as having different and conflicting interests from the people who created them. In fact, as I will show, a better approach, which aligns with the trajectories of harm identified by epigenetic changes, is to argue that the well-being of future generations is impacted by social inequality (*intra*-generational inequality) as well as specific individual harms. This gives rise to a duty on the State to protect the well-being of future generations by assisting the existing person whose future progeny may be harmed by their unequal treatment. This would also unburden the pregnant person or potentially pregnant person from sole or even primary culpability and instead equip them with a claim themselves for legal remedies that demand State protection from the risk of harm to the health and well-being of their prospective children. In what follows, I draw on the research being undertaken in the fields of DOHaD and epigenetics to make a case for a legal duty that is owed *to* parental actors rather than *by* them for the harms caused by hostile, degrading, and discriminatory environments.

9.2 Law's Reliance on Discourses of Epigenetics

9.2.1 Expert Evidence and Epigenetic Narratives in Law

The term epigenetics has been slow to enter the legal lexicon in Australia. A review of Australian legislation turns up almost no mention of epigenetics or epigenetic processes in bills, Acts, regulations, and subordinate legislation [28, 29].[4] A quick search of Australian case law, however, identifies a small bundle of cases where the word epigenetics has crept in once or twice. These cases evidence the slow but definite infiltration into the law of a particular aspect of this scientific narrative that speaks to the intergenerational impact of trauma. While these were only single paragraphs or sentences in lengthy judgements that turned on many factors, their appearance is a sign that this relatively new and highly contentious scientific discourse seeking to explain the DOHaD is slowly finding its way into legal decision-making.

One example from Australian administrative law is a 2017 Coronial Inquest[5] examining the deaths of 13 Aboriginal children and young persons in the Kimberley region[6] of Western Australia. Epigenetics was referred to in that report to highlight the collective impact of intergenerational trauma. The inquest was initiated because 'there were similar circumstances, life events, developmental experiences and behaviours that appear to have contributed to making [the 13 children] vulnerable to suicide' [30, para 1]. It is further commented that

> To focus only upon the individual events that occurred shortly before their deaths would not adequately address the circumstances attending the deaths. The tragic individual events were shaped by the crushing effects of intergenerational trauma and poverty upon entire communities. That community-wide trauma, generated multiple and prolonged exposures to individual traumatic events for these children and young persons. [30, para 3]

---

[4] With an all-Australian legislation database search in Austlii, only the one following mention of epigenetics was found: *NSW Greyhound Racing Rules 2022* (NSW) r 150(1)(e) which prohibits 'the administration of any gene editing agents designed to alter genome sequences and/or the transcriptional or epigenetic regulation of gene expression'.

[5] A coronial inquest is a formal hearing where the coroner exercises various powers to investigate a death and consider evidence to determine the identity of the deceased and the date, place, manner, and cause of death of the deceased.

[6] The Kimberley region is the northernmost area of Western Australia. Approximately 40 per cent of the population is of Aboriginal descent.

Dr Paul Simons, the Kimberley region's child and adolescent psychiatrist draws on epigenetics to support his argument that the poor health and well-being of Indigenous young people in the Kimberly region is, in part, due to ongoing trauma resulting from colonisation and forced family separation. He states:

> Before birth, some children are exposed to high levels of stress and trauma, to alcohol and drugs, and poor nutrition; high levels of stress hormones in utero can affect the expression of genes, and these *epigenetic* processes can affect brain development, such that babies can be born hardwired to preferentially employ 'fight and flight' coping strategies as they develop, at the cost of executive brain functioning, which facilitates emotional regulation. [30, para 195] (my emphasis)

Scholars Warin, Kowal, and Meloni have cautioned that the use of epigenetic discourses by Indigenous scholars and activists may result in a different kind of determinism tied to 'milieu, history, and social and physical location (molecularly incorporated into the body)' [31]. The danger here is that the focus will not be on the environment that creates the harm but on the individual who has been harmed, undermining possible remedies and declaring them redundant. While this is a concern, there is the possibility of a different response, and in the 2017 Coronial Inquest, the evidence led to a recommendation for training in intergenerational trauma for those working with Indigenous youth in the Kimberley region.

On the other hand, there are other areas of law where there is frustration that this evidence is not being more thoroughly incorporated and considered. I consider three areas briefly below.

9.2.2 Environmental Law

In the field of environmental law, there is a tendency to regulate to limit rather than prohibit polluting agents. Eisen et al., for example, suggest that Canada and the United States have a permissive approach to chemical regulation 'in which the burden of proof falls on those trying to show that chemicals are harmful' [20, p. 13]. This needs to change as evidence of long-term effects accumulates. Eisen et al. point out that there 'is increasing scientific support for the theory that children, even grandchildren, of those exposed to brominated flame retardants (BFRs) and phthalates [ubiquitous chemicals in household furniture and products] may incur health consequences' [20, pp. 10, 17].

Legal scholars are drawing on epigenetic claims to argue that environmental protection needs to be crafted around the potential intergenerational and early-life impact of toxic environments, understood as incorporating both physical and psychosocial harms. As Rothstein et al. point out, systemic disadvantage increases the potential for harm from polluted environments. They state that

> It is well-known that disadvantaged populations with poor nutrition, substandard or nonexistent healthcare, stress from factors such as housing instability and fear of violence, and high-risk lifestyle factors increase susceptibility to environmental exposures. [33, p. 4]

In the case of chemical pollutants, for example, Scott et al. argue that 'BFRs can be thought to create a fleshy material archive of one's social location, practices, and movements. Not only are bodies embedded in social contexts and structures, but the social is also embedded, literally, in material bodies' [34, p. 333]. Thus, the presence of BFRs does not just tell us about immediate harm but also about the likely location of that harm and the social circumstances that led to its magnitude. *Inter*generational harm is thus integrally linked to *intra*-generational inequality. Epigenetics too suggests that people are integrated into harmed communities and are subject to multiple networks of harming effects that are passed on to existing children and future generations, distributing the responsibility for the harm across communities and the State. These realisations demand a conceptual change to law's traditional approach of assigning responsibility by tracing an uninterrupted line of cause and effect.

9.2.3 Tort Law

US tort law offers another example where the traditional response to these kinds of harms fails to protect those who are harmed. In torts, remediable transgenerational epigenetic effects do not generally include those that manifest in the first *unexposed* generation because the line of causation is narrowly cast and cannot accommodate multiple forms of insult. The classic example is the case of diethylstilboestrol known as DES, the drug that was given to women from the 1940s up to the 1970s to prevent miscarriage. It was withdrawn from the market after it was found to cause vaginal cancer. The children who were in utero when the drug was given were also found to have a higher incidence of cancer and infertility as were the children of those children [35]. However, the US Courts limited claims to the mothers directly given the drug and their children who had been exposed in utero, disallowing claims beyond first-generation exposure because of what they called 'victim attenuation' – namely, the difficulty of connecting, causally and temporally, the tortious conduct, and the injured victim [29, 33, 35].

In other words, the greater the distance in time between the offence and the victim's injury, the greater the possibility for potentially unknown causal acts to have been responsible or even partly responsible. However, as we have seen above, even when there is direct exposure there is also a network of other environmental influences and effects that may make one more susceptible to the harm. Individuals are exposed to thousands of different toxins from multiple sources throughout their lifecourse. The likely scenario where those who are most disadvantaged economically and socially are also those who will be most harmed, allows for the argument that the identification of a single responsible agent is untenable, leaving generations of victims with no recourse. On the other hand, scholars such as Doci et al. argue that 'individuals who are affected by epigenetic side effects should have a right to obtain justice and to present an epigenetic case within a legal system which is suited to handle it' [29, p. 274].

9.2.4 Regulating Reproductive Bodies

On the other side of the coin is the willingness of law to identify a cause and effect when it comes to the putative pregnant person. The proximity of a pregnant person to their fetus appears to create a sufficiently *un*-attenuated line of causation that justifies pre-emptive hyper-surveillance of their behaviour from policymakers, public health institutions, and sometimes legal actors. While the scientific literature is contested, it nevertheless offers an alternate narrative that can be used to insist on a more complex and contingent account of responsibility and harm. However, rather than cautiously drawing on the scientific claims emerging in the fields of epigenetics and DOHaD that trace a physical harm from psychosocial sources such as stress, trauma, violence, and abuse against the pregnant or potentially pregnant person, public health initiatives tend to focus instead on the aspect of DOHaD research that identifies the pregnant woman as the locus of harm. Pregnant women and those seen as of reproductive age are schooled to modify their behaviour to counter some of these societal and environmental effects.

One example of such schooling is the US Centre for Disease Control (CDC) guidelines on preconception care, for example, that were published in 2006 but are still referred to in the literature. These guidelines have as their first recommendation that there should be individual responsibility across the lifespan. They describe the 'target population' as women from 'menarche to menopause who are capable of having children, even if they do not intend to conceive' [36]. These women are told that they should be conscious of their genetic factors and cumulative risks and modify their diets accordingly. Among the lengthy list of things for women to avoid while pregnant is a caution to be aware of 'fetal exposures to teratogens'. In the plain English version on their website, the CDC warns women to avoid harmful chemicals at work and at home. Perhaps unsurprisingly, there is thus considerable concern among feminist legal scholars that more research in the field of DOHaD and epigenetics will see women subjected to more scrutiny. Take, for example, studies such as that of Roberts et al. linking maternal exposure to child abuse with a higher rate of autism in their offspring, or Slykerman et al.'s study linking depression in early adolescence with stress during pregnancy [37, 38]. These are just two examples among many [39].

Outside the discipline of law, scholars such as Sarah Richardson and Megan Warin have cautioned against an approach that places women at the centre of this harm. Richardson asks, for instance, whether there is 'potential for this research to heighten public health surveillance and restrictions on pregnant women and mothers through a molecular policing of their behaviour?'[40, p. 210] Warin et al. argue that 'A new and powerful meta-discourse has emerged in which women are blamed for both their reproductive physiology and their social role as mothers, thus constructing women as potentially contaminating future generations by creating obesity lineages' [41, p. 361]. This they say, 'coupled with a neoliberal agenda that emphasises self-governance and individual responsibility', individualises the responsibility for harm, and it does so in a gendered manner [41, p. 361]. In such a discourse, the responsibility for harm is shifted back to the individual who must, it seems, find a way to protect her offspring from the harms to which she herself has been subjected. A collection of cases where women have been prosecuted for neglect and abuse in raising obese children or not protecting their children from an abusive partner speak to the concern that epigenetics will be used to increase the scope of that responsibility, not delimit it [43, 44]. Contrary to such cases, feminist challenges suggest the need for an approach that recognises systemic injustices that create, as stated above, *networks* of harming effects.

Interestingly, scholars Loi, Del Savio, and Stupka optimistically suggest that we should look forward to 'a society in which people can be informed by their family physician of the accumulation of risk due to specific environmental insults, including those arising prenatally and in early childhood for which people cannot be held responsible' [45, p. 143]. Unfortunately, however, their assumption that women will not be held responsible is not borne out by recent history and is likely to be significantly amplified in the next few years with the recent development of so-called *epigenetic* tests. According to Dupras, Beauchamp, and Joly, these tests 'may provide sensitive information about individuals, not only their increased risks of diseases but also about their exposures and lifestyles' [46]. They list some of those exposures as comprising smoke, stress, alcohol, and other 'toxic chemicals' and describe the tests as potentially 'uncovering new layers of sensitive information about individuals that were not made accessible by genetic tests' [46]. Dupras et al. note the burgeoning industry specifically in the unregulated field of direct-to-consumer epigenetic tests with companies such as Chronomics, EpigenCare, Muhdo, MyDNAge and TruMe now offering them.

Arguably, women could be pressured to use direct-to-consumer epigenetic tests and, depending on the outcome, be held responsible for the 'harms' that follow. Dupras et al. indicate that one of the present uses of direct-to-consumer epigenetic testing is to reveal a person's smoke exposure history. In the traditional legal framing of individual responsibility, this might be an area where a regulatory response is triggered. Typically, women are viewed as culpable for harm if they smoke while pregnant, and while they might not be morally condemned for unwittingly exposing themselves to secondhand or environmental smoke, should they undergo a test that identifies their level of exposure to such smoke, a new responsibility arises to respond to the information provided by that test, and with it, a choice to either terminate an affected pregnancy or not move forward with plans to become pregnant. This new burden of responsibility is further complicated by the context of anthropogenic climate change, as demonstrated by epigenetic studies on smoke exposure undertaken in the wake of the Australian bushfires of 2019, which tracked the increased risk of adverse pregnancy and fetal outcomes for pregnant women who were exposed to bushfire smoke [47]. Viewing exposure through the prism of the individual maternal body in such studies highlights how social responsibility for harm can be masked and neutralised by such testing regimes [47].

Developing an alternate approach entails recrafting laws and public policy to recognise the network of harming effects. Ideally such an approach would distribute responsibility across the community and demand State action and responsibility, as I will examine in more detail below.

9.3 How Can Law Respond?

Because epigenetics blurs the distinction between the physical and the psychological by revealing a physical register for psychological harm through changes to methylation and the epigenome, it is possible to show how social adversity has physical effects. This kind of evidentiary trail is particularly appealing to law.

9.3.1 Legal Orthodoxy and the Autonomous Individual

Legal systems found in most common law countries operate within an orthodoxy which, to differing degrees, centres on the self-determining, independent, and autonomous individual both in terms of who it is aimed to protect and to whom it attributes responsibility. At the same time and perhaps ironically, law is sometimes used to assign responsibility to the harmed individual by characterising it as a failure of self-care and self-regulation. This accords with a contemporary neoliberal ideology where, as Robertson puts it,

> notions of individual autonomy, the free market and limited government are related, in a mutually producing and sustaining way, to the imperatives of 'self-care' – in the form of self-surveillance and self-regulation. [47]

It is clear then that we cannot understand or develop a response to epigenetic harms derived from psychosocial adversity and their intergenerational impact without revising these underlying ideological limitations.

Feminist legal scholar Jennifer Nedelsky argues for an alternative model for law that foregrounds our relational status. She states that 'human beings are in a constant process of becoming in interaction with the many layers of relationship in which they are embedded' [49, p. 38] and 'a relational self requires relational conceptions of values, which then require appropriate forms of law and rights built around those conceptions' [49, p. 5]. This relational model is one alternative. Another is Fineman's model of universal vulnerability, a model that demands that laws are refashioned around people as 'embodied creatures who are inexorably embedded in social relationships and institutions' and 'experience the world with differing levels of resilience' [49, pp. 1–7]. 'Resilience' according to Fineman is not an inherent trait but rather a resource that is unequally distributed. This occurs, as I have said elsewhere, 'when the "assaults" of inequality turn ordinary vulnerability (and dependency) into a politically amplified source of embodied and abiding psychosocial harm' [11, p. 1121].

In this vein, epigenetics offers us both a scientific account of cause and effect and a model for a conceptual shift to the relational self as an animating architecture around which to construct laws (rights, duties, and responsibilities). While there is a risk that foregrounding epigenetics can lead to a new form of stigma – the epigenetically disadvantaged – I argue that epigenetic processes nevertheless offer a constructive metaphor for rethinking legal rights and responsibilities. This is because epigenetic discourses reveal the impossibility of the autonomous, self-sufficient individual of liberal legalism.

Laws and public policy that are reworked to recognise *the network* of harming effects, however, must also be conscious of assumptions around what constitutes a harm. Assertions of 'harm' are inevitably entangled in prescriptions about what is normal, and therefore to talk about harm risks further stigmatising diverse embodiment. As such, a disability studies critique must also be mapped over the top of any legal remedies that are proposed to ensure that we do not simultaneously and unthinkingly instantiate inherited difference as self-evidently a harm. (See also Azevedo et al. in this volume.) Rosemarie Garland-Thomson has argued, for example, that feminist disability studies 'questions our assumptions that disability is a flaw, lack or excess' [51, p. 1157]. Eisen et al. argue too that 'critical disability studies scholarship calls on us to confront evocations of "anomalous bodies" as emblems of a tragic or dystopian future as constituting a distinct set of harms with their own distinct intertemporal dimensions' [20, p. 40]. They go on to note, quoting Alison Kafer, that the critical disability studies literature frames disability as relational and 'that individuals inhabit: the social institutions, laws, and policies within which they are embedded and that regulate their daily interactions and encounters; and the "social patterns that exclude or stigmatize particular kinds of bodies, minds and ways of being."' [20, p. 40]. Clearly, then, any invocation of relational accounts of harm and responsibility must not degrade anomalous embodiment and determine it as presumptively harmed.

9.3.2 Bioinequality and the Dismantling of the Individual in Law

Creating a new conceptual apparatus for legal action requires a linguistic device that names the previously unnamed. Karen O'Connell and I have developed the term bioinequalities, a concept that ties together biology and inequality to offer a language in which legislative life can be given to a harm previously unnamed in the law: the bodily effects of unequal treatment [25]. What is understood by unequal treatment is not simply different treatment but disadvantageous treatment in a system of oppression and subordination based on gender, race, socio-economic status, and ability among other traits. Bioinequalities suggest material harms tied to systemic injustices that inhere in bodies that occupy those systems both now and in the future. By taking account of the growing literature suggesting that trauma associated with unequal treatment affects us materially in our molecular biology and may be transmitted intergenerationally, it can be argued that a legal response that provides only an individual remedy to an individual incident of harm is insufficient. Instead, what is needed are positive legal obligations to protect communities (and in particular disadvantaged communities) from harmful bioinequalities that are shared among them both intra-generationally and intergenerationally.

Harmful environments in the workplace, in public spaces, in educational institutions, and in private corporations currently operate within a cultural milieu that upholds certain hierarchies of power and subordination that favour some individuals over others. Treating harms as environmental anomalies only, and not pervasive, entrenches bioinequalities by masking the way environments are reflections of cultural values and standards of oppression. It fails to identify the cultural framework of inequality that informs law and infiltrates legal processes and systems rendering the harms invisible to normative (dominant group) legal thinking.

Currently, where law provides redress, it tends to do so on the basis that the incident is resolved once the finding is made. The possibility that the harm continues materially and internally is not addressed I have argued throughout this chapter that DOHaD's version of an interconnected and entangled human provides a unique counter to the reductive individualised notion of legal subjectivity that currently pervades common law systems. Legal thinkers must address the claim that the psychosocial harms of systemic oppression cause harmful epigenetic changes in individuals and their progeny (both gestating and not yet conceived), creating intergenerationally harmed communities. Only by doing so can we craft real protective legal action that acknowledges that people are not just harmed as individuals but are always situated inside an epigenetic logic of relational, vulnerable, and continuous entanglement with others.

References

1. Sen A, Heredia N, Senut MC, Land S, Hollocher K, Lu X, et al. Multigenerational epigenetic inheritance in humans: DNA methylation changes associated with maternal exposure to lead can be transmitted to the grandchildren. Sci Rep 2015; 5(1): 14466–75.

2. Blaze J, Roth TL. Evidence from clinical and animal model studies of the long-term and transgenerational impact of stress on DNA methylation. Semin Cell Dev Biol 2015; 43: 76–84.

3. Yehuda R, Lehrner A. Intergenerational transmission of trauma effects: Putative role of epigenetic mechanisms. World Psychiatry 2018; 17(3): 243–57.

4. Scorza P, Duarte CS, Hipwell AE, Posner J, Ortin A, Canino G, et al. Research review: Intergenerational transmission of disadvantage: Epigenetics and parents' childhoods as the first exposure. J Child Psychol Psychiatry 2019; 60(2): 119–32.

5. McCrory C, Fiorito G, Ni Cheallaigh C, Polidoro S, Karisola P, Alenius H, et al. How does socio-economic position (SEP) get biologically embedded? A comparison of allostatic load and the epigenetic clock (s). Psychoneuroendocrinology 2019; 104: 64–73.

6. Singh G, Morrison J, Hoy W. DOHaD in Indigenous populations: DOHaD, epigenetics, equity and race. J Dev Orig Health Dis 2019; 10(1): 63–4.

7. Volpe VV, Dawson DN, Laurent HK. Gender discrimination and women's HPA activation to psychosocial stress during the postnatal period. J Health Psychol 2022; **27**(2): 352–62.

8. Mansfield B. Race and the new epigenetic biopolitics of environmental health. BioSocieties 2012; **7**(4): 352–72.

9. Kuzawa CW, Sweet E. Epigenetics and the embodiment of race: Developmental origins of US racial disparities in cardiovascular health. Am J Hum Bio 2009; **21**(1): 2–15.

10. Radtke KM, Ruf M, Gunter HM, Dohrmann K, Schauer M, Meyer A, et al. Transgenerational impact of intimate partner violence on methylation in the promoter of the glucocorticoid receptor. Transl Psychiatry 2011; **1**(7): e21–6.

11. Karpin I. Vulnerability and the intergenerational transmission of psychosocial harm. Emory LJ 2018; **67**(6): 1115–34.

12. Day J, Savani S, Krempley BD, Nguyen M, Kitlinska JB. Influence of paternal preconception exposures on their offspring: Through epigenetics to phenotype. Am J Stem Cells 2016; **5**(1): 11–8.

13. Hehar H, Ma I, Mychasiuk R. Intergenerational transmission of paternal epigenetic marks: Mechanisms influencing susceptibility to post-concussion symptomology in a rodent model. Sci Rep 2017; **7**(1): 7171–84.

14. Hutchison A. The Whanganui River as a legal person. Alternative Law Journal 2014; **39**(3): 179–82.

15. Rowlands M. Can Animals Be Persons? New York: Oxford University Press, 2019.

16. Garland-Thomson R, Reynolds JM. Rethinking fetal personhood in conceptualizing Roe. Am J Bioeth 2022; **22**(8): 64–8.

17. Assisted Reproductive Technology Act 2007 (NSW) s 3(b)(1).

18. National Health and Medical Research Council. Ethical Guidelines on the Use of Assisted Reproductive Technology in Clinical Practice and Research. Canberra: National Health and Medical Research Council, 2017.

19. Weiss EB. In Fairness to Future Generations: International Law, Common Patrimony, and Intergenerational Equity. New York: Transnational Publishers, 1989.

20. Eisen J, Mykitiuk R, Scott DN. Constituting bodies into the future: Toward a relational theory of intergenerational justice. UBC L Rev 2018; **51**(1): 1–54.

21. Greally JM. A user's guide to the ambiguous word 'epigenetics'. Nat Rev Mol Cell Biol 2018; **19**(4): 207–8.

22. Buss C, Davis EP, Muftuler LT, Head K, Sandman CA. High pregnancy anxiety during mid-gestation is associated with decreased gray matter density in 6–9-year-old children. Psychoneuroendocrinology 2010; **35** (1):141–53.

23. Ng SF, Lin RCY, Laybutt DR, Barres R, Owens JA, Morris MJ. Chronic high-fat diet in fathers programs β-cell dysfunction in female rat offspring. Nature 2010; **467**(7318): 963–6.

24. Weder N, Zhang H, Jensen K, Yang BZ, Simen A, Jackowski A, et al. Child abuse, depression, and methylation in genes involved with stress, neural plasticity, and brain circuitry. J Am Acad Child Adolesc Psychiatry 2014; **53**(4):417–24.e5.

25. Karpin I, O'Connell K. The challenge of bioinequality: Addressing the health impact of unequal treatment on gendered bodies through law. Special Issue Med Law Rev. 2022. fwac035. https://doi.org/ 10.1093/medlaw/fwac035

26. Krieger N. Measures of racism, sexism, heterosexism, and gender binarism for health equity research: From structural injustice to embodied harm – An ecosocial analysis. Annu Rev Public Health 2020; **41**: 37–62.

27. Karpin IA. Taking care of the health of the preconceived embryos or constructing legal harm. In: Nisker J, Baylis F, Karpin I, McLeod C, Mykitiuk R, eds. The

'Healthy' Embryo: Social, Biomedical, Legal and Philosophical Perspectives. Cambridge: Cambridge University Press. 2009; 136–50.

28. *NSW Greyhound Racing Rules 2022* (NSW) r 150(1)(e)

29. Doci F, Venney C, Spencer C, Diemer K. Epigenetics and law: The quest for justice. In: Crawford M, ed. Epigenetics in Society. Windsor: Emerging Scholars' Press. 2015; 257–77.

30. *Thirteen Children and Young Persons in the Kimberley Region; Inquest into the Deaths of 13 Children and Young Persons in the Kimberley Region* (Ref No: 25/2017) [2019] WACorC 5 (7 February 2019).

31. Warin M, Kowal E, Meloni M. Indigenous knowledge in a postgenomic landscape: The politics of epigenetic hope and reparation in Australia. Sci Technol Human Values 2019; 45: 87.

32. *Hauraki v Steinhoff Asia Pacific Limited trading as Freedom Furniture* [2021] ACTSC 54.

33. Rothstein MA, Harrell HL, Marchant GE. Transgenerational epigenetics and environmental justice. Environ Epigenet 2017; 3(3): 1–12.

34. Scott DN, Haw J, Lee R. 'Wannabe toxic-free?' From precautionary consumption to corporeal citizenship. Env Polit 2017; 26(2): 322–42.

35. Fox D. Causation and compensation for intergenerational harm. Chi-Kent L Rev 2022; 96(1): 129–44.

36. CDC preconception guidelines. Centre for Disease Control and Prevention. Recommendations to improve preconception health and health care – United States: A report of the CDC/ATSDR Preconception Care Work Group and the Select Panel on Preconception Care. Atlanta (GA): MMWR (US); 2006 Apr 21. 23 p. Report No.: RR-6.

37. Roberts AL, Lyall K, Rich-Edwards JW, Ascherio A, Weisskopf MG. Association of maternal exposure to childhood abuse with elevated risk for autism in offspring. JAMA Psychiatry 2013; 70(5): 508–15.

38. Slykerman RF, Thompson J, Waldie K, Murphy R, Wall C, Mitchell EA. Maternal stress during pregnancy is associated with moderate to severe depression in 11-year-old children. Acta Paediatrica 2015; 104 (1): 68–74.

39. Cao-Lei L, Laplante DP, King S. Prenatal maternal stress and epigenetics: Review of the human research. Curr Mol Bio Rep 2016; 2: 16–25.

40. Richardson SS. Maternal bodies in the postgenomic order: Gender and the explanatory landscape of epigenetics. In: Richardson SS, Stevens H, eds. Postgenomics: Perspectives on Biology after the Genome. Durham, NC: Duke University Press. 2015; 210–31.

41. Warin M, et al., Mothers as smoking guns: Fetal overnutrition and the reproduction of obesity, 361. Fem Psychol, 2012: 22(3): 360.

42. Khazan O. The second assault. *The Atlantic* [Internet]. December 16, 2015. www.theatlantic.com/health/archive/2015/12/sexual-abuse-victims-obesity/420186/ accessed 28/08/2022.

43. Zivkovic T, Warin M, Davies M, Moore V. In the name of the child: The gendered politics of childhood obesity. J Sociol 2010; 46(4): 375–92.

44. Mahoney A. How failure to protect laws punish the vulnerable. Health Matrix 2019; 29: 429–62.

45. Loi M, Del Savio L, Stupka E. Social epigenetics and equality of opportunity. Public Health Ethics 2013; 6(2): 142–53.

46. Dupras C, Beauchamp E, Joly Y. Selling direct-to-consumer epigenetic tests: Are we ready? Nat Rev Genet 2020; 21: 335–6.

47. Kumar R, Eftekhari P, Gould GS. Pregnant women who smoke may be at greater risk of adverse effects from bushfires. Int J Environ Res Public Health 2021; 18(12): 6223–6.

48. Robertson A. Risk, biotechnology and political rationality: Lessons from women's accounts of breast cancer risks. In: Mykitiuk R, Miller F, Weir L, eds. The Gender of Genetic Futures: The Canadian Biotechnology Strategy, Women and

Health. Proceedings of the National Strategic Workshop on Women and the New Genetics. 2000 Nov 2; Toronto: NNEWH Working Paper Series, 2000; 64–75.

49. Nedelsky J. Law's Relations: A Relational Theory of Self, Autonomy, and Law. New York: Oxford University Press, 2011.

50. Fineman MA. Introduction. In: Fineman MA, Mattsson T, Andersson U, eds. Privatization, Vulnerability, and Social Responsibility: A Comparative Perspective. New York: Taylor & Francis. 2016; 1–7.

51. Garland-Thomson R. Feminist disability studies. Signs 2005; 30(2): 1557–87

Lifecourse

Mark Tomlinson, Amelia van der Merwe, Marguerite Marlow, and Sarah Skeen

10.1 Introduction

Lifecourse theory was developed in the last 50 years, combining neurobiology, child psychology, developmental psychopathology, sociology, population sciences, and increasingly genetics [1]. Up to the latter part of the twentieth century, the focus was largely on the treatment of infectious diseases, acute illness, and injury within single-cause, simple biomedical models [2]. This was followed by a growing awareness of the roles of social and behavioural influences on illness, and revised bio-psychosocial models were developed that focused on managing chronic diseases over time and shifting unhealthy lifestyle choices [2]. However, health and social services continued to largely function separately, and the integration of physical and psychological health programmes was limited [2].

Lifecourse models take into account the influences of multiple risk and protective factors, operating across health trajectories or pathways throughout the lifespan and across generations [2]. The principles of lifecourse theory include: human agency in the construction of lives, timing (the developmental consequences of life transitions or events, which depend on when they take place in an individual's life), linked or interdependent lives (social and historical impacts are expressed through shared relationships), and human lives in historical time and place [3]. Developmental psychology contributed to the concepts of life stages and turning points, while sociology added the contributions of history, social conditions, and adaptation [1]. Genetics has contributed numerous concepts such as differential susceptibility [4]. A proliferation of research conducted during the early twenty-first century, including a large number of longitudinal studies that monitored continuity and change across the lifecourse, has prompted new ways of thinking about developmental trajectories and entrenched the lifecourse perspective in developmental research [1].

The lifecourse perspective overlaps with a number of theoretical traditions, including sociocultural perspectives that emphasise the social meaning of age and developmental stages, such as the socially defined, age-graded meanings associated with the biological facts of birth, puberty, or death, for example [5]. The concept of the lifecourse can also be historically linked to particular social transitions and to the meanings associated with a specific cohort [5]. Lifecourse theory incorporates some of the principles of interactionist thinking, particularly its emphasis on the interactions between the person and context, and the organisation and shifts in the organisation of social structures and pathways through the lifecourse [5]. Lifecourse theory is also based on Bronfenbrenner's concepts of the ecology of human development, including multi-level influences from the environment, extending from micro- to macro-level influences. The individual lifecourse furthermore shares conceptual premises with developmental science with its focus on developmental trajectories and the dynamic interactions between events and processes that occur across time frames in multiple contexts [5].

Previously, studies focusing on continuity and change from childhood and adulthood tended to include only correlational and regression analyses of patterns between measures of outcomes at two time points, typically childhood and adulthood [5]. There was very little exploration of what happened in between and what the mechanisms of change and continuity were. Furthermore, there was limited awareness of individuals as agents of change in their lives [5]. The lifecourse focus brought this into sharp relief and replaced child-based, growth-oriented (ontogenic) explanations of development with theories that account for development and ageing over the lifecourse. This focus emphasised how human lives are organised over time, including patterns of continuity and change, which focus on the developmental effects of social change and transitions [5]. In this chapter, we explore the issues of continuity and change across the lifecourse, developmental trajectories, and a lifecourse theory to investigate how exposures and experiences influence different individuals in different ways, with some more vulnerable or susceptible to risk than others, resulting in significant variability in developmental outcomes.

10.2 Lifecourse Approach to Health

Modern healthcare systems need to synthesise prevention, treatment, and health promotion and set in motion more integrated and networked strategies for designing and implementing multi-level interventions that move beyond the individual to include populations [2]. The lifecourse development perspective shifts our understanding from simple, linear, mechanistic, and reductionist models to models that acknowledge that the development of health is complex, interactive, holistic, and adaptive [2]. It also shifts our focus to inclusive explanations about the developmental origins of health, how stress influences current and future health, and the outcomes associated with dynamic interactions between individuals and their multiple environments across time [6]. Lifecourse perspectives provide a conceptual bridge between constructs that have until recently been assumed to be opposites, such as nature and nurture, mind and body, individual and population, and short-term and long-term change [2].

The lifecourse perspective incorporates pathways, which are constructed by the choices and actions that form individual lifecourses, and their developmental implications and consequences, including potential resources and constraints [5]. Rutter and colleagues argue that pathways involve dependent sequences, to include an exposure/experience at one point in the lifecourse, how it affects the likelihood of others occurring later in the lifecourse, and how this in turn influences health and developmental outcomes, including chains of risk [7]. A number of concepts are relevant to pathways, such as latency, which refers to the association between an exposure or experience at one point in the lifecourse and the related developmental outcome years or decades later, despite the presence of intervening exposure or experience [7]. Cumulative risk is another relevant concept that describes multiple exposures, either to a recurrent single factor or sequential exposures to different factors over the lifecourse, which combine to influence development [7]. These factors relate reciprocally, so that children with multiple exposures (to, for example, low socio-economic status [SES], poor parenting style, and residential instability) are likely to have more difficult trajectories than those exposed to single-risk factors [7]. These constructs tend to coexist in the real world. In fact, research conducted by Hertzman and colleagues in 2001 has demonstrated a strong relationship between latency, pathways, and cumulative factors in childhood and self-rated health at age 33 [7]. The current extensive focus on adverse child experiences (ACEs, see also chapter Kenny and Müller) [8] is the next logical step building on the work of Sameroff [9] and Hertzman [7].

Social interactions that are sustained by their consequences (cumulative) and behavioural styles that tend to evoke maintaining reactions from the environment (reciprocal) lead to behavioural continuities across the lifecourse [5]. Thus, both cumulative continuity and reciprocal continuity result in the cumulation of experiences that maintain and further the same behavioural outcome [5]. Conversely, transitional experiences disrupt continuity through individual agency, dispositions, situational constraints and opportunities, and previous experiences that accompany individuals to new situations [5]. This can bring about a significant change in behavioural trajectories and constitute a turning point [5].

10.3 Developmental Origins of Health and Disease (DOHaD)

Research focusing on the Developmental Origins of Health and Disease (DOHaD) began to emerge in the 1970s [10]. Subsequently, researchers began to integrate the new 'fetal origins', and later DOHaD, research outcomes, with results from lifecourse sociology and psychology to create newer lifecourse models of health and disease [2]. The theories on which these models draw, such as evolutionary life-history theory, propose that development during fetal life is designed to prepare the infant for a particular external environment, and so, when conditions in utero match the conditions in infancy, development occurs along pathways originating in utero [11]. However, when a mismatch occurs between the intrauterine and postnatal environments, certain dimensions of development may be compromised, or disadvantaged; for example, when intrauterine undernutrition is followed by an oversupply of nutrients postnatally, it poses risks for metabolic health [11].

The centrality of maternal and child healthcare in DOHaD focuses research and intervention on health trajectories that can improve child health outcomes, as well as health development across the lifespan, and possibly even into subsequent generations [2]. There is substantial research evidence for the notion that maternal physiology, body composition, diet, and lifestyle during pregnancy significantly influence the health of the infant throughout their life, including the presence of cardiovascular and metabolic illnesses (such as hypertension, obesity, and type 2 diabetes), atopic conditions, cancer, and neurological impairment [12].

10.3.1 Biological Embedding and Differential Susceptibility

DOHaD research, framed by a lifecourse perspective, can account for how both ordinary and extraordinary experiences may 'get under the skin' by altering biological functions during developmental windows of opportunity, which can ultimately shift lifecourse trajectories and influence intergenerational health patterns [7]. There are four systems that have the features of biological embedding: the HPA axis and the associated secretion of cortisol; the autonomic nervous system and its relation to epinephrine and norepinephrine; the development of the prefrontal cortex (including memory, attention, etc.); the primitive amygdala and locus coeruleus, and associated higher order cerebral connections, mediated by serotonin and other important hormones that are involved in systems of social affiliation [7]. For example, poor nurturance, through the mediation of gene expression, may lead to a disturbed HPA axis, impaired capacity for complex learning, and high age-related declines in learning and memory capacity [7].

Chronic stresses cause wear and tear on the HPA axis, which leads to dysregulation. This, in turn, may result in either hypo- or hypersecretion of cortisol with lifelong implications for health [13, 14]. It is also clear that it isn't either genes or the environment, or even genes and the environment, but gene-by-environment interactions that affect developmental trajectories [7]. Epigenetic processes – for example, DNA methylation – have been identified as important processes through which early environmental signals are altered into conditionally adaptive shifts in key functions in metabolic, endocrine, and neuroregulatory pathways [7, 15]. These changes produce systematic developmental biases towards more adaptive functioning in terms of growth, metabolism, immune responsivity, developmental pace, and behaviour, although changes are not uniformly protective [7]. Epigenetic changes, which occur in response to environmental cues, also play a role in the development of psychopathology and chronic medical conditions [7].

Exposures and experiences affect individuals differently, and there is significant variability in developmental outcomes. Approximately 15 per cent of children may be more biologically reactive to their immediate social environment than other children [7]. The effect of this on pathological outcomes is bivalent, as it can be protective or risk-enhancing depending on context [7]. This has been described as differential susceptibility, which refers to the risk-enhancing or risk-abating character of the social contexts children inhabit [16]. Experimental studies have shown that the majority of children with low autonomic reactivity have only slightly more symptoms in families with high family conflict, while the high-reactivity children display a combination of significantly more symptoms in high-conflict families but markedly fewer symptoms than peers in families with low levels of conflict [16]. As a result the 15–20 per cent of study children with the highest levels of reactivity either demonstrated the worst outcomes or the best outcomes, as a function of the level of conflict in their families [17]. It has been argued that more reactive children were more sensitive to both positive and negative social influences, while children who were low in reactivity were able to function adequately in a variety of contexts [18, 19]. Boyce and Ellis (2005) outline the following principles:

A. Exposure to high-stress childhood environments enhances biological sensitivity to context and increases the child's capacity to identify and respond to environmental threats;

B. Exposure to particularly supportive childhood environments also enhances biological sensitivity to context and increases receptiveness to social supports and resources; and

C. The majority of children are not exposed to environments that are either very stressful or very supportive, which reduces biological sensitivity to context and protects them against stressors [20].

Differential susceptibility is a useful concept to bear in mind when attempting to account for why environmental and intervention effects have been shown to be both variable and typically modest in published studies [21]. This is possibly a function of samples including both more and less susceptible individuals, which renders the average effect across all participants an invalid index of intervention effectiveness [16]. For example, distinguishing between short-allele and long-allele carriers was significant in determining the effectiveness of a maternal–infant attachment intervention. Specifically, for infants with one or two copies of the short allele of 5HTTLPR, the intervention improved attachment quality dramatically and significantly, while for those with only the long allele, the intervention produced no significant changes [4]. Differential susceptibility demonstrates in this way that averaging across all participants does not produce meaningful results [4]. Adverse social conditions such as socio-economic disadvantage increase the risk for various and multiple types of pathology by producing a generalised susceptibility [7]. Typically, social adversities include feedback loops that result in one stressful or traumatic event following another, resulting in extremely negative social contexts [22].

Although preconception and intrauterine experience have demonstrated marked effects on later health outcomes, there is a huge body of research that shows that childhood is a critical period for preventive and intervention efforts [16, 23]. Neurobiological susceptibility is not categorical and should be viewed as occurring on a continuum [16]. It is also important to bear in mind that less susceptible individuals may benefit from more intense intervention efforts to obtain results similar to those who are more susceptible [16]. Furthermore, less susceptible individuals may not always stay that way, and individuals may be more or less susceptible in different stages across the lifespan [16]. For this reason, and because equity matters as much as intervention efficacy, certain groups should not be excluded from supportive services [16]. This is in addition to population-level interventions advocated by the lifecourse health perspective to prevent poor developmental outcomes, such as folic acid supplementation during pregnancy. One cross-cutting risk factor that results in a generalised susceptibility or vulnerability to risk which is broadly pathogenic and presents a host of challenges occurring at multiple ecological levels, is socio-economic disadvantage (SED).

10.3.2 A Cross-Cutting Theme: Socio-economic Disadvantage and Exposure to Adverse Childhood Events

Socio-economic disadvantage early in life has repeatedly and robustly been shown to influence health outcomes across the lifespan, even when considering later SES. Socio-economic disadvantage in infancy is associated with higher infant mortality and adverse birth outcomes [24]. In both childhood and adolescence, SED has been linked to an increased risk for asthma, dental problems, and physical inactivity [24]. In terms of psychological health outcomes, a range of researchers have shown that SED is linked to poor language, cognitive deficits, and behavioural difficulties during childhood and higher rates of substance abuse, disruptive behaviours, and depression in adolescents [24].

Heightened stress levels appear to be the most important mediating mechanism underlying the influence of socio-economic disadvantage on health development [24]. Childhood socio-economic disadvantage is linked to greater exposure to stressors, including harsh parenting, exposure to violence, separation from parents, lower school quality, negative peer relations, substandard housing, pollutants, noise, and crowding [24]. Meijer and colleagues have also demonstrated that neighbourhood deprivation poses risks, including a lack of access to physical and cultural resources such as fresh fruits and vegetables, open space and other recreational amenities, libraries, and transportation, in addition to higher levels of exposure to violence and crime [25]. Those who have been exposed to SED are significantly more likely to encounter multiple, chronic, and severe stressors, which over time disables individuals' capacity to cope [24].

Exposure to ACEs such as those associated with socio-economic disadvantage is robustly associated with a range of childhood outcomes, including impaired physical growth and cognitive development, higher risks for childhood obesity, asthma, infections, non-febrile illnesses, disordered sleep, delayed menarche, and non-specific somatic complaints [26]. Although these health conditions vary according to ACE characteristics, age of occurrence, and specific types of exposures, it is clear that the more ACEs the child is exposed to, the more likely she or he will have complex health problems, with multiple needs across developmental, physical, and mental health domains [26]. Among ACEs, caregiver mental health is particularly important in terms of child health outcomes and is especially important for children aged under 5 years [26]. Retrospective studies have shown that ACEs also increase the risk of chronic non-communicable diseases, substance abuse, sexual risk-taking behaviours, suicide, domestic violence, and impaired physical and mental health, which may lead to the transfer of ACEs to the next generation [26].

Chronic exposure to cumulative risk factors linked to socio-economic disadvantage 'gets under the skin', by leading to dysfunction in the brain and associated physiological systems, and these dysfunctions impact the likelihood of physical and psychological illnesses [24]. Neurobiological mechanisms of stress emphasise three areas of the brain that are involved in stress perception, appraisal, and regulation, namely, the amygdala, hippocampus, and medial prefrontal cortex [27]. Ulrich-Lai and Herman argue that the purpose of these areas of the brain is to regulate the physiological stress systems, especially the hypothalamus-pituitary-adrenal axis and autonomic nervous system [27]. Chronic exposure to adversity exceeds the neuroendocrine system's ability to maintain homeostasis and, particularly during life stages associated with greater neuroplasticity (from pregnancy to early childhood), influences important components of brain development involved in cognition, self-regulation, and physical and mental health [26]. As we have noted, chronic exposure to stressors can result in hyper- or hypo-responsivity of the HPA axis, which represents impaired adaptation and results in a higher likelihood of eventual exhaustion. Lopez and colleagues cite a multitude of studies that show that HPA-axis dysregulation has far-reaching effects on young children and may manifest as both internalising and externalising behaviours [26].

The allostatic load model is important in this regard, as it suggests that exposure to chronic stress may result in wear and tear in primary stress regulatory systems (the hypothalamus-pituitary-adrenal axis and autonomic nervous system) and, consequently, in secondary physiological stress systems (metabolic processes, inflammatory and immune responses, and cardiovascular responses), which may lead to long-term damage and impairment [24]. Dysregulation of these physiological systems, which is understood in terms of allostatic load, is a strong indicator of health development outcomes in adulthood, including cardiovascular disease, diabetes, as well as cognitive impairment and premature mortality [24].

10.4 Limitations and Future Directions

Although there have been major strides in lifecourse health research, there continue to be significant gaps and limitations in the available research, particularly in terms of translation to policy and practice [6, 28]. Much of the research on the early biological origins of later health outcomes is based on animal studies, there are few longitudinal studies on preconception and pregnancy, and three-generational data are limited [6]. In addition, most lifecourse and developmental research is based on studies that have not been designed for this specific purpose [6, 28]. Banati (2018) argues, in reference to the cross-sectional measurement of the Sustainable Development Goals, that longitudinal data add depth and complexity in understanding the lifecourse and provide answers to 'why', which is crucial to the nature and timing of interventions [1]. A number of important lifecourse constructs – such as stress, weathering, and allostatic load – are not consistently defined or measured, and we lack knowledge of how these constructs could be best operationalised across different life stages, such as childhood and adolescence [29].

In spite of progress, much of the available research still uses reductionist statistical approaches that focus on isolating causal variables [6, 28]. More sophisticated statistical methods, such as longitudinal growth models to explore health trajectories, and multi-level modelling to better understand contextual contributors to health status, as well as decomposition methods to determine the influence of multiple risk and protective factors at different life stages on future health outcomes are necessary [6, 28]. New methods of analysis based on dynamic systems approaches are more suited to the complexity of the lifecourse health framework, but these have been limited in their application to understanding the roots of health disparities [6, 28]. Dynamic systems methods differ from correlational and regression approaches and include a number of computational approaches that can be applied to model dynamic and shifting interactions between individuals and their multiple environments, as well as complex processes such as feedback loops and non-linear relations [6, 28].

Despite the focus of lifecourse health research on structural and upstream policy and community-level factors influencing health status disparities, most research continues to examine downstream determinants, for example, health behaviours and healthcare [6, 28]. There is still limited knowledge of how complex processes resulting from dynamic interactions between biological, environmental, social, and behavioural factors over time produce disparities in population health [6]. Many debates are unresolved, such as the relative importance of early vs. later exposures and the timing and plasticity of sensitive periods in development [6, 28].

The lifecourse health framework offers a foundation for more integrated, preventative, and developmentally prepared health systems that are developed around the central notion of advancing health and health-promoting environments across the lifespan and across generations [6, 28]. Cross-disciplinary knowledge can only be generated when there is an integration of lifecourse research, greater cooperation, and more collaboration and synthesis of disciplines [6, 28] to allow the development of a common set of principles that promote resilience under stress [30]. This requires integrated, transdisciplinary funding opportunities and research agendas [31].

A lifecourse perspective is relevant to all dimensions of health but is most relevant to health equity [32]. A lifecourse perspective allows us to examine and understand how health disparities develop, are amplified or mitigated, as well as reproduced across generations, which may allow us to intervene more effectively [32]. Specifically, this perspective helps us understand how social risks and opportunities create vulnerability or resilience at each life stage, and how they accumulate, or are reduced across lives and generations [32]. The lifecourse perspective highlights stark disparities – children from relatively more wealthy contexts have benefitted the most, while there has been a limited impact on the poorest, who continue to need more resources and safety nets to mitigate the effects of the multiple vulnerabilities they face [1].

In this chapter, we have drawn attention to how socio-economic disadvantage contributes to pathology across the lifecourse and beyond. The findings have far-reaching implications for policymakers and interventionists. In the spirit of equity, the lifecourse perspective and DOHaD theory suggest that early, population-level intervention (at critical or sensitive periods) may prevent the consequences of exposure to socio-economic disadvantage and all its associated risks. In addition, and perhaps in combination with population-level interventions, the concept of differential susceptibility suggests the importance of identifying risk indicators that render some more vulnerable than others and the urgency of conducting more research on the factors that influence responsivity to interventions. Identifying indicators that point to both additional risk or vulnerability and heightened responsivity to intervention will allow for the more efficient implementation of targeted services. This approach may be our best chance at addressing the probability of socio-economically linked disease outcomes and its repercussions, which are likely to be felt across multiple lifetimes.

References

1. Banati P. Bringing life course theory to the sustainable development goals. In: Verma S, Petersen A, editors. Developmental Science and Sustainable Development Goals for Children and Youth. Cham, Switzerland: Springer International Publishing; 2018. pp. 313–328.

2. Halfon N, Larson K, Lu M, Tullis E, Russ S. Lifecourse health development: Past, present and future. Matern Child Health J. 2014;18(2):344–65.

3. Elder GH. The life course as developmental theory. Child Dev. 1998;69 (1):1–12.

4. Morgan B, Kumsta R, Fearon P, Moser D, Skeen S, Cooper P, et al. Serotonin transporter gene (SLC6A4) polymorphism and susceptibility to a home-visiting maternal-infant attachment intervention delivered by community health workers in South Africa: Reanalysis of a randomized controlled trial. PLoS Med. 2017;14(2): e1002237.

5. Elder GH, Shanahan MJ. Handbook of Child Psychology. Lerner RM, editor. New Jersey: John Wiley & Sons; 2006.

6. Halfon N, Forrest CB, Lerner RM, Faustman EM, Tullis E, Son J. Introduction to the Handbook of Life Course Health Development. In: Christopher B. Forrest, Neal Halfon, and Richard M. Lerner, editors. Handbook of Life Course Health Development. Cham, Switzerland: Springer; 2018. pp. 1–18.

7. Hertzman C, Boyce T. How experience gets under the skin to create gradients in developmental health. Annu Rev Public Health. 2010;31:329–47

8. Hughes K, Bellis MA, Hardcastle KA, Sethi D, Butchart A, Mikton C, et al. The effect of multiple adverse childhood experiences on health: A systematic review and meta-analysis. Lancet Public Health. 2017;2(8):e356–e66.

9. Sameroff A. A unified theory of development: A dialectic integration of nature and nurture. Child Dev. 2010;81 (1):6–22.

10. Barker DJP. The origins of the developmental origins theory. J Intern Med. 2007;261(5):412–7.

11. Salsberry P, Tanda R, Anderson SE, Kamboj MK. Pediatric Type-2 Diabetes: Prevention and Treatment Through a Life Course Health Development Framework. In: Christopher B. Forrest, Neal Halfon, and Richard M. Lerner, editors. Handbook of Life Course Health Development. Cham, Switzerland: Springer; 2018. pp. 197–236.

12. Fleming TP, Watkins AJ, Velazquez MA, Mathers JC, Prentice AM, Stephenson J, et al. Origins of lifetime health around the time of conception: Causes and consequences. Lancet. 2018;391 (10132):1842–52.

13. McEwen BS. Protective and damaging effects of stress mediators. N Engl J Med. 1998;338(3):171–9.

14. McEwen BS. Effects of adverse experiences for brain structure and function. Biol Psychiatry. 2000;48 (8):721–31.

15. de Kloet ER, Fitzsimons CP, Datson NA, Meijer OC, Vreugdenhil E. Glucocorticoid signaling and stress-related limbic susceptibility pathway: About receptors, transcription machinery and microRNA. Brain Res. 2009;1293:129–41.

16. Ellis BJ, Boyce WT, Belsky J, Bakermans-Kranenburg MJ, van Ijzendoorn MH. Differential susceptibility to the environment: An evolutionary – Neurodevelopmental theory. Dev Psychopathol. 2011;23 (1):7–28.

17. Boyce WT. Epigenomic susceptibility to the social world: Plausible paths to a 'Newest Morbidity'. Acad Pediatr. 2017;17(6):600–6.

18. Boyce WT, Ellis BJ. Biological sensitivity to context: I. An evolutionary-developmental theory of the origins and

19. Boyce WT. The Orchid and the Dandelion: Why Sensitive People Struggle and How All Can Thrive. London: Pan MacMillan; 2019.

20. Boyce WT, Ellis BJ. Biological sensitivity to context: I. An evolutionary-developmental theory of the origins and functions of stress reactivity. Development and Psychopathology. 2005;17:271–301.

21. Ellis BJ, Boyce WT, Belsky J, Bakermans-Kranenburg MJ, Van IJzendoorn MH. Differential susceptibility to the environment: An evolutionary-neurodevelopmental theory. Development and Psychopathology. 2011;23(1):7–28.

22. Masten A, Cicchetti D. Developmental cascades. Dev Psychopathol. 2010;22 (3):491–5.

23. Patton GC, Olsson CA, Skirbekk V, Saffery R, Wlodek ME, Azzopardi PS, et al. Adolescence and the next generation. Nature. 2018;554 (7693):458–66.

24. Kim P, Evans GW, Chen E, Miller GE, Seeman T. How socioeconomic disadvantages get under the skin and into the brain to influence health development across the lifespan. In: Halfon N, Forrest CB, Lerner RM, Faustman EM, editors. Handbook of Life Course Health Development. Berlin: Springer; 2018. pp. 463–97.

25. Meijer M, Röhl J, Bloomfield K, Grittner U. Do neighborhoods affect individual mortality? A systematic review and meta-analysis of multilevel studies. Soc Sci Med. 2012;74:1204–12.

26. Lopez M, Ruiz MO, Rovnaghi CR, Tam GK, Hiscox J, Gotlib IH, et al. The social ecology of childhood and early life adversity. Pediatr Res. 2021;89(2):353–67.

27. Ulrich-Lai YM, Herman JP. Neural regulation of endocrine and autonomic stress responses. Nat Rev Neurosci. 2009;10(6):397–409.

28. Halfon N, Forrest CB, Lerner RM. Life Course Research Agenda (LCRA), Version 1.0. In: Halfon N. FC, Lerner R.,

Faustman E., editors. Handbook of Life Course Health Development. Cham, Switzerland: Springer; 2018. pp. 623–45.

29. Halfon N, Forrest CB. The emerging theoretical framework of life course health development. In: Halfon N, Forrest CB, Lerner RM, Faustman EM, editors. Handbook of Life Course Health-development Science. Berlin: Springer; 2017. pp. 19–43.

30. Ungar M. Systemic resilience: Principles and processes for a science of change in contexts of adversity. Ecol Soc. 2018;23(4).

31. Suleiman AB, Dahl RE. Leveraging neuroscience to inform adolescent health: The need for an innovative transdisciplinary developmental science of adolescence. J Adolesc Health. 2017;60 (3):240–8.

32. Braveman P. What is health equity: and how does a life-course approach take us further toward it? Matern Child Health J. 2014;18(2):366–72.

Chapter

11

Syndemics

Edna N. Bosire, Michelle Pentecost, and Emily Mendenhall

11.1 Introduction

Recognising how early experiences frame and impact later health is a central focus of DOHaD. However, rarely in DOHaD studies are the synergistic characteristics of diseases throughout the lifecourse a central focus. Syndemic theory can enhance our understanding of health over the lifecourse by integrating a more synergistic understanding of early stressors and long-term adverse health, often caused by the interactions of health and social conditions. Syndemic theory posits that disease concentrations (where diseases cluster together) and disease interactions (what adverse effects result from the clustering) cause more health adversity due to their synergistic dynamics. Moreover, because the clusters and interactions of health conditions share upstream drivers, designing interventions to mitigate one condition may have larger-scale impacts on health and well-being. In this way, syndemic theory can contribute meaningfully to DOHaD studies because it considers how and why diseases occur, cluster, and interact across the lifecourse. Further, DOHaD thinking is inherent to syndemic theory, which recognises how chronic stress and inflammation over the lifecourse can play central roles in the interaction and exacerbation of certain infectious and/or non-infectious health conditions. Recognising how and why health conditions cluster together, and what factors from early life through adolescence may have a major impact on adult multi-morbidities, can advance both DOHaD and syndemic thinking.

In this chapter, we consider how syndemic thinking can advance DOHaD scholarship by critically engaging with the synergistic underlying conditions of early life that profoundly affect health and disease in later life. In what follows, we describe the history of the syndemics framework and provide a few examples of how the framework has been used in other studies. We discuss the synergies of syndemic and DOHaD theory. We draw on our work with the 'Birth to Thirty' birth cohort based at the Developmental Pathways for Health Research Unit (DPHRU) at the University of the Witwatersrand to provide some examples of how social, psychological, and biological factors cluster and drive health and disease over a lifetime, and demonstrate how the syndemic framework may benefit DOHaD research.

11.2 History of Syndemic Theory

The term syndemics was first proposed by Merrill Singer [1] to demonstrate how socio-economic, political, or environmental factors influenced the frequently co-occurring problems of substance abuse, violence, and HIV. Singer and Clair [2] defined syndemics as a set of intertwined and mutually enhancing epidemics involving disease interactions at the biological level that develop and are sustained in a community/population because of harmful social conditions and injurious social connections. Singer argued that the *synergies* of epi*demics* are crucial for understanding what diseases emerge, where, and why. Specifically, syndemics theory focuses on disease concentration (the where) and disease interactions (the how) and provides a framework for understanding what drives disease clusters and for designing interventions that might mitigate these effects. Others have described syndemics by thinking about interactions of 'people, place, and time' and as a 'constellation of affliction' [3]. In many ways, the syndemics framework provides a clear way of thinking about disease: rarely does an individual or population experience a disease in isolation from other conditions – such as social, political, or historical contexts where people live.

Singer first proposed the SAVA Syndemic, showing how substance abuse, violence, and AIDS cannot be understood in isolation among inner-city residents of Hartford, Connecticut. Singer argued that the local HIV epidemic could not be dissociated from the local epidemic of substance abuse and that the pathways of transmission were inextricably linked and deepened by structural violence [1]. In this way, Singer emphasised that understanding local history and social context was fundamental for understanding the social life of an infectious disease. The SAVA syndemic framework is now widely used to develop interventions in the field of HIV/AIDS, while recognising that the interactions between and concentration of diseases have a history and may share an origin. This framing provides clear pathways for intervention, such as through integrating mental health and substance use interventions for the prevention of and living with HIV.

Three rules frame syndemic thinking [1, 2], and these rules are crucial for defining what comprises a syndemic and what does not [4]. First, two or more diseases concentrate within a population. In many cases, this relationship is well documented in the epidemiological literature, often cited as a comorbid or multi-morbid relationship. Second, disease interactions are measurable through bio-bio, bio-social, or bio-psychological pathways, which may include anything from well-documented interactions in biology (such as inflammation) to cultural dynamics (like stigma). Third, macro-scale forces precipitate disease clustering, framed by factors at the macro-level (such as structural violence) to meso-level (such as immigration or gender-based policy) and micro-level (such as interpersonal violence or chronic food insecurity). DOHaD takes a similarly integrative approach, recognising how early exposures to adversity and chronic stress, particularly in relation to nutrition, can profoundly shape disease risk later in life. It is this adversity and the diseases that emerge that often become syndemic; chronic stress and inflammation are closely linked to non-communicable diseases, and these conditions increase the risk for or compromise health when one confronts infections like HIV. It is these underlying conditions, and the weakening of immune function, that compromise one's ability to fight off or live well when multiple serious conditions concentrate together within individuals and communities. The elevated risk of morbidity and mortality among people with such conditions, who are socially and economically marginalised, was exemplified by the recent COVID-19 crisis.

Another example is the syndemic of violence, racist immigration policy, diabetes, depression, and abuse (verbal, emotional, physical, or sexual) among Mexican immigrant women living in the Chicago metropolitan area, as described by Emily Mendenhall [5]. In a mixed-methods study consisting of data collected through life history narrative interviews, biological specimens, and validated psychiatric instruments, Mendenhall describes how interpersonal violence and fear (bound to immigration policy) drove distress. These experiences linked stress and trauma from undocumented migration and navigating a racist immigration system to the deleterious effects of living with chronic illness (type 2 diabetes) amidst financial uncertainty. In this case, the adverse health effects of these larger forces, often obscured, could be observed in the epidemiological data demonstrating the close biological and psychological links between depression and type 2 diabetes [5, 6]. A central focus of this work was to describe how study participants, despite seeking care for diabetes or being identified by the state as having diabetes (e.g. via Medicaid), could not become well without psychological healing and overcoming structural barriers like a lack of safety and food [7]. In this way, their diabetes was entangled in a feedback loop with traumatic memories, family stress, chronic financial uncertainty, and untreated depression that required nuanced care and support from the clinic, their community, and their families [5].

These examples illustrate how syndemic co-factors build throughout a lifetime. DOHaD studies can emphasise at what time and in what ways interventions for one aspect of a syndemic may elevate overall health and well-being by lessening the interactions within and among syndemic problems [8] – in this way, syndemic and DOHaD theories are complementary and synergistic.

11.3 How Syndemics Thinking and DOHaD Studies Are Inherently Synergistic

Understanding the social and biological histories of people is as fundamental to the syndemic framework as it is for DOHaD studies. Histories of disease have long engaged with a 'disease biography' approach – where diseases are viewed as biological entities, overlooking how diseases become interconnected and co-occur through social and political processes [9, 10]. Thinking about the rise and decline of syndemics across time, as well as intergenerationally, provides an opportunity to recognise the fundamental role of contexts and driving forces that underlie how and why diseases interact within bodies and populations in a certain time and place. Studies central to driving DOHaD scholarship, such as of the 1944 Dutch Hunger Winter famines [11] and other famines such as in China and Nigeria [12, 13], can provide situational evidence for why and how socio-political contexts may have affected biological risk for disease later in life or across generations. DOHaD studies emphasise how experiences of deprivation can provoke multiple and overlapping chronic conditions later in life, but rarely do they emphasise how these synergistic interactions occur and why. In many ways, DOHaD studies are already thinking syndemically, but making these links clearer, with a focus on interactions that perpetuate disease experiences, can provide clearer modes for intervention [14]. Using syndemic theory in DOHaD research could push forward an understanding of the connectedness of synergistic conditions through time and across space. This allows for syndemics to be studied historically and may allow researchers to fundamentally understand current syndemics and anticipate future ones.

Another attractive aspect of syndemics framework is its broad applicability to conditions or diseases that commonly cluster together such as malnutrition, obesity, and diabetes; HIV and TB; and HIV and non-communicable diseases such as diabetes and mental health [15]. This provides a chance to develop interventions that respond to these diseases concurrently and in an integrative manner as opposed to dealing with individual diseases. Further, preventing syndemics requires not only prevention or control of each disease, respectively, but also understanding and controlling the forces that tie the diseases together. Insights gained from understanding syndemics (e.g. HIV syndemics research) can then be transferred and applied to other syndemics.

Syndemics often emphasise how deleterious social and political conditions such as poverty, food insecurity, inequalities, or political instabilities expose populations to disease clustering and interactions across the lifecourse [16]. These factors further shape disease burden, from immune responses to healthcare access. The reverse is also true; disease burden and limited access to healthcare may influence social and economic conditions or processes [17]. For DOHaD research, the syndemic framework may allow researchers to understand diseases holistically by examining how biological synergisms cluster and are worsened by social and structural forces. In other words, the syndemics framework may shed some light on inequalities in diseases and health and why some people suffer more than others within or outside the same geographical locations. For instance, although conditions like type 2 diabetes have been associated with old age [18], we know that insulin resistance can emerge and afflict younger people in part because economic pressures and intensified economic inequalities cause increasing stress, and viral and metabolic conditions are increasingly linked [19–22]. This may best be exemplified in countries such as South Africa that have experienced extraordinary social and political changes [23]. Metabolic disease appears to emerge at earlier ages in South Africa and makes people sicker faster compared to other developed countries [24, 25].

While DOHaD interventions often focus on child, maternal, and preconception health as influential for health across the lifecourse, a syndemic lens is useful to foreground the social or environmental challenges that interact in the early life period to influence well-being. For example, part of our collaborative work in South Africa under the Healthy Life Trajectory Initiative (HeLTI) has suggested that women suffer considerably because of long-term exposure to hardships, poverty, and intergenerational conflicts at home [26]. Women may also frequently parent alone, in part due to parental separations and the early departure of the father in the context of women giving birth before marriage [26]. Women with girl children, fearing for their daughters' futures, sometimes exert undue pressure on their children to achieve educational goals and find secure employment before marriage or childrearing, but this can lead to significant intergenerational tensions. Daughters express stress, anger, anxiety, depression, and suicidal ideations [26], which may affect the risk of early pregnancy [27]. Patriarchal culture plays a crucial role in girls' experiences, where a hierarchy of power and privilege that typically favours men over women, and boys over girls, affects access to food, school, jobs, emotional support, and other crucial aspects of well-being. This then reinforces a systemic inequality that undermines the rights of women and girls and restricts the opportunity for women, men, and gender minorities to express their authentic selves.

This example illustrates the complex social dynamics that affect young people's health, from ways of thinking about sexuality and power to financial security, emotional support, and conceptualisations of a healthy life and well-being. Social, psychological, and biological conditions emerge and interact in different ways throughout the lifecourse. By disentangling how conditions interact and perpetuate one other, clinical programmes can integrate mental and physical healthcare, and policymakers can also prioritise community-based interventions, given that, as we have found in Soweto, people engage in health-seeking far beyond the clinic and can improve their overall health and well-being by engaging in activities that may be religious or relational [28].

Moreover, syndemic theory can advance DOHaD studies as it highlights where, when, and how disease concentration or interaction is likely to occur across the lifecourse. For example, households that are exposed to violence (e.g. gender-based violence including intimate partner violence, child maltreatment, or early marriages) may have consequential impacts in later life. Studies have shown that children born in households that experience violence may have developmental delays first seen in infancy; anxiety and mood disorder symptoms and poor peer relationships first seen in childhood; substance use, abuse, or addiction or a diagnosis of substance use disorder often first seen in adolescence; and increased risk for personality and other psychiatric disorders and relationship problems during adulthood [29]. Other research shows that among people exposed to major psychological stressors in childhood, there are elevated rates of morbidity and mortality from chronic diseases of ageing [30]. Understanding such factors can enable the development of timely interventions to ensure that disease clustering does not happen.

In sum, syndemic thinking in DOHaD studies can illuminate how macro-scale factors such as structural violence, meso-level factors such as health policies, and micro-level factors such as intimate partner violence influence disease clustering and interactions and produce poor health outcomes.

11.4 Conclusion

Syndemic theory facilitates an understanding of the cumulative effects of social and environmental influences, and how these interact with other variables such as demographic, biological, genetic, and epigenetic factors across the lifecourse. The syndemic framework underscores a need to focus on social inequality as a root cause of syndemic clustering and interactions and demonstrates that population-level disease prevention can only occur by addressing the large-scale social and structural forces that shape both individual and population health. In addition, addressing harmful or injurious forces at family, community, and population levels can help reduce disease clustering or interactions now and later in life. In this sense, the syndemic framework can highlight 'hotspots' where there is a high likelihood of disease clustering now or in the future and provide an opportunity to intervene before the clustering and interaction take place. Finally, the syndemic framework provides an avenue for interdisciplinary research – as it focuses on multi-layered factors that shape disease distribution at the population level. Thus, integrating syndemics in DOHaD studies may enhance cross-disciplinary research. The framework also enables researchers to address one of the greatest barriers to health improvements: the failure to examine linked phenomena. Syndemic theory allows researchers to move beyond understanding the proximate causes of diseases and draws attention to the processes that create clusters of disease and noxious living conditions for particular populations, affected by a particular condition. It is therefore imperative for DOHaD to think syndemically to understand disease patterns across different time periods.

References

1. Singer M. A dose of drugs, a touch of violence, a case of AIDS: Conceptualizing the SAVA syndemic. Free Inq Creat Sociol. 1996;24(2):99–110.

2. Singer M, Clair S. Syndemics and public health: Reconceptualizing disease in bio-social context. Med Anthropol Q. 2003;17(4):423–441.

3. Milstein B. An introduction to the syndemics: Implications for health promotion. Syndemics prevention network, centers for disease control and prevention. (2006). Available from: www

.google.de/?gws_rd=ssl#q=Milstein +Introduction+to+syndemics

4. Tsai AC. Syndemics: A theory in search of data or data in search of a theory? Soc Sci Med. 2018;206:117–122.

5. Mendenhall E. Syndemic Suffering: Social Distress, Depression, and Diabetes among Mexican Immigrant Women. Routledge, New York; 2012.

6. Lynch EB, Fernandez A, Lighthouse N, Mendenhall E, Jacobs E. Concepts of diabetes self-management in Mexican American and African American low-income patients with diabetes. Health Educ Res. 2012;27(5):814–824.

7. Mendenhall E, Seligman RA, Fernandez A, Jacobs EA. Speaking through diabetes: Rethinking the significance of lay discourses on diabetes. Med Anthropol Q. 2010;24(2):220–239.

8. Soepnel LM, McKinley MC, Klingberg S, et al. Evaluation of a text messaging intervention to promote preconception micronutrient supplement use: Feasibility study nested in the healthy life trajectories initiative study in South Africa. JMIR Form Res. 2022;6(8):e37309.

9. Proctor DA. Testing the waters: Syndemic gastrointestinal distress in Lambaréné, Gabon, 1926–1932. Soc Sci Med. 2022;295:113405.

10. Newfield T. Syndemics and the history of disease: Towards a new engagement. Soc Sci Med. 2022;295:114454.

11. Roseboom T, de Rooij S, Painter R. The Dutch famine and its long-term consequences for adult health. Early Hum Dev. 2006;82(8):485–491.

12. Heijmans BT, Tobi EW, Stein AD, et al. Persistent epigenetic differences associated with prenatal exposure to famine in humans. Proc Natl Acad Sci USA. 2008;105(44):17046–17049.

13. Song S, Wang W, Hu P. Famine, death, and madness: Schizophrenia in early adulthood after prenatal exposure to the Chinese Great Leap Forward Famine. Soc Sci Med. 2009;68(7):1315–1321.

14. El Hajj N, Schneider E, Lehnen H, Haaf T. Epigenetics and life-long consequences of an adverse nutritional and diabetic intrauterine environment. Reproduction. 2014;148(6):R111–R120.

15. Mendenhall E. Rethinking Diabetes: Entanglements with Trauma, Poverty, and HIV. Cornell University Press, Ithaca, NY; 2019.

16. Manderson L, Ross FC. Publics, technologies and interventions in reproduction and early life in South Africa. Humanit Soc Sci Commun. 2020;7(1):40.

17. Douglas-Vail M. Syndemics theory and its applications to HIV/AIDS public-health interventions. Int J Med Sociol Anthropol. 2016;6(1):001–010.

18. Kalyani RR, Golden SH, Cefalu WT. Diabetes and aging: Unique considerations and goals of care. Diabetes Care. 2017;40(4):440–443.

19. Mendenhall E, Richter LM, Stein A, Norris SA. Psychological and physical co-morbidity among urban South African women. PLoS One. 2013;8(10):e78803.

20. Hardin J. Faith and the Pursuit of Health: Cardiometabolic Disorders in Samoa. Rutgers University Press, New Brunswick; 2019.

21. Gálvez A. Eating NAFTA: Trade, Food Policies, and the Destruction of Mexico. University of California Press, Berkeley; 2018.

22. Yates-Doerr E. The Weight of Obesity: Hunger and Global Health in Postwar Guatemala. University of California Press, Berkeley; 2015.

23. Moodley G, Christofides N, Norris SA, Achia T, Hofman KJ. Obesogenic environments: Access to and advertising of sugar-sweetened beverages in Soweto, South Africa, 2013. Prev Chronic Dis. 2015;12:E186.

24. Barnett K, Mercer SW, Norbury M, Watt G, Wyke S, Guthrie B. Epidemiology of multimorbidity and implications for health care, research, and medical

education: A cross-sectional study. Lancet. 2012;380(9836):37–43.

25. Gluckman PD, Hanson MA, Mitchell MD. Developmental origins of health and disease: Reducing the burden of chronic disease in the next generation. Genome Med. 2010;2(14):1–3.

26. Cohen E, Ware LJ, Prioreschi A, Draper C, Bosire E et al. Material and relational difficulties: The impact of the household environment on the emotional well-being of young Black women living in Soweto, South Africa. J Fam Issues. 2020; 41 (8):1307–1332

27. Bouvette-Turcot AA, Unternaehrer E, Gaudreau H, et al. The joint contribution of maternal history of early adversity and adulthood depression to socioeconomic status and potential relevance for offspring development. J Affect Disord. 2017;207:26–31.

28. Bosire EN, Cele L, Potelwa X, Cho A, Mendenhall E. God, Church water and spirituality: Perspectives on health and healing in Soweto, South Africa. Glob Public Health. 2022;17(7):1172–1185.

29. Norman RE, Byambaa M, De R, Butchart A, Scott J, Vos T. The long-term health consequences of child physical abuse, emotional abuse, and neglect: A systematic review and meta-analysis. PLoS Med. 2012;9(11):e1001349.

30. Miller GE, Chen E, Parker KJ. Psychological stress in childhood and susceptibility to the chronic diseases of aging: Moving toward a model of behavioral and biological mechanisms. Psychol Bull. 2011;137(6):959–997.

Chapter

12

Embodiment

Ziyanda Majombozi and Mutsawashe Mutendi

12.1 Introduction

Embodiment is an established concept within the fields of medical anthropology and other social sciences. It has been used as a way of thinking and writing about the body and bodily experiences that challenge dualistic assumptions about the mind and the body. This chapter explores the various ways in which the concept of embodiment has been used in the social sciences and health sciences research with a particular focus on the 'first 1000 days' and the Developmental Origins of Health and Disease (DOHaD). By drawing on case studies and ethnographic data, this chapter illustrates how the concept of embodiment can be used as a heuristic or analytical tool to challenge the way we understand the body – particularly the ailing body, the sick body, and the birthing body. We draw on examples that illustrate how the concept of embodiment has the potential to contribute to DOHaD research. Using the concept of embodiment as a tool within DOHaD research allows us to show the ways in which challenging social environments and stressors have long-term effects on health and biology [1].

12.2 What Is Embodiment?

According to Musolino et al. [2], the conceptual framing of embodiment came into social science writing as a critique of the highly contested theory of Cartesian dualism, which continues to be the dominant approach to understanding and treating the body in other disciplines. René Descartes's theory of dualism asserts that the mind and the body are separate entities that exist independently of one another and that could not exist in unity. Descartes believed that '...Mind was unextended, an immaterial but thinking substance and body was an extended, material but unthinking substance' [3]. This theory had implications for science and, of interest to this paper, the practice of medicine. In medicine, the body is often portrayed as a biological fact, an object, a collection of cells and tissue, a '... machine, void of mind or soul' [4]. This can mean that the mind and its significance in one's experiences of health and illness are not accounted for. However, since the 1970s, anthropologists and other social scientists have challenged Cartesian dualism and have suggested different ways to think about the body, one of which is the concept of embodiment.

While the concept of embodiment has been used differently within various disciplines, we will draw on three notions of embodiment that are of particular relevance to DOHaD: first, the political economy approach within critical medical anthropology [5]; second, the phenomenological approach conceptualised by Csordas [6]; and finally, the biosocial approach, drawing on Nancy Krieger's work [7]. Thus, the first part of the chapter is a survey of how embodiment has been theorised and used within the social sciences. In the second half of the chapter, we argue that DOHaD should embrace social science concepts as biosocial collaboration compels cross-disciplinary legibility and a shared vocabulary. We provide a discussion of why embodiment (conceptualised in the three ways we present) is a useful theoretical tool for DOHaD science. In doing so, we illustrate why it is important to integrate concepts/tools from social sciences, in this case embodiment, to deepen our awareness and understanding of the kind of influence environmental experiences can have on the development of health and disease over the lifecourse. We suggest that employing the embodiment concept can make DOHaD research and interventions more socially just and socially sensitive.

12.3 Approaches to Embodiment

The political economy approach to embodiment is best described by Nancy Scheper-Hughes and Margaret Lock. In their seminal essay, *The mindful body: A prolegomenon to future work in medical anthropology*, Nancy Scheper-Hughes and Margaret Lock [5] conceptualise the body as something that is 'simultaneously a physical and symbolic artifact, as both natural and culturally produced, and as securely anchored in a particular historical moment' [5]. They propose the idea of three bodies. Firstly, the 'individual body' represents one's personal experiences, perception, and consciousness of their body. Secondly, the 'social body' focuses on the messages that the body sends and how the body is perceived and analysed by others. Thirdly, the 'political body' focuses on the regulation, control, and surveillance of bodies. This way of thinking about the body challenges the view that the body is simply a biological fact. The idea of the three bodies not only challenges mind–body dualism but also opens up a new lens of analysis in which illness is not experienced solely in the mind or the body but is crucially shaped by social and political structures. This is best illustrated by their concluding words:

> What we have tried to show in these pages is the interaction among the mind/body and the individual, social and body politic in the production and expression of health and illness. Sickness is not just an isolated event, nor an unfortunate brush with nature. It is a form of communication – the language of organs – through which nature, society and culture speak simultaneously. The individual body should be seen as the most immediate, proximate terrain where social truths and contradictions are played out, as well as a locus of personal and social resistance, creativity, and struggle [5]

The phenomenological approach to embodiment conceptualised by Thomas Csordas has also been widely influential within anthropology and social sciences discourses. Csordas [6] proposed the idea of phenomenological embodiment to move away from discourses that frame the body as a passive subject. Instead, he advocates for a conceptual framework that captures human existence as relational, temporal, embodied, and situated [8]. Csordas [6] sees the body as 'a biological raw material' that 'inherits its culturality through the process of embodiment'. This approach has allowed scholars to illuminate how culture and history shape bodily experiences. Used in this way, the concept of embodiment provides us with useful tools for thinking about everyday taken-for-granted bodily practices, about how bodily knowledge is acquired, and about how, in turn, this acquisition accounts for the differences in how people hold and use their bodies (gestures or accents) [2, 9].

The biosocial approach to embodiment goes beyond 'considering' how culture and politics influence health and illness experiences to show the detrimental implications of not considering embodiment. A failure to consider embodiment can lead to deeply unjust experiences of health and illness as the social becomes biological. Scholars such as Nancy Krieger have described embodiment as 'a concept referring to how we literally incorporate, biologically, the material and social world in which we live, from conception to death; a corollary is that no aspect of our biology can be understood absent knowledge of history and individual and societal ways of living' [7]. Embodiment for epidemiology grapples with the implications of how global and local social, political, and economic structures shape people's lives and become embodied in individual sickness and suffering [10].

We now move onto three case studies that illustrate the usefulness of the above approaches to embodiment. It is important to note that we do not advocate for any one approach to embodiment; we see all the approaches we have surveyed here are equally useful. The case studies below show us an alternative to the DOHaD tendency to individu-alisation and blame that is often directed towards women for negative outcomes with regard to reproduction. For example, Manderson and Ross [11] suggest that DOHaD research and the interventions born from it tend to over-emphasise the maternal role in keeping the fetus safe and healthy. As a result, there is a tendency to focus interventions on women with the assumption that a woman's body is 'an incubator of population health, both in the immediate present and, according to current understandings of epigenetics, for two generations (at least) into the future' [11]. This has the unintended consequence of leaving other bodies such as those of men underexamined and puts the responsibility of the health and well-being of future generations solely on women, leading to the surveillance of particular bodies in order to control population health [11]. The following case studies provide insight into how the experience of pregnancy cannot be adequately grasped by focusing on the individual mother. Instead, they illustrate how an embodiment approach can better illuminate the environmental and structural conditions surrounding pregnancy.

12.4 Case Studies

Anthropologist Emily Yates-Doerr's [12] work in Guatemala effectively illustrates how health and illness are shaped by social and political structures. Yates-Doerr [12] provides an insightful multi-layered analysis using embodiment to trace the relations and material conditions that shape the worlds of mothers and their infants. In 2006, the Central American Free Trade Agreement came into effect. This resulted in Guatemalan markets importing an influx of US market foods, which included unhealthy and highly processed foods that were not a staple commodity prior to the implementation of the international trade agreement. Furthermore, the liberalisation of the Guatemalan food economy meant it became more expensive for the country to locally produce staple commodities, thus resulting in the proliferation of supermarkets that could mass import food into the country. Yates-Doerr [12] notes that the rising rates of diabetes, heart disease, hyperten-sion, and other illnesses associated with dietary practice within the country are in part due to the transformation of the region's food economy brought about by the inter-national trade agreements [12, 13]. Like Yates-Doerr, many other scholars have noted that the introduction of the Western diet, especially the emergence of highly processed foods in particular countries, corresponds to the rising rates of cardiovascular diseases and hypertension [14]. Thus, in the case of Guatemalan women, the high rates of obesity and diabetes in infants cannot be solely blamed on a mother's individual lifestyle choices. The political economy of Guatemala is embodied in the lives and bodies of women and their infants; in Rubin and Hines' words [15], political economy 'enters the body', transforming the bodies of women and their infants, and affects their health outcomes.

The second example we draw on is from Mutsawashe Mutendi's [16] work on maternal health among South African platinum mineworkers. Mutendi [16] shows how platinum mining makes mineworkers vulnerable to various occupational health-related problems, particularly reproductive health-related problems. The exposure to toxic chemicals while mining underground can potentially be harmful to the health of pregnant women and the health of the fetus. Her work shows how women opt to evade mining policies that stipulate that when a female mineworker discovers that she is pregnant, she should report her pregnancy to human resources so that an alternative and safer job can be found for her. Under such policies, if the number of pregnant women exceeds the number of available alternative jobs on the surface, the remaining pregnant mineworkers are sent home by the mining company until they give birth. In such cases, women will only be compensated for four months of maternity leave, as stipulated by the Basic Conditions of Employment Act (BCEA) of 1997, Section 25 [17]. Hence, pregnant mineworkers in this context opt to conceal their pregnancies and continue working underground despite the reproductive dangers that this potentially poses to the mineworkers, their fetuses, and subsequent generations. Mutendi highlights the complex political and economic realities and multiple forms of vulnerability faced by female mineworkers during pregnancy. These include how pregnancy, mining policies, the fear of being economically redundant, motherhood, exposure to toxins, and the in utero experience shape one another.

Some of the groundbreaking research conducted on the biosocial approach builds on Krieger's work on embodiment, to show how racial inequality can result in poor health outcomes for particular groups of people (see Meloni et al. in this volume). For instance, the work of neonatologists David and Collins [18] illustrates how racial oppression can be embodied and influence the health outcomes of infants. In *Disparities in infant mortality: what's genetics got to do with it?*, David and Collins explore the differences between infants of African American women and white women in the United States, with a particular focus on the disparities in low birth weight between the two racial groups. Their research shows that low birth weights of infants were not a result of genetic predisposition but rather the socio-economic and environmental influences that African-born women were exposed to, which changed their biology, putting them at a higher risk of birthing infants with low birth weight. Their research speaks to the ways in which structural racism is embodied: it enters the bodies of women of colour, and the stressors associated with racism lead to women having unfavourable maternal health outcomes and their infants also having bad outcomes such as low birth weight and premature birth. Thus, the social issue of racism manifests itself in biological ways. Although research that is framed within the biosocial approach of embodiment is largely Euro-American as is shown in the example above, there have been some recent strides in this topic within South Africa. Kim et al. [19] look at the intergenerational mental health impacts of prenatal stress in South Africa, focusing on a longitudinal birth cohort in South Africa called Birth to Twenty Plus (Bt20++). Their research illustrates how the trauma caused by apartheid conditions, coupled with other societal ills such as poverty and inequality, can be inherited and embodied by children in utero and affect their mental health in the future. Kim et al.'s key findings are that trauma and stressors caused by apartheid conditions have had enduring biological effects that continue to influence socio-emotional behaviour and mental health across the lifecourse [19].

12.5 Discussion

As the definitions and case studies that we have used in this chapter make clear, the conceptual framework of embodiment allows us to connect the subjective experiences of the body to broader social contexts and also shows us how the body is inscribed with history, politics, and culture. That is, individual bodily experiences are shaped by social, political, historical, and cultural forces [5, 20]. Furthermore, the concept of embodiment has allowed social scientists and health scientists to incorporate more nuanced approaches to quantify stress or other social, cultural, and material circumstances that could influence one's illness or sickness [21]. As Buklijas et al. mention in this volume, DOHaD research is based on the premise that conditions experienced in the womb, infancy, and childhood could potentially predict adult biological and health outcomes [21]. In the same vein, Krieger [7] argues that the clues to the current changing health population patterns can be found in the dynamic social, material, and ecological contexts in which people are born into, develop, and interact within.

While the focus is on interventions that aim to modify the behaviour and lifestyle of pregnant women might be useful, there are much larger structural forces at work beyond the control of the mother. The case studies we have presented demonstrate that we cannot divorce the body from politics and cultural context. Thus, to understand health and disease, DOHaD research needs to go beyond looking at what is present in the body, or the personal decisions made by an individual. Considering these case studies, we would want to look beyond the pregnant women who choose to work underground or pregnant women who eat processed food. Instead we want to consider the amalgamation of socio-economic-political factors that influence the decision-making of pregnant women and, ultimately, their health and that of their unborn babies. Such a deepened awareness can bring about more socially aware representations of women in DOHaD research and more socially just DOHaD interventions. In the Kim et al. case, for example, the health outcomes of pregnant women and future generations must be understood in the context of the racial inequality and injustice that occurred during apartheid South Africa; these have biological implications for Black maternal bodies. This awareness of how racial inequality and injustice can be embodied demands DOHaD research and interventions that take seriously the health impacts of racial inequality. In bringing attention to broader contexts, an embodiment approach would also encourage DOHaD interventions to focus on other reproductive actors and caregivers beyond pregnant women, including men and adolescents, as well as attending to broader contexts.

Adopting an embodiment approach in DOHaD research is challenging but vital. Such an approach widens the scope and focus of intervention, takes racial discrimination, political issues, and structural violence into consideration, and investigates how those socio-economic-political issues may enter the body and cause disease. An embodiment approach to DOHaD research navigates questions such as: how do bodies experience pregnancy and childbirth? How do certain contexts produce particular kinds of experiences of pregnancy? How do the circumstances under which women are pregnant enter their bodies and cause disease or ill health? Under what circumstances are bodies learning how to be pregnant and how to then feed an infant? How do others relate to certain pregnant bodies? What kind of power relations play out in the pregnant body, and how does this affect the health outcomes of the mother and child? Our hope is that using embodiment as a tool will help DOHaD researchers heed Krieger's call in her latest work, to use what we know about how injustice and inequalities shape people's health to guide our actions and direct resources into 'prevention, redress, accountability and change' [22].

12.6 Conclusion

This chapter has defined and illustrated embodiment as a crucial concept for theorising the body and illness in social and health sciences. These perspectives highlight that the body is relational, temporal, embodied, and situated. Using embodiment as a conceptual tool allows us to go beyond highlighting how structural inequality can literally be embodied and trigger sickness and move towards emphasising the transgenerational implications of health as a result of the previous generation/s embodying social ills. DOHaD science provides the scientific backing for the embodiment concept as it clearly shows that environmental factors impact health. This chapter calls for DOHaD research and interventions that not only acknowledge the environmental impact on health but also consider and include that wider environment and wider social structures in the interventions proposed. Embodiment is an insightful analytical tool that allows for conducting DOHaD research that can attend to social, political, cultural, and material processes and ultimately produce socially aware and socially just research and interventions. Embracing social science concepts such as embodiment also allows for shared vocabulary between DOHaD scientists and social scientists, which is vital for biosocial collaboration.

References

1. Clarkin PF. The embodiment of war: Growth, development, and armed conflict. Annual Review of Anthropology. 2019 21 Oct;48(1):423–42.

2. Musolino CM, Warin M, Gilchrist P. Embodiment as a paradigm for understanding and treating SE-AN: Locating the self in culture. Frontiers in Psychiatry. 2020 Jun 12;11:534.

3. Mehta N. Mind-body dualism: A critique from a health perspective. Mens Sana Monographs. 2011 Jan;9(1):202.

4. Goldberg L. Rethinking the birthing body: Cartesian dualism and perinatal nursing. Journal of Advanced Nursing. 2002 Mar;37(5):446–51.

5. Scheper-Hughes N, Lock MM. The mindful body: A prolegomenon to future work in medical anthropology. Medical Anthropology Quarterly. 1987 Mar;1(1):6–41.

6. Csordas TJ, Harwood A, editors. Embodiment and Experience: The Existential Ground of Culture and Self. United Kingdom: Cambridge University Press; 1994 17 Nov.

7. Krieger N. Theories for social epidemiology in the twenty-first century: An ecosocial perspective. International Journal of Epidemiology. 2001;30(4):668–77.

8. Zigon J, Throop J. Phenomenology. The Cambridge Encyclopaedia of Anthropology. 2021 Aug. http://doi.org/10.29164/21phenomenology

9. Bourdieu P. Outline of a Theory or Practice. Trans. Richard Nice. Cambridge: Cambridge University Press; 1977:21–2.

10. Gravlee CC. How race becomes biology: Embodiment of social inequality. American Journal of Physical Anthropology. 2009 May;139(1):47–57.

11. Manderson L, Ross FC. Publics, technologies and interventions in reproduction and early life in South Africa. Humanities and Social Sciences Communications. 2020;7(1):1–9.

12. Yates-Doerr E. Bodily betrayal: Love and anger in the time of epigenetics. A Companion to the Anthropology of the Body and Embodiment. 2011:292–306.

13. Groeneveld IF, Solomons NW, Doak CM. Nutritional status of urban schoolchildren of high and low socioeconomic status in Quetzaltenango, Guatemala. Revista Panamericana de Salud Pública. 2007;22:169–77.

14. Hall KD. Challenges of human nutrition research. Science. 2020 20 Mar;367 (6484):1298–300.

15. Rubin SE, Hines J. 'As long as I got a breath in my body': Risk and resistance in Black maternal embodiment. Culture, Medicine, and Psychiatry. 2022 6 Apr;47 (2):495–518.

16. Mutendi M. 'Making a Plan to Keep My Baby': Navigating Maternal Health Policy Among South African Mineworkers. Bodies of Knowledge: Children and Childhoods in Health and Affliction. 2021 1 Dec:227–248.

17. South Africa. Basic Conditions of Employment Act 75 of 1997

18. David R, Collins J Jr. Disparities in infant mortality: What's genetics got to do with it? American Journal of Public Health. 2007 Jul;97(7):1191–7.

19. Kim AW, Mohamed RS, Norris SA, Richter LM, Kuzawa CW). Psychological Legacies of Intergenerational Trauma under South African Apartheid: Prenatal Stress Predicts Increased Psychiatric Morbidity during Late Adolescence and Early Adulthood in Soweto, South Africa. medRxiv. 2021.

20. Foucault M. Discipline and punish: The birth of the prison (Trans A. Sheridan). New York: Vintage Books. 1977 (Original work published 1975).

21. Kuzawa CW, Sweet E. Epigenetics and the embodiment of race: Developmental origins of US racial disparities in cardiovascular health. American Journal of Human Biology: The Official Journal of the Human Biology Association. 2009 Jan;21(1):2–15.

22. Krieger N. Ecosocial Theory, Embodied Truths, and the People's Health. USA: Oxford University Press; 2021.

Chapter

Causal Crypticity

Sarah S. Richardson

Causal crypticity is an epistemic norm in the field of maternal–fetal effects science. That is, fetal origins researchers assert causal hypotheses about links between small permutations in the gestational environment and later life outcomes. The causes and effects of these permutations are typically not directly observed but are inferred from variations in developmental outcomes or health risks that occur later in life, often along a decades-long chain of other exposures and experiences. To advance these hypotheses requires field-wide epistemic norms that accept, in most cases, an ineliminable crypticity – meaning both subtlety and elusiveness – in the causes and effects under study.

This feature of Developmental Origins of Health and Disease (DOHaD) science is not the perception of hard-nosed sceptics. Many DOHaD researchers are frank about its causal dilemmas [1–3]. DOHaD scientists have faced fierce criticisms of their theories and findings by scientists who doubt the plausibility of their causal claims [4–7], and scientists in the varied research streams that comprise fetal origins/maternal effects science have been openly debating the question of causality for decades. The search for causal mechanisms propelled the entry of epigenetic methodologies into the field and contributed to the pioneering of new inference causal testing models such as Mendelian randomisation to attempt to examine the plausibility and strength of hypothesised causal relations [8–12].

The crypticity of causality in DOHaD is no standard-issue causality conundrum. As I argued in *The Maternal Imprint: The Contested Science of Maternal-Foetal Effects* (2021), from the field's inception, causal crypticity has been deeply carved into the historical development of the field and will likely continue to be a persistent feature of any research in maternal–fetal effects science, regardless of the amount of data acquired or the sophistication of computational methods employed [13]. Nods to the context-specificity and complexity of causal attributions in DOHaD science do not sufficiently acknowledge the persistent, intransigent crypticity of causality in maternal–fetal effects science, nor do they capture the social dimension of its function as an epistemic style in DOHaD discourse.

High tolerance for causal crypticity can be defined as a field-defining epistemic norm that accepts a persistent state of indeterminacy about the empirical reality, strength, and magnitude of hypothesised causal phenomena that are the object of study. Causal crypticity distinguishes approaches to causal reasoning within DOHaD from certain ideals of scientific inference prising replicable experiments, intervenability demonstrating causal invariability across conditions, and identification of a physiological mechanism [14]. But this does not imply that causal crypticity is particularly epistemically suspect compared to other causality-seeking knowledge projects. Causal crypticity is not a term intended to pinion the scientific merit or rigour of DOHaD science but to characterise its epistemic norms to better understand the field's theories, its evidential base, and the judgements that undergird its inferences. My claim is descriptive, not evaluative: causal crypticity operates as an epistemic norm in DOHaD science.

In this chapter, I explicate and develop the concept of causal crypticity, first introduced in Richardson (2021). Causal crypticity can be understood in three ways: as an epistemic norm; as a boundary-delimiting signature of field culture or epistemic style; and as a promissory mode. Contending with causal crypticity as a norm-shaping feature of the knowledge landscape of maternal–fetal effects science, I conclude, demands reflection on strategies for ethical and accountable practices of claimsmaking in DOHaD science, in a world where its findings are received as carrying social implications in arenas ranging from reproductive autonomy to efforts to redress the health implications of racism and intergenerational trauma.

13.1 Crypticity

The term 'cryptic' has multiple connotations, which I embrace. Something that is cryptic may be real but difficult to decode or retrieve. Equally, something that is cryptic can be unclear, and whether it is real or not can be impossible to discern. Phenomena that are cryptic are elusive, shape-shifting, and impermanent in form. DOHaD science connects cryptic effects with cryptic causes. *Cryptic effects* are findings of health outcomes in exposed compared to unexposed populations that are small in effect size and that present inconsistently across different study cohorts; moreover, such crypticity in reported outcomes is persistent and unresolved despite expanding volumes of data. Cryptic effects are typified by DOHaD studies reporting small absolute changes in risk factors for common diseases among populations of healthy, average births exposed to a hypothesised intrauterine variable.

The field's tolerance for causal crypticity is in clear evidence, for instance, in the Dutch famine studies, a touchstone in DOHaD research. The Dutch famine studies are often presented as definitively demonstrating a causal link between nutrition in the womb and obesity and related metabolic conditions, including high blood pressure, diabetes and insulin resistance, and cardiovascular disease. These metabolic outcomes are based on measures taken from a small sample of 422 survivors, in their fifties, who were gestationally exposed to the famine (and matched siblings) during the four months of the acute famine of 1944–1945 in the Netherlands [15]. As researchers will readily agree when queried, the findings from these studies are much less generalisable, and much more contingent and uncertain, than portrayed in the standard textbook narrative. Famine survivors have been found to have, on average, modestly elevated blood pressure compared to non-survivors [16]. Women gestated during the Dutch famine have, on average, an extra few centimetres around the waist, at age 59, than their non-exposed sisters [17]. However, the effect sizes in such findings are small. They are also unstable, appearing and disappearing across different age cohorts and genders/sexes within the study populations. Critical reviews demonstrate that the Dutch famine studies have shown a few, if any, stable metabolic outcomes of significant effect size specifically correlated with in utero exposure to famine [18].

Other statements frequently reiterated in the literature, such as that early exposure to famine doubles the risk of obesity, are, upon examination, not supported by current evidence but are statistical relics of dated metrics of what constitutes abnormally overweight body composition from the 1970s [19]. Furthermore, researchers have struggled to identify biological mechanisms that could account for the purported specific causal effects of famine exposure during gestation. A much-celebrated early finding of epigenetic changes in the insulin-like growth factor 2 (IGF2) gene among famine survivors has never been replicated [20, 21]. Subsequent studies attempting to find epigenetic mediators of triglyceride levels among survivors have not withstood causality inference testing [3]. Yet even as effects are causally cryptic – effect sizes remain small, findings are contested and conflicting, and mechanisms are elusive – the Dutch famine studies are presented in the literature as a foundation and model for future work [22], and scientific publications, textbooks, and popular media frequently feature studies of health outcomes among ageing members of the cohort of infants gestated during the Dutch famine as a gold-standard example of the promise of developmental origins science [23].

Causal crypticity characterises the explanations for *cryptic effects* because such cryptic effects are unstable and variable, such that they make non-ideal observations for substantiating a link to a specific cause. In the case of maternal intrauterine effects, in which the direct effects of perturbations during gestation are already challenging to observe, measure, or quantify, causal crypticity is particularly amplified. This is because, due to the many environmental and genetic confounders of early human development, in nearly every case the cryptic maternal effect is an endpoint of complex, multiply confounded causal chains, frequently occurring at a significant temporal distance from the hypothesised initial exposure, which itself is sometimes a confounded, variably defined, difficult-to-measure 'cryptic cause' such as 'stress' or 'metabolic dysregulation'.

Such crypticity is apparent even within maternal–fetal programming science that is often presented as most foundational, most settled, and as presenting the most extreme exposures, the largest effects, and the most incontrovertible findings, as in the Dutch Hunger Winter studies. The field's high tolerance for causally cryptic findings as constituting knowledge helps us understand how such findings, which at best offer support for what may be model-theoretically *plausible* or physiologically *possible*, become concretised as a textbook, settled science, and as known or proven facts within the field of DOHaD.

13.2 Causal Crypticity as an Epistemic Style and Promissory Mode

Tolerance for causal crypticity, as a feature of the DOHaD field's culture, norms, standards, or epistemic style, is apparent in the forms of evidence accepted within the DOHaD field as contributions to scientific knowledge and reflected in its shared assumptions about the questions and objects of interest. For example, the quality of crypticity is arguably constitutive of what makes something a developmental or maternal *effect* rather than, for instance, a birth defect or anomaly. Causal crypticity is, furthermore, integral to the central questions and problems that the DOHaD field addresses and to how it goes about addressing them. As Gemma Sharp, Debbie Lawler, and I have argued, the question of whether maternal–fetal programming effects are *real* is in many senses not a question for researchers in the DOHaD field. For DOHaD researchers, it is indisputable that programmable maternal–fetal effects are real [24]; the question is only whether we can see and prove them, given that the biology involved must be very complex and that the pragmatics of studying maternal–fetal effects in human populations is challenging.

Scientific fields are social formations. Sociologists and historians of science posit that scientific fields function most efficiently to advance empirical understanding of phenomena when there is a shared culture of sorts and when the field agrees on its core questions. As a part of this boundary-defining work, fields typically close down or defer certain questions as well as certain epistemological considerations [25–28]. Causal crypticity can be tolerated, one might hypothesise, when it serves other important functions for the field as a social formation. Following scholars of scientific hype [29, 30], one speculation is that causal crypticity may function to keep fetal origins science at the centre of controversy, with findings persistently described as emergent, yet to be validated, still being tested, and even essentially contested. In part because of this, causal crypticity could work cathectically to draw intrigue and to construct a continually self-replicating arc of future speculation and possibility. In this way, causal crypticity may function as an electric current that both makes the field of maternal–fetal effects a flashpoint and draws curious researchers to it.

In this sense, causal crypticity can be understood as a promissory discourse that conveys causal-ish claims that generate excitement and interest [29]. Thus, although the field is now more than three decades old, its claims are frequently presented as offering a new, emergent, and provocative resource for science. It is commonplace to read in publications, to hear at an academic conference on DOHaD, or to find in a media presentation of DOHaD research a statement such as: 'In recent years, research from the field of the Developmental Origins of Health and Disease (DOHaD) has suggested that events before birth can have life-long consequences' [31]. Such broad statements suggesting a powerful causal relation between intrauterine environment and later life health are, technically speaking, perfectly consistent with a collection of unreplicated findings that intrauterine exposure X is associated with small effects on offspring outcome Y in study population Z, yet it also implies stronger and more widely validated causal effects actionable for public health and in the clinic than present evidence can support.

Specifically, causal crypticity may function socially and discursively to generate excitement and interest in the scientific field by pointing towards a future in which knowledge of such cryptic patterns could be harnessed to optimise health outcomes [32]. Notably, cryptic patterns of perturbations linked to outcomes do not promise control or prediction for any particular individual, but at best speak to patterns and trends and to risk categories and potential problems at the level of population groups [33]. These patterns and risk categories generate uncertainty and require *concern* and ongoing *monitoring*.

In a world rife with crises, risk, and uncertainty, the potential for cryptic sources of fetal developmental perturbation requiring ongoing tracking is everywhere. We thus see speculation about the relevance of developmental origins theories to nearly every area of social anxiety and uncertainty, including natural disasters and political or economic crises, from the 9/11 attacks [34–36] to climate change [37–39], to most recently, the COVID-19 pandemic [40–42]. Writing in 2021, Tessa Roseboom and colleagues warned in the *Journal of the Developmental Origins of Health and Disease* that 'the legacy of this pandemic looms large for unborn babies … These individuals, being unseen and unheard, are likely to go unprotected'. The implications of experiencing the pandemic while in the womb, these authors assert, will affect an entire generation and 'all of our future societies': 'Today's (unborn) children will drive growth and development in our future societies. [. . .] We must now act to prevent further scarring of the life chances of a generation' [41]. The potential for harm to the 'unborn' is pervasive, as in Figure 13.1, which conceptualises the mother's work, daily hassle, and even the condition of pregnancy itself, as health-imperilling stressors transmuted to the fetus through the mother [42].

DOHaD science on maternal–fetal effects promises to inform public policy to improve future outcomes, but causal crypticity entails that DOHaD research is not, by and large, likely to produce interventions driven by the reversal of biochemical mechanisms at the moment or site of programming [33]. In a field of inquiry characterised by the epistemic style and promissory mode of causal crypticity, interventions, while hoped-for, are ultimately less the order of the day than *demonstrating the possibility or plausibility of harm*. In the case of DOHaD, this harm is conceptualised as a limitation on future potential. That is, DOHaD findings of cryptic effects deliver evidence of limitations or lesions in the potential for life flourishing, from early mortality to educational achievement. Powerful ableist, Western norms and pressures to optimise birth outcomes, complemented by globalist, development economics frameworks for measuring human capital in the metrics of health and at the level of the body, help sustain this promissory mode in maternal–fetal effects science [43–46]. The range of possible future adverse outcomes is so wide that the full implications of the developmental harm can never be fully grasped, only proxied by limited quantitative physiological measures such as adiposity or blood pressure. Moreover, it is argued that these harms are set so early in development that compensating for or redressing the harms will be challenging. DOHaD researchers frequently suggest that early developmental harms might only be redressed in future generations by removing or waiting out the scourge of trauma, poverty, or metabolic deprivation.

13.3 Causal Crypticity in the Context of Big Data and Postgenomic Science

While DOHaD science has long operated with a high tolerance for causal crypticity, the epistemic norm of causal crypticity, as I have characterised it here, increasingly might be said to characterise the knowledge claims and knowledge practices endemic to data-rich, twenty-first-century postgenomic biomedical life sciences, particularly those endeavours operating in complex biosocial causal spaces. Indeed, as commentators have pointed out [47], in many areas of postgenomic biomedicine, causal claims are *not expected* to result from investigations. It is expected that the strength of findings will vary depending on contextual factors and that findings will not replicate across all datasets. Even as researchers strive to validate causal connections, a tolerance for a certain permissiveness with implying the likely causality of observed correlations is increasingly integrated into the norms and culture of postgenomic biomedicine.

There is a broader social context for these shifts in knowledge paradigms in the postgenomic life sciences. The epistemic style of causal crypticity is primed to flourish in a knowledge culture defined by massive information. The epistemology of massive information is defined by constructs such as 'search', trending ideas, chatter, pattern recognition, the notion of 'data mining', network, and systems-like ideas about the

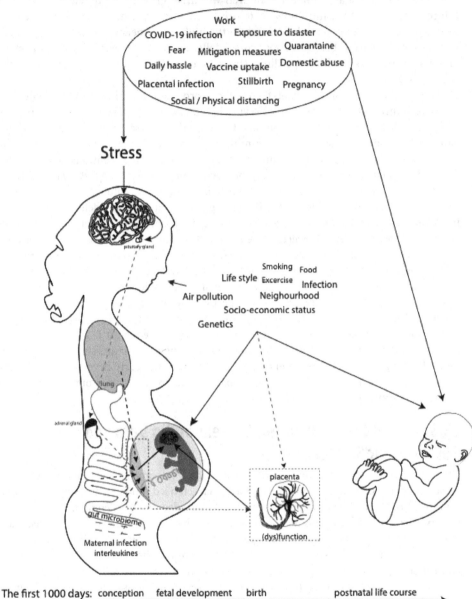

The first 1000 days during the COVID-19 era

Work
COVID-19 infection   Exposure to disaster
Fear   Mitigation measures   Quarantaine
Daily hassle   Vaccine uptake   Domestic abuse
Placental infection   Stillbirth   Pregnancy
Social / Physical distancing

Stress

pituitary gland

Smoking   Food
Life style   Excercise   Infection
Air pollution   Neighourhood
Socio-economic status
Genetics

lung

adrenal gland

placenta

gut microbiome

(dys)function

Maternal infection
interleukines

The first 1000 days: conception   fetal development   birth   postnatal life course

Early life course medicine

Figure 13.1 'Overview of potential maternal prenatal stressors during the current COVID-19 pandemic as part of the early life course medicine'.
Source: Schoenmakers et al. [42]

connectivity of all things, total information, emergence, and surveillance [48]. This epistemology contrasts sharply with 'magic bullet' or 'master molecule' approaches to knowledge that are oriented towards control, intervention, and cure [49]. In a knowledge culture embracing causal crypticity, grievance or evidence of harm is not expected to surface as a gaping wound – acute, localisable, and repairable – but as a population-level signal – subtle, elusive, and with harms and benefits of uncertain interpretation.

Similarly in postgenomic science, signals are not expected to be single-gene lesions [50], but polygenic scores or risk calculi that must be carefully contextualised against a backdrop of population genetic structure, developmental context, and social conditions. These sciences, underpinned by genome-wide association studies, multidimensional forms of social data, and AI-informed analytics, are made up of statistically sophisticated evidence of correlations between biological and social outcomes. While these correlations themselves do not support causal inference, causal crypticity enables a presumption of the likelihood of causality. Findings are narrated within a larger frame that implies a strong assumption that such correlations, summed in their entirety, are evidence supporting an intuition of causality. This shift in epistemic norms is collapsing the twentieth-century oppositional distinction between the complexity-affirming 'dissident' anti-genetic determinist sciences and the reductionist and determinist gene-centric biological sciences [51].

In sum, causal crypticity is an epistemic norm that aligns with the speculative and promissory mode of today's transnational, big data-crunching science, which proposes to mine previously undetected patterns across populations, unlocking a key to who we are and where we are going in our uncertain era of demographic transformation in lifespans and family size, technological change, and environmental crisis. Like these fields, DOHaD pleads for a deferral of judgement and for more space for free investigation, by implicitly suggesting that cryptic patterns long postulated or hypothesised, and for which current evidence is trace-like at best, will soon be detectable as meaningful sources of human variation in health – once we have the data and the proper data mining tools to retrieve those patterns. In this way, within the postgenomic life sciences, DOHaD science offers an index case of the leading edge of a broadening trend of embracing the bold pursuit of cryptic causes.

13.4 Ethical and Accountable Claimsmaking in DOHaD Science under Conditions of Causal Crypticity

In *The Maternal Imprint*, I traced the history of attempts to empirically confirm speculations about the long-term or permanent effects of experiences or exposures in the womb [13]. The book followed three intertwining threads within this history: First, discourses about maternal agency and responsibility for reproductive outcomes. Second, progressive, anti-genetic determinist constructs of the biosocial body position the maternal–fetal relation as a particularly heightened space for the inscription of social and environmental context on the body. Third persistent and unresolved questions about the limits of empirical science in confirming the causal effects of intrauterine perturbations on disease distribution in human populations.

This third, seemingly epistemic dimension, I argued, cannot be fully pulled apart from the other two. This is because bold causal claims in the absence of consistent and convincing evidence of predictive, intervenable effects can only persist if there is a powerful social and scientific imaginary carrying them forward. The churning, resilient, charged space of maternal responsibility for optimising reproductive outcomes and the subversive, hopeful, riveting, intuitive, and narratively compelling picture of bodies embedded in environments and social systems are two such imaginaries.

The subtle effect sizes and complex confounding typical of causal claims in DOHaD science are not simply an everyday causal challenge but rather function as both a defining epistemic norm of the field and a future-oriented social discourse. The concept of 'causal crypticity' directs attention to the links between causal crypticity as an epistemic norm, the production of risk categories, and the promissory hype cycle of science.

Fields such as DOHaD are defining the epistemic terrain of postgenomic inquiry, particularly at the interface of the genetic and social sciences [51]. For some DOHaD scientists, the concept of causal crypticity as I have motivated it here may at first provoke defensiveness. Most scientists understand themselves instead to be seeking – even if not always finding – causal relations grounded only on rigorous empirical inference. However, embracing this feature of DOHaD research could make DOHaD a laboratory for grappling with causal crypticity in a reflective and forthcoming manner. This surely includes strengthening frameworks for making causal inferences in the face of causal crypticity, as some already are [2, 52]. But it also includes practices such as rigorously placing risk claims emerging from such sciences in context, in particular through collaboration with social scientists exploring the socio-structural dimensions of health and lifecourse development [53], accurately characterising the degree of uncertainty in scientific findings in this area [54], and educating the consumers of such science in the features of reasoning in a field defined by causal crypticity.

References

1. Heijmans BT, Mill J. The seven plagues of epigenetic epidemiology. International Journal of Epidemiology. 2012;41 (1):74–8.

2. Lawlor DA, Relton C, Sattar N, Nelson SM. Maternal adiposity – A determinant of perinatal and offspring outcomes? Nature Reviews Endocrinology. 2012;8 (11):679–88.

3. Richmond R, Relton C, Davey Smith G. What evidence is required to suggest that DNA methylation mediates the association between prenatal famine exposure and adulthood disease. Scientific Advances. 2018;eLetter to eaao4364.

4. Paneth N, Susser M. Early origin of coronary heart disease (the 'Barker hypothesis'). British Medical Journal. 1995;310(6977):411–12.

5. Lancet. An overstretched hypothesis? Lancet. 2001;357(9254):405.

6. Geronimus AT. Deep integration: Letting the epigenome out of the bottle without losing sight of the structural origins of population health. American Journal of Public Health. 2013;103:S56.

7. Wilcox AJ. On the importance – and the unimportance – of birthweight. International Journal of Epidemiology. 2001;30(6):1233–41.

8. Birney E, Smith GD, Greally JM. Epigenome-wide association studies and the interpretation of disease -omics. PLOS Genetics. 2016;12(6):e1006105.

9. Davey Smith G, Hemani G. Mendelian randomization: Genetic anchors for causal inference in epidemiological studies. Human Molecular Genetics. 2014;23(R1):R89–R98.

10. Langley K, Heron J, Smith GD, Thapar A. Maternal and paternal smoking during pregnancy and risk of ADHD symptoms in offspring: Testing for intrauterine effects. Am Journal of Epidemiology. 2012;176(3):261–8.

11. Lawlor DA, Timpson NJ, Harbord RM, Leary S, Ness A, McCarthy MI, et al. Exploring the developmental overnutrition hypothesis using parental-offspring associations and FTO as an instrumental variable. PLoS Medicine. 2008;5(3):e33.

12. Richmond RC, Timpson NJ, Felix JF, Palmer T, Gaillard R, McMahon G, et al. Using genetic variation to explore the causal effect of maternal pregnancy adiposity on future offspring adiposity: A Mendelian Randomisation Study. PLoS Medicine. 2017;14(1):e1002221.

13. Richardson SS. The Maternal Imprint: The Contested Science of Maternal-fetal Effects. Chicago: University of Chicago Press; 2021. 310 p.

14. Woodward JF. Making Things Happen: A Theory of Causal Explanation. New York: Oxford University Press; 2003. vi, 410 p.

15. Lumey LH, Stein AD, Kahn HS, van der Pal-de Bruin KM, Blauw GJ, Zybert PA, et al. Cohort profile: The Dutch Hunger Winter families study. International Journal of Epidemiology. 2007;36 (6):1196–204.

16. Stein AD, Zybert PA, van der Pal-de Bruin K, Lumey LH. Exposure to famine during gestation, size at birth, and blood pressure at age 59 y: Evidence from the Dutch famine. European Journal of Epidemiology. 2006;21(10):759–65.

17. Rundle A, Stein AD, Kahn HS, van der Pal–de Bruin K, Zybert PA, Lumey L. Anthropometric measures in middle age after exposure to famine during gestation: Evidence from the Dutch famine. The American Journal of Clinical Nutrition. 2007;85(3):869–76.

18. Lumey LH, Stein AD, Susser E. Prenatal famine and adult health. Annual Review of Public Health. 2011;32(1):237–62.

19. Ravelli GP, Stein ZA, Susser MW. Obesity in young men after famine exposure in utero and early infancy. New England Journal of Medicine. 1976;295(7):349–53.

20. Heijmans BT, Tobi EW, Stein AD, Putter H, Blauw GJ, Susser ES, et al. Persistent epigenetic differences associated with prenatal exposure to famine in humans. Proceedings of the National Academy of Sciences. 2008;105(44):17046–9.

21. Tobi EW, Slieker RC, Luijk R, Dekkers KF, Stein AD, Xu KM, et al. DNA methylation as a mediator of the association between prenatal adversity and risk factors for metabolic disease in adulthood. Science Advances. 2018;4(1): eaao4364.

22. Roseboom TJ. Epidemiological evidence for the developmental origins of health and disease: Effects of prenatal undernutrition in humans. Journal of Endocrinology. 2019;242(1):T135–T44.

23. Zimmer C. The famine ended 70 years ago, but Dutch genes still bear scars. *The New York Times.* 2018 31 Jan.

24. Sharp GC, Lawlor DA, Richardson SS. It's the mother!: How assumptions about the causal primacy of maternal effects influence research on the developmental origins of health and disease. Social Science & Medicine. 2018;213:20–7.

25. Bourdieu P. The specificity of the scientific field and the social conditions of the progress of reason. Social Science Information. 1975;14(6):19–47.

26. Panofsky A. Misbehaving Science: Controversy and the Development of Behavior Genetics. Chicago: The University of Chicago Press; 2014.

27. Kuhn TS. The Structure of Scientific Revolutions. Chicago: University of Chicago Press; 1962. xv, 172 p.

28. Knorr-Cetina K. Epistemic Cultures: How the Sciences Make Knowledge. Cambridge, MA: Harvard University Press; 1999. xiii, 329 p.

29. Fortun M. Promising Genomics: Iceland and deCODE Genetics in a World of Speculation. Berkeley: University of California Press; 2008.

30. Caulfield T. Spinning the genome: Why science hype matters. Perspectives in Biology and Medicine. 2018;61:560–71.

31. Jacob CM, Hanson M. Implications of the Developmental Origins of Health and

Disease concept for policy-making. Current Opinion in Endocrine and Metabolic Research. 2020;13:20–7.

32. Heeney C. Problems and promises: How to tell the story of a Genome Wide Association Study? Studies in History and Philosophy of Science Part A. 2021;89:1–10.

33. Penkler M. Caring for biosocial complexity. Articulations of the environment in research on the Developmental Origins of Health and Disease. Studies in History and Philosophy of Science. 2022;93:1–10.

34. Berkowitz GS, Wolff MS, Janevic TM, Holzman IR, Yehuda R, Landrigan PJ. The world trade center disaster and intrauterine growth restriction. JAMA: Journal of the American Medical Association. 2003;290(5):595–6.

35. Engel SM, Berkowitz GS, Wolff MS, Yehuda R. Psychological trauma associated with the World Trade Center attacks and its effect on pregnancy outcome. Paediatric and Perinatal Epidemiology. 2005;19(5):334–41.

36. Ohlsson A, Shah PS, the Knowledge Synthesis Group of Determinants of Preterm LBWb. Effects of the September 11, 2001 disaster on pregnancy outcomes: A systematic review. Acta Obstetricia et Gynecologica Scandinavica. 2011;90(1):6–18.

37. Wesselink AK, Wellenius GA. Impacts of climate change on reproductive, perinatal and paediatric health. Paediatric and Perinatal Epidemiology. 2022;36(1):1–3.

38. Cao-Lei L, de Rooij SR, King S, Matthews SG, Metz GAS, Roseboom TJ, et al. Prenatal stress and epigenetics. Neuroscience and Biobehavioral Reviews. 2017;117:198–210.

39. Derfel A. Prenatal stress from extreme weather is having negative effect on babies. *The Montreal Gazette.* 2009 31 Jan;Sect. News.

40. Forestieri S, Pintus R, Marcialis MA, Pintus MC, Fanos V. COVID-19 and developmental origins of health and disease. Early Human Development. 2021;155:105322.

41. Roseboom TJ, Ozanne SE, Godfrey KM, Isasi CR, Itoh H, Simmons R, et al. Unheard, unseen and unprotected: DOHaD council's call for action to protect the younger generation from the long-term effects of COVID-19. Journal of Developmental Origins of Health and Disease. 2021;12(1):3–5.

42. Schoenmakers S, Verweij EJ, Beijers R, Bijma HH, Been JV, Steegers-Theunissen RPM, et al. The impact of maternal prenatal stress related to the COVID-19 pandemic during the first 1000 days: A historical perspective. International Journal of Environmental Research and Public Health. 2022;19(8):4710.

43. Valdez N. Weighing the Future: Race, Science, and Pregnancy Trials in the Postgenomic Era. Oakland: University of California Press; 2022. pages cm p.

44. Murphy M. The Economization of Life. Durham, NC; London: Duke University Press; 2017. ix, 220 p.

45. Baedke J, Nieves Delgado A. Race and nutrition in the New World: Colonial shadows in the age of epigenetics. Studies in History and Philosophy of Science Part C: Studies in History and Philosophy of Biological and Biomedical Sciences. 2019;76:101175.

46. Reiches M. Reproductive justice and the history of prenatal supplementation: Ethics, birth spacing, and the 'Priority Infant' model in The Gambia. Signs: Journal of Women in Culture and Society. 2019;45(1):3–26.

47. Richardson SS, Stevens H. Postgenomics: Perspectives on Biology after the Genome. Durham, NC: Duke University Press; 2015. ix, 294 p.

48. Stevens H. Networks: Representations and tools in postgenomics. In: Richardson SS, Stevens H, editors. Postgenomics: Perspectives on Biology after the Genome. Durham: Duke University Press; 2015. p. 0.

49. Keller EF. The Century of the Gene. Cambridge, MA: Harvard University Press; 2000. 186 p.

50. Boyle EA, Li YI, Pritchard JK. An expanded view of complex traits: From

polygenic to omnigenic. Cell. 2017;169 (7):1177–86.

51. Richardson SS. Maternal bodies in the postgenomic order: Gender and the explanatory landscape of epigenetics. In: Richardson SS, Stevens H, editors. Postgenomics: Perspectives on Biology after the Genome. Durham, NC: Duke University Press; 2015. pp. 210–31.

52. Gage SH, Munafo MR, Davey Smith G. Causal inference in Developmental Origins of Health and Disease (DOHaD) Research. Annual Review Psychology. 2016;67:567–85.

53. Müller R, Hanson C, Hanson M, Penkler M, Samaras G, Chiapperino L, et al. The biosocial genome? EMBO Reports. 2017;18(10):1677–82.

54. Richardson SS, Daniels CR, Gillman MW, Golden J, Kukla R, Kuzawa C, et al. Society: Don't blame the mothers. Nature. 2014;512(7513):131–2.

Chapter 1

Intergenerational Trauma

Jaya Keaney, Henrietta Byrne, Megan Warin, and
Emma Kowal

14.1 Introduction

The term intergenerational trauma describes how trauma experienced in one generation
can lead to trauma in the lives of descendants. For scholars and practitioners of
Developmental Origins of Health and Disease (DOHaD), intergenerational trauma is
an important aspect of human experience that can shape physiological development and
influence individual, family, and community health across generations. In a DOHaD
model, parental and community experiences of trauma can be transmitted in utero and
in early life, having a cumulative physiological effect such that historical experiences are
embodied in the present. In this chapter, we provide a conceptual overview of 'intergenerational trauma' in the interdisciplinary field of DOHaD research. The concept has
been variously defined in relation to other disciplines and implicitly or explicitly drawn
on other concepts such as historical trauma, transgenerational trauma, and post-
traumatic stress disorder (PTSD). Intergenerational trauma is of interest to many
disciplines and frameworks in part because it lends itself to 'biosocial' understandings
of violence and discriminatory social contexts as physiologically embodied. Yet, intergenerational trauma also presents challenges for scientific study due to the difficulties
inherent in stabilising it as a scientific object. As a group of social theorists working
across anthropology, gender studies, and science and technology studies (STS), we attend
in this chapter to both the operationalisation of intergenerational trauma in DOHaD
research (including the increasing importance of epigenetic mechanisms) and the particularities of how intergenerational trauma is enacted as a supposedly stable entity in
science. Given the growing public interest in intergenerational trauma, and its increasing
clinical uptake for the care of marginalised communities, this chapter also considers a
range of important questions related to policy translation, biopolitics, and social justice.

14.2 What Is Intergenerational Trauma?

Broadly speaking, intergenerational trauma can be understood as 'emotional and psychological wounding that is transmitted across generations' [1]. It is entangled with the allied
concepts of historical trauma and transgenerational trauma. While often used synonymously with intergenerational trauma, we distinguish historical trauma here through its
connection to large-scale historical violence 'such as enslavement, colonization, and genocide' [1, 2]. While this understanding of historical trauma falls within the remit of
intergenerational trauma, the latter can also encompass traumatising experiences that do
not register in large-scale histories of global violence but occur on more personal and

micro-scales, such as interpersonal violence. 'Transgenerational trauma' is another term that is often used synonymously with intergenerational trauma (e.g. [1, 3]); however, in the DOHaD field, the term 'transgenerational' has a specific meaning that pertains to epigenetic mechanisms of transmission to two or more subsequent generations (as discussed in more detail later in this chapter). As we define it here, intergenerational trauma does not imply a particular kind of violence or a particular biological mechanism of transmission.

A capacious concept, intergenerational trauma has captured the attention of theorists, clinicians, and writers across innumerable fields. These range from Indigenous studies [2, 4], psychology and psychiatry [5–7], social work [3], and public health, to literature [8], queer studies [9], and memory studies [10]. Scholars across these fields differently approach intergenerational trauma as a useful concept for thinking through human relatedness, collective identity formation, and the channels through which histories and legacies are embodied, suturing us across time and space. Theories of *how* intergenerational trauma is inherited vary widely across these different approaches – from attention to narratives and material culture shared in families [3], to artistic texts and collective remembrance practices through which new generations are enculturated [10], to somatic mechanisms of implicit or bodily memory held by individuals [3, 7].

While social environments were key to early formulations of DOHaD [11], the increasing molecularisation of the environment has narrowed the focus to biological mechanisms of transmission. This includes two important junctures. The first is the transmission to a fetus of a pregnant person's real-time experience of a traumatic event/ environment or its after-effects. Developmental programming in utero and in early life in response to trauma can foster a greater propensity for stress and mental health challenges [12] and can contribute to low birth weight, preterm birth, chronic disease, and immune and metabolic dysfunction later in life [13–15]. The second juncture is the effects of patterns of parental care behaviours, including breastfeeding, nutrition, and emotional responsiveness [16]. Here, the destructive effects of trauma in caregivers' own lives, often compounded by material disadvantage and ongoing discrimination, can lead to the re-creation of traumatising contexts for children. Manifesting as developmental challenges, sustained distress, and detachment from caregivers, communities, and culture, this is often referred to as the 'cycle of trauma'. Here, trauma is both cause and effect. Past traumas suffered by parents, communities, or ancestors may be an origin of an individual's present-day health challenges and may also manifest as personal experiences or psychological symptoms of trauma.

The scholarly genealogy of intergenerational trauma and its potential mechanisms is often traced to empirical studies of the effects of the Holocaust on children of survivors [16, 17]. These studies found that the children of Holocaust survivors experienced mental health challenges characteristic of those who experienced trauma directly [1, p. 2]. The application of the concept has since broadened considerably, including to explore the impacts of colonisation on First Nations communities [2, 4]; the effects of forced displacement and armed conflict on survivors and refugee populations [18–20]; intergenerational harms among African American communities wrought by trans-Atlantic slavery and enduring racism [21, 22]; and the embodied legacies of systemic gender-based violence [19, 23].

While 'trauma' is deployed as a stable biomedical entity in DOHaD-informed studies, defining and measuring trauma scientifically is a complex endeavour always entangled with social worlds. Far from a 'timeless unity' [24, p. 3], trauma is made measurable within diagnostic categories and measurement tools that stabilise it as a pathological disease entity. Chief among these are the diagnosis of PTSD, which was added to the Diagnostic and Statistical Manual (DSM) in the 1980s and has been critical to studies and therapeutic interventions for trauma; and measurement tools such as the Adverse Childhood Experiences scale [25, 26], which aims to quantify experiences of trauma through scales tabulating challenging events and living conditions.

Such tools conceptualise and enact trauma differently from one-another and in context-dependent ways [27]. For example, the association between context, symptom, and relationship is differently assembled in individual study designs. As Judy Atkinson and co-authors [28, p. 289] have written, trauma is variously conceived as an 'event, environment, or reaction'. Trauma is often implicitly conceptualised as an event itself, for example, a collective historical trauma or a set of adverse childhood experiences. Yet in other contexts, it is defined as the distress exhibited *in response to* an event or situation [1, p. 16]. These slippages have a significant impact on understanding what trauma is, who is affected, and the scales of intervention. Defining trauma with reference to a particular historical event such as colonisation, for example, risks homogenising members of a group by assuming they all experienced the event as similarly traumatising [6]. As Andrew Kim [29] writes, studies of stress and trauma can also often result in researchers assessing whether a given event is traumatic according to their own worldview rather than through deep engagement with the worldview and reference points of the participants. Furthermore, studies that focus conceptualisations of trauma on an event can make it challenging to attend to heterogenous groups for whom traumas are compounding or not easily delineated as discrete events. As Cerdeña et al. [1, p. 2] note, one of the reasons that Latinx communities are underrepresented in the literature on intergenerational trauma may be due to their significant heterogeneity and the multiple overlapping sources of trauma, including diverse forms of colonisation, political oppression within Latin America, dangerous passages of international migration, and systemic racism.

14.2.1 DOHaD Research, Epigenetics, and Transgenerational Trauma

As discussed above, much of the early scholarly literature surrounding DOHaD has focused on historical cohorts that have experienced trauma from war and nutritional deprivation (particularly famine – for example, the Biafran (1967–70) or Chinese famine (1959–61)). The oft-cited Dutch Winter famine from the Second World War is perhaps the best known: a period of severe malnutrition forced on Dutch families by Nazi occupiers in the western part of the Netherlands in 1944–45. Pregnancy data, birth records (including placental weights and birth weights), and daily food ration cards were collected from women across differing trimesters in order to map any developmental 'insults' from 'hostile environments'. The perinatal and gestational data collected (including data from fathers) have been tracked across the lifecourse of the children as they progressed into adult life. Thirty thousand people died as a result of malnutrition and extreme cold, and the children conceived and born during the famine were found to have disproportionally higher rates of adult disease risk, such as diabetes, coronary heart disease, and cancer (with different outcomes dependent on respective trimesters in utero during the famine) [30, 31]. Researchers claim the Dutch Winter famine cohort as an example of intergenerational transmission of adverse exposures that is linked to epigenetic changes.

In the DOHaD context, much attention has been given to epigenetics in relation to transgenerational trauma. Broadly defined, epigenetics is the study of how various external factors, including food, stress, and toxins, alter genetic expression. While interest in the 'science' of trauma was strongly rooted in neurology and neurobiology in the 1980s [24], epigenetics has recently emerged as a popular concept when it comes to attempts to codify trauma in a scientific or biological frame. Epigenetic studies look at how the epigenome is impacted by various factors that modify DNA and the proteins it binds to, therefore affecting how genes are expressed. The most widely studied mechanism through which this occurs is DNA methylation. DNA methylation is often described through the metaphor of a volume knob on a stereo, operating by 'turning down (or even off) certain genes in some cases and turning up other genes in other cases' [32, p. 200–1]. Epigenetics offers a biological pathway for the transmission of impacts of traumatic events from one generation to the next, and also potentially between *more than two* generations (known as '*trans*generational transmission'). Transgenerational epigenetic transmission is established in some non-human models, such as the nematode *C. Elegans* [33, 34], drosophila [35, 36], honeybees [37], and rodents [38–40]. Though well understood in animal models, transgenerational epigenetic transmission in humans is heavily debated. Despite this contestation though, the theory itself – that multiple generations of families and communities hold the epigenetic 'marks' of previous social environments and experiences – is widely discussed in relation to trauma both within and beyond the field of DOHaD.

14.3 Critiques of Trauma: Biopolitics and Pathologisation

Given the rising public and scholarly interest in epigenetic mechanisms of trauma transmission and intergenerational trauma more broadly, it is important to consider some questions related to policy translation, biopolitics, and social justice. While trauma-informed approaches have become increasingly important in DOHaD science and therapeutic interventions globally, researchers must also pay attention to cultural specificity and the limitations of cross-cultural translation. Trauma manifests in bodies in ways that are deeply localised, framed by situated histories, cultures, and modes of embodiment [29]. While instruments to measure stress and trauma are often adapted for local contexts, this is not always effective, with localised idioms of pain and distress rendered illegible [1, 41, p. 18]. Non-Western theories of intergenerational trauma and the holistic epistemologies of embodiment that they derive from, such as 'blood memory' among Native American communities [42] or 'communal wounds' [43] and 'trauma trails' [3] among Indigenous Australians, may likewise be rendered illegible by biomedical definitions and measures that place emphasis on the individualised scale of the patient. Differing cultural concepts of time, reproduction, and kinship that do not rely on colonial imperatives of linear temporalities also need to be considered. Compounding these challenges is the difficulty of measuring trauma when it is ongoing, without a clear beginning or end. For many communities that face intergenerational trauma, violent forces such as colonisation, racism, and socio-economic inequality are not only formations connected to historical events but are ongoing structures of devastation with deeply felt daily impacts.

One of the most pressing interrelated questions around invoking intergenerational trauma in DOHaD is how to effectively translate this into policy in such a way that avoids pathologising individuals and instead addresses ongoing structural inequalities. In the Australian context, with which the authors are most familiar and from where we write, there is considerable concern that 'trauma' and associated concepts such as intergenerational trauma and trauma-informed care are becoming 'buzzwords' that are used in policy discussions but do not lead to any concrete policy changes. Instead, invoking 'trauma' can obfuscate the need to direct attention to specific socio-environmental situations that need to be urgently addressed. The use of 'intergenerational trauma' in particular can lend to a sense that the marginalisation and discrimination that continue to impact the lives of many people are somehow inevitable and fixed [44].

For example, prominent Aboriginal scholar Chelsea Watego recently contended that the strikingly high rate of incarceration of Indigenous people in Australia, which is often described as an 'intergenerational trauma issue', is in fact an 'institutional racism issue' [45]. As seen in this example, there is a risk that trauma is being used as a vague umbrella term that does not name or make explicit the proximate sources of trauma. 'Trauma' can be a euphemism for the experience of forces like racism, poverty, and domestic violence, erasing the perpetrators (individual and/or state) and placing attention on the 'recipient' of the trauma and their capacity to 'manage', rather than on structural injustice and policy failures that need correcting. In the case of DOHaD, where the concept of intergenerational trauma is often invoked in relation to parenting, we are concerned that discourses of trauma can perpetuate increased surveillance of the ability of parents to cope with 'their trauma', rather than keeping the lens squarely focused on the structural conditions that lead to circumstances of difficulty in which families live.

Further, this focus on individual risk factors and parenting is often directed towards women and mothering. In their review of literature on intergenerational trauma in Latinx communities, Cerdeña et al. [1] found that, of the many mechanisms of inter-generational trauma transmission, the 'vast majority center around disrupted maternal behaviour (e.g. maternal distress, maternal substance abuse, harsh parenting) and impaired attachment'. They describe this focus on maternal behaviour as a 'weakness' in DOHaD literature on intergenerational trauma as it fails to account for structural barriers [1, p. 17]. This slippage or trick is a common problem in studies of trauma, and in the DOHaD field more generally. Here, theories attuned to the biosocial are engaged to bring to light structural inequalities and marginalisation at socio-ecological levels (e.g. intergenerational trauma). Yet through the research process the undue focus on individual (and most often, maternal) behaviour as the scale of inquiry routinely propagates reductive frames of individual responsibility.

14.4 Conclusion

Intergenerational trauma is a powerful concept within the scientific fields that contribute to DOHaD research, and within a range of academic disciplines in the humanities and social sciences. The reach and utility of intergenerational trauma is a strength, allowing concepts from DOHaD research to travel far beyond the field and, in turn, to be influenced by many other disciplines concerned with biopolitics and social justice. However, with these strengths come inevitable weaknesses. Intergenerational trauma can be used to denote a cause, a mechanism, an effect, or all three at once. This capaciousness of the concept increases its usefulness to a range of scholars but decreases its precision. When there are attempts to operationalise intergenerational trauma through more precise definitions (e.g. PTSD diagnosis) and measurements (e.g. ACE scales), these can erase certain experiences of trauma, for example, those derived from a range of chronic experiences of racism and marginalisation rather than a discrete historical event. Further, focusing on the effects of intergenerational trauma on individuals often leads to a focus on interventions that seek to improve individual coping mechanisms rather than interventions that address the structural causes of trauma for marginalised groups. This can cause pathologising treatment of these groups as 'inherently' traumatised, paradoxically compounding the effects of intergenerational trauma. Similarly, a focus on pregnancy and maternal care as a mechanism of the transmission of intergenerational trauma can lead to the pathologisation of mothers as inherently risky to their children and as a site of surveillance and interventions.

For intergenerational trauma to be an empowering concept that leads to structural, collective change rather than punitive measures towards individuals, the tendency of DOHaD research and media reporting of this research to focus on mothers' individual behaviours needs to be challenged (see [46–48]). Similarly, the keen interest in intergenerational trauma in DOHaD research should be balanced by stories of survivance and strength from communities that face intergenerational marginalisation. The growing interest in intergenerational trauma among a wide range of scholarly and clinical practitioners provides an opportunity for DOHaD researchers to exert a wide influence. The onus is on DOHaD researchers to ensure this influence leads to outcomes that promote social and reproductive justice.

References

1. Cerdeña J, Rivera L, Spak J. Intergenerational Trauma in Latinxs: A Scoping Review. Social Science & Medicine 2021; 270: 113662.

2. Bombay A, Matheson K, Anisman H. The Intergenerational Effects of Indian Residential Schools: Implications for the Concept of Historical Trauma. Transcultural Psychiatry 2014; 51(3): 320–38.

3. Atkinson J. Trauma Trails, Recreating Song Lines: The Transgenerational Effects of Trauma in Indigenous Australia. Australia: Spinifex Press; 2002.

4. Redvers N, Yellow Bird M, Quinn D, Yunkaporta T, Arabena K. Molecular Decolonization: An Indigenous Microcosm Perspective of Planetary Health. International Journal of Environmental Research and Public Health 2020; 17(12): 4586.

5. Scorza P, Duarte CS, Hipwell AE, Posner J, Ortin A, Canino G, Monk C. Program Collaborators for Environmental influences on Child Health Outcomes. Research Review: Intergenerational Transmission of Disadvantage: Epigenetics and Parents' Childhoods as the First Exposure. Journal of Child Psychology and Psychiatry 2019; 60(2): 119–32.

6. Gone JP, Kirmayer LJ. Advancing Indigenous Mental Health Research: Ethical, Conceptual and Methodological Challenges. Transcultural Psychiatry 2020; 57(2): 235–49.

7. Van Der Kolk B. The Body Keeps the Score: Mind, Brain and Body in the Transformation of Trauma. 1st ed. London: Penguin Press; 2015.

8. Caruth C. Unclaimed Experience: Trauma, Narrative and History. Baltimore: Johns Hopkins University Press; 1996.

9. Cvetkovich A. An Archive of Feelings: Trauma, Sexuality, and Lesbian Public Cultures. Durham, NC: Duke University Press; 2003.

10. Hirsch M. The Generation of Postmemory: Writing and Visual Culture After the Holocaust. New York: Columbia University Press; 2012.

11. Warin M, Moore V, Zivkovic T, Davies M. Telescoping the Origins of Obesity to Women's Bodies: How Gender Inequalities Are Being Squeezed Out of Barker's Hypothesis. Annals of Human Biology 2011; 38(4): 453–60.

12. Yehuda R, Lehrner A. Intergenerational Transmission of Trauma Effects: Putative Role of Epigenetic Mechanisms. World Psychiatry 2018; 17(3): 243–57.

13. Singh G, Morrison, J, Hoy, W. DOHaD in Indigenous Populations: DOHaD, Epigenetics, Equity and Race. Journal of Developmental Origins of Health and Disease 2019; 10(1): 63–64.

14. Phillips-Beck W, Sinclair S, Campbell R, Star L, Cidro J, Wicklow B, Guillemette M, McGavock M. Early-Life Origins of Disparities in Chronic Diseases among Indigenous Youth: Pathways to Recovering Health Disparities from Intergenerational Trauma. Journal of Developmental Origins of Health and Disease 2019; 10(9): 115–22.

15. Lewis AJ, Austin E, Galbally. Prenatal Maternal Mental Health and Fetal Growth Restriction: A Systematic Review. Journal of Developmental Origins of Health and Disease 2016; 7(4): 416–28.

16. Conching AKS, Thayer Z. Biological Pathways for Historical Trauma to Affect Health: A Conceptual Model Focusing on Epigenetic Modifications. Social Science & Medicine 2019; 230: 74–82.

17. Kellerman NP. Psychopathology in Children of Holocaust Survivors. Israel Journal of Psychiatry Related Science 2001; 38(1): 36–46.

18. Clarkin, PF. The Embodiment of War: Growth, Development, and Armed Conflict. Annual Review of Anthropology 2019; 48(1): 423–42.

19. Uwizeye G, Thayer Z, DeVon H, McCreary L, McDade T, Mukamana D, Park C, Patil CL, Rutherford JN. Double Jeopardy: Young Adult Mental and Physical Health Outcomes Following Conception via Genocidal Rape during the 1994 Genocide against the Tutsi in Rwanda. Social Science & Medicine 2021; 278: 113938.

20. Perroud N, Rutembesa E, Paoloni-Giacobino A. The Tutsi Genocide and Transgenerational Transmission of Maternal Stress. World Journal of Biological Psychiatry 2014; 15: 334–45.

21. Kuzawa CW, Sweet E. Epigenetics and the Embodiment of Race: Developmental Origins of US Racial Disparities in Cardiovascular Health. American Journal of Human Biology 2009; 21(1): 2–15.

22. Grossi E. New Avenues in Epigenetic Research on Race: Online Activism around Reparations for Slavery in the United States. Social Science Information 2020; 59(1): 93–116.

23. Karpin I. Vulnerability and the Intergenerational Transmission of Psychosocial Harm. Emory Law Journal 2018; 67(6): 1115–134.

24. Leys R. Trauma: A Genealogy. Chicago: University of Chicago Press; 2000.

25. Leitch L. Action Steps Using ACEs and Trauma-Informed Care: A Resilience Model. Health & Justice 2017; 5(1): 5.

26. Müller R, Kenney M. A Science of Hope? Tracing Emergent Entanglements between the Biology of Early Life Adversity, Trauma-informed Care, and Restorative Justice. Science, Technology, & Human Values 2020; 46(6): 1230–260.

27. Dubois M, Guaspare C. From Cellular Memory to the Memory of Trauma: Social Epigenetics and Its Public Circulation. Social Science Information 2020; 59(1): 144–83.

28. Atkinson J, Nelson J, Atkinson C. Trauma, Transgenerational Transfer and Effects on Community Wellbeing. In: Purdie N, Dudgeon P, Walker R, editors. Working Together: Aboriginal and Torres Strait Islander Mental Health and Wellbeing Principles and Practice. Australia: Telethon Institute of Child Health Research and Australian Government Department of Health and Ageing; 2010.

29. Kim A. How Should We Study Intergenerational Trauma? Reflections on

a 30-Year Birth Cohort Study in Soweto, South Africa. Somatosphere, June 16, 2020, http://somatosphere.net/2020/intergenerational-trauma-birth-cohort-study-south-africa.html/. (Accessed 30 June, 2022).

30. Painter RC, Osmond C, Gluckman P, Hanson M, Phillips DIW, Roseboom TJ. Transgenerational Effects of Prenatal Exposure to the Dutch Famine on Neonatal Adiposity and Health in Later Life. BJOG: An International Journal of Obstetrics & Gynaecology 2008; 115(10): 1243–249.

31. Heijmans BT, Tobi EW, Stein AD, Putter H, Blauw GW, Susser ES, Eline Slagboom P Lumey PH. Persistent Epigenetic Differences Associated with Prenatal Exposure to Famine in Humans. Proceedings of the National Academy of Sciences 2008; 105(44): 17046–7049.

32. Sullivan S. Inheriting Racist Disparities in Health: Epigenetics and the Transgenerational Effects of White Racism. Critical Philosophy of Race 2013; 1(2): 190–218.

33. Woodhouse R, Ashe, A. How Do Histone Modifications Contribute to Transgenerational Epigenetic Inheritance in C. elegans? Biochemical Society Transactions 2020; 48(3): 1019–1034

34. Frolows N, Ashe A. Small RNAs and Chromatin in the Multigenerational Epigenetic Landscape of Caenorhabditis elegans. Philosophical Transactions of the Royal Society B 2021; 376(1826): 20200112.

35. Xing Y, Shi S, Le L, Lee CA, Silver-Morse L, Li WX. Evidence for Transgenerational Transmission of Epigenetic Tumor Susceptibility in Drosophila. PLOS Genetics 2007; 3(9): 1598–606.

36. Ciabrelli F. Transgenerational Epigenetic Inheritance: A Drosophila Tale. Heredity Genetics Current Research, 4th International Congress on Epigenetics and Chromatin, 2018; 7.

37. Remnant EJ, Ashe A, Young PE, Buchmann G, Beekman M, Allsopp M, Suter CM, Drewell R, Oldroyd BP. Parent-of-Origin Effects on Genome-Wide DNA Methylation in the Cape Honey Bee (*Apis mellifera capensis*) May Be Confounded by Allele-Specific Methylation. BMC Genomics 2016; 17: 226.

38. Horsthemke B. A Critical View on Transgenerational Epigenetic Inheritance in Humans. Nature Communications 2018; 9: 2937.

39. Miska EA, Ferguson-Smith AC. Transgenerational Inheritance: Models and Mechanisms of Non-DNA Sequence-based Inheritance. Science 2016; 354: 59–63.

40. Gapp K, Jawaid A, Sarkies P, Bohacek J, Pelczar P, Prados J, Farinelli L, Miska E, Mansuy IM. Implication of Sperm RNAs in Transgenerational Inheritance of the Effects of Early Trauma in Mice. Nature Neuroscience 2014; 17: 667–69.

41. Mendenhall E, Kim AW. How to Fail a Scale: Reflections on a Failed Attempt to Assess Resilience. Culture, Medicine, and Psychiatry 2019; 43(2): 315–25.

42. Thunderbird Partnership Foundation. Indigenous Knowledge & Epigenetics. AFN Mental Wellness Forum 2019.

43. Gilbert S. Ways of Seeing: An Insight into Aboriginality. 2017. www.newcastle.edu.au/profile/stephanie-gilbert (Accessed 30 January 2022).

44. Pentecost M. The Politics of Trauma: Gender, Futurity, and Violence Prevention in South Africa. Medical Anthropology Quarterly 2021; 35(4): 441–57.

45. Watego C. 30 July 2020 tweet. Accessed 15 February 2022. https://twitter.com/drcwatego/status/1288674559852294145

46. Lappé M. Epigenetics, Media Coverage and Parent Responsibilities in the Post-Genomic Era. Current Genetic Medicine Reports 2016; 4(3): 92–97.

47. Warin M, Zivkovic T, Davies M, Moore V. Mothers as Smoking Guns: Fetal Overnutrition and the Reproduction of Obesity. Feminism and Psychology 2012; 22(3): 360–75.

48. Richardson S, Daniels C, Gillman M, Golden J, Kukla R, Kuzawa C, Rich-Edwards J. Don't Blame the Mothers. Nature 2014; 512: 131–32.

Chapter

15

Bioethnography

Elizabeth F.S. Roberts, Jaclyn M. Goodrich, Erica C. Jansen, Belinda L. Needham, Brisa N. Sánchez, and Martha M. Téllez Rojo

Critical social scientists and scholars in medical anthropology, sociology, geography, science technology studies, and feminist theory had hoped that, by moving past genetic reductionism, DOHaD and allied postgenomic frameworks might become a bridge between life and social sciences [1–5]. DOHaD research, however, especially within biomedical paradigms, has often retained a reductive focus on the behaviour of individuals, especially mothers, instead of on the larger political-economic processes and environments that contribute to poor health and exacerbate inequality [6–10]. Additionally, DOHaD researchers, who tend to reside in high-resource environments, often universalise their own experience as they develop research questions and test hypotheses, rather than identifying the most relevant research questions for people living within circumstances quite different from their own.

DOHaD researchers can counteract this reductionism and universalism by incorporating more open-ended, iterative, observational methods into their investigations. Our multidisciplinary team engaged in an environmental health birth cohort study in Mexico City has been developing one such tool, 'bioethnography', which provides DOHaD with an even more powerful and sensitive framework for understanding the relationship of the environment to health outcomes and disease burdens. Our bioethnographic approach combines methods and data from both ethnography and the life sciences to arrive at a better understanding of the larger histories and life circumstances that shape health, disease, and inequality. Unlike most mixed or biocultural methods, where ethnographers are often asked to consult on data after its collection, bioethnography

The authors are deeply grateful for ELEMENT PI, Karen Petersen's support and encouragement in developing this paper, and our bioethnographic approach over the last decade. The various projects described in this paper were made possible by members of the ELEMENT team in Mexico and the United States: Libni Avib Torres Olascoaga, Luis Bautista, Astrid Zamora, Laura Arboleda Merino, Ana Benito, and Adriana Mercado. The team from the NESTSMX project also provided insight and support for practising and theorising bioethnography: David Palma, Mary Leighton, Ernesto Martinez, Alyssa Huberts, Hannah Marcovitch, Faith Cole, Zoe Boudart, Paloma Contreras, Krista Wigginton, Branko Kerkez, and Lesli Scott. This chapter is much stronger through conversations with the editors of this handbook – Michelle Pentecost, Jaya Keaney, Tessa Moll, and Michael Penkler – as well as our workshop exchange buddies Chris Kuzawa and Ayuba Issaka, with members of the Biosocial Birth Cohort Network led by Sahra Gibbon. The bioethnographic efforts we describe here were funded and supported by the Instituto Nacional de Salud Pública, the National Institute of Health, the National Science Foundation, the Wenner Gren, and the University of Michigan through the Institute for Research on Women and Gender, the College of Letters Arts and Sciences, and the Institute for Social Research Center for Group Dynamics.

makes open-ended ethnography a first step, which provides the capacity to generate better hypotheses and better data about the developmental origins of disease.

Ethnographers usually reside long term with or near the people they are learning from, so that they can observe the dynamic environments that shape research participants' lives. Additionally, ethnography tends to entail a wider aperture than focus groups or interviews, because the ethnographer does not predetermine a list of 'standardised' questions in advance. In its beginning stages, ethnography fosters what can seem like an excessive initial vagueness to scientists who are accustomed to deductively posing hypotheses in advance. By approaching a study population in a non-hypothesis-driven fashion, ethnography allows for deeper insights into how, where, when, and why people do what they do. Open-ended observations about a group can provide the basis for collecting more relevant and accurate environmental, quantitative, and biomarker data. While ethnographic findings are produced from a small sample size, they can guide the development of context-specific epidemiological hypotheses and appropriate data collection procedures to test them. In other words, ethnography can be used to generate empirically grounded theories and hypotheses about environmental causal mechanisms, which can then be tested in larger, population-representative samples [11].

A short example of how we have used bioethnography to understand sleep illustrates the process. In 2016, birth cohort researchers began designing a new adolescent sleep survey that asked cohort participants, now teenagers, about length of sleep, perceived sleep quality, technology use before bedtime, and sleep difficulties, which would be combined with accelerometer data. At the initial survey design meetings, the ethnographer, who had lived near and worked with cohort families, noticed that the life science researchers assumed that participants had their own bedrooms, or at most shared them with one other person. Even though the ethnographer had never explicitly studied sleeping arrangements among project participants, she knew that in most participant homes, bedrooms accommodate up to eight people at once. This insight allowed the researchers to include survey questions about bedroom sharing. When the team analysed the data, they found that adolescents who shared a bedroom had lower levels of mental/emotional sleep disturbances than adolescents who did not share a bedroom, which complicates the assumptions embedded in research conducted among middle-class populations that bedroom sharing negatively impacts sleep quality [12, 13]. This collaborative experience prompted the team to design a new bioethnographic sleep study that seeks to characterise the complex social, chemical, and economic ecology of sleep within households in Mexico City.

15.1 Bioethnography's Background

Since 1994, researchers involved in the longitudinal birth cohort study, Early Life Exposures in Mexico to ENvironmental Toxicants (ELEMENT), have carried out chemical or molecular analysis of blood, urine, breast milk, hair, toenails, bone, and teeth, as well as administered questionnaires and psychometric testing on over 1,000 mother-child pairs, mostly living in working-class neighbourhoods in Mexico City [14]. These women and children return for periodic follow-up visits. Initially, ELEMENT researchers focused on the effects of early-life lead exposure on neurological development in childhood (Tellez-Rojo et al., 2002). Over time, ELEMENT expanded to include additional metals, and other chemical exposures, that might affect conditions like diabetes, obesity, menopause, and sleep. Many ELEMENT researchers deploy a DOHaD framework, investigating whether chemical, dietary, or social 'exposures' during pregnancy, infancy, and puberty impact health outcomes [15]. In 2014, a medical anthropologist (Roberts, first author) began collaborating with ELEMENT to carry out long-term ethnographic observations with ELEMENT participants. Roberts aimed to combine her ethnographic findings about the lives of working-class participants with ELEMENT biomarker data. The goal of this 'bioethnographic' process was to ask questions more specific to the study population and to produce better knowledge about dynamic and situated bodily processes in a highly unequal world.

In 2014–2015, Roberts carried out long-term ethnographic work with a subset of six ELEMENT participant families, gathering extensive qualitative data on their everyday lives. This research involved living in participant neighbourhoods and spending three to six hours at a time with specific families, returning multiple days each week over the course of a year, and then follow-up visits ever since. During these visits, Roberts participated in and documented the families' daily routines, including neighbourhood activities, such as festivals and political events, through field notes, photographs, and recordings, which were later thematically coded [16]. After this initial intensive field work year, Roberts began working with ELEMENT researchers to combine ethnographic and biomarker data in projects focused on nutrition, sleep, and household water infrastructure in order to ask research questions that could not be answered through any one data source alone.

Bioethnography then is the combination of two different methodologies – ethnographic observation and biochemical sampling – in an analysis that understands environment–body interactions as always relational, contingent, and constructed phenomena. This combination of methods might sound like other mixed-methods approaches, but bioethnography is more open-ended than combining focus groups or interviews with quantitative data, where the focus and questions have been decided in advance. Additionally, bioethnography avoids designating biomarker data as 'biological' and ethnographic observations as 'social'. Avoiding these domain designations makes it easier to grasp how phenomena like diabetes are produced together through class hierarchy, epigenetic processes, international trade agreements, household organisation, body mass index (BMI), and zoning laws, which are all parts of an 'environment'.

The team's experience with the iterative design and counter-intuitive results of the sleep study described above also demonstrated that bioethnography can reduce one of the biggest unseen challenges to DOHaD and health science investigations more generally. Euro-American researchers tend to be from middle-class backgrounds, which emphasise individual autonomy, while their study subjects tend to be from communities designated as, in some way, marginalised. Without knowing they are doing so, middle-class researchers tend to universalise their own experience and often do not know how to identify the important environmental drivers of the developmental origins of disease. Instead, many focus on what can be easily measured, like the characteristics of individuals (e.g. mother's education or lack of it) or seemingly individual behaviours like sleep or eating, which, in practice, are deeply social.

Our bioethnographic collaborations have allowed us to develop three principles that guide our ongoing research projects: (1) individuals are not necessarily the most meaningful unit of analysis when, beyond households and neighbourhoods, nation-states and political and economic processes shape bodily conditions [17]; (2) biological conditions are as dynamic and historically shaped as any other process; and (3) an open-ended, ethnographically inductive stage before narrowing the aperture to a specific and testable hypothesis is a powerful means of generating robust research questions about the relationship of environment to disease. In the next section, we lay out how these principles can be applied to DOHaD-focused research by using examples from our bioethnographic work within ELEMENT, focused on eating and nutrition.

15.2 A Bioethnographic Approach to Eating and Nutrition

Throughout its first decades, ELEMENT researchers collected data about the diet and nutritional intake of ELEMENT mothers and children through standard methods, including semi-quantitative Food Frequency Questionnaires (FFQs). ELEMENT researchers published papers analysing prenatal and early childhood consumption patterns with health outcomes in adolescence, including body weight, metabolic markers, and timing of sexual maturation [18–20]. In order to understand what biological mechanisms could explain how maternal nutrition during gestation influences children's health, the ELEMENT team examined links between maternal diet and the epigenome (DNA methylation) of the children [21]. In 2013, this research took on additional urgency when the WHO designated Mexico the world's most obese industrial nation.

Soon after this designation, Roberts commenced ethnographic fieldwork in the households of ELEMENT participants and their neighbours. Much of her research focused on how ELEMENT families and their neighbours purchased, prepared, served, shared, and ate food. Roberts' ethnographic findings affirmed what most ethnographies of food have long demonstrated about many non-elite communities: that eating is intrinsically collective [22, 23]. Few eat alone, and food is rarely measured, controlled, organised, or experienced as pertaining to individual health. Eating and sharing food reinforces collective survival, especially in economically precarious environments [24, 25]. In addition, girth and fat are often valued among groups who have experienced past deprivation, and sharing food is a common and potent way to care for others, especially children [26–28].

In light of the importance of shared eating, public messaging on billboards and public-service announcements decrying junk food, especially soda, as unhealthy seemed particularly tone-deaf to how participant households and their neighbours shared food and ate with others. The ubiquity of soda and the need to demonstrate love outweighed health education messages about the harms of soda. By ethnographically following study participants from their households and neighbourhoods to ELEMENT study visits, it was clear that ELEMENT study participants likely underreported consumption of FFQs, especially soda, because participants knew that soda was considered unhealthy by those administering the survey. Likewise, when sugar-sweetened beverages were banned from schools, women hid soda in their children's lunches by putting clear soda in single-use water bottles [28]. These ethnographic observations demonstrated that questionnaire items, such as 'how much soda did you consume last week?', are not likely to produce accurate data. Instead, researchers might develop surveys and questionnaires that ask respondents to describe the crucial elements of different meals or eating/drinking events throughout the day. Or perhaps: who shares in a meal? What do people ideally drink at meals? Who buys it? How much does it cost? Which household members drink what beverages? All of these questions might provide a better portrait of when, how, and why soda is consumed. Additionally, if DOHaD researchers built in ethnographic research early on, even before the recruitment of pregnant women, they would know more about the environments of their study participants, which could help them avoid the unintended moralism so common to survey data collection.

Ethnography also made it easier to see how the abundance of pleasurable foods available to share in working-class households in Mexico City is produced through global processes and trade agreements. Retail and census data have demonstrated that the North American Free Trade Agreement (NAFTA) inundated Mexico City's food landscape with cheap, mass-marketed goods. Following NAFTA, Mexico overall registered increases in caloric intake, particularly for low-income households [29]. In addition, government subsidies in the form of tax incentives, sugar subsidies, and water rights have made soda nearly as cheap as purchased water, and Mexico is now one of the largest per capita soda consumers on earth [30]. Public health researchers' response to this rise in soda consumption continues to focus on individual behaviour as driving this change, in effect continuing to designate mothers (i.e. their soda consumption patterns during pregnancy and the amount of soda they provide to their children) as the relevant environment to understand children's health and development. But what if, instead, DOHaD researchers used longitudinal surveys and biomarker data before and after NAFTA to test the hypothesis that trade agreements like NAFTA are environmental processes that impact disease incidence?

Ethnographic findings about study participants' food environments allowed the team to carry out a new ELEMENT diet and nutrition analysis. In one paper, our bioethnographic team compared ethnographic data about eating with the FFQ data of 550 cohort adolescents to reassess assumptions about diet patterns that standard epidemiological studies correlate with the nutrition transition [31]. The nutrition transition tends to be understood as a process in which people 'choose' to forsake traditional diets for Western diets, which are categorised as distinct dietary patterns. Our bioethnographic approach to understanding eating among cohort participants told a different story.

We found that rather than moving from one dietary pattern to another, the patterns we identified likely reflected the economic status of a household. If we had only carried out an epidemiological analysis, we might have characterised participants with a higher score on the plant-based and lean protein dietary pattern as choosing to follow an overall 'healthy' or 'traditional' diet. By including ethnographic data, we found, however, that adolescents with a higher score on this pattern likely lived in more economically stable households, where there were enough resources to prepare a large afternoon meal for sharing, with leftovers remaining for subsequent days. Furthermore, it was evident that in all household diets and meals there were elements of 'Westernised' and 'traditional' foods. This co-occurrence suggests that instead of adopting a more 'Westernised' pattern of eating and living, households may simply be incorporating available and affordable 'Western' foods into their typical meals. In sum, our bioethnographic findings challenged understandings about the nutrition transition as coming from individual preference or that families make clear-cut distinctions between traditional and Western foods. Importantly, our findings allowed us to call for more attention to how economic processes alter eating.

In another paper, we examined the range of other factors besides maternal body mass (understood in DOHaD terms as the outcome of biology and behaviour) that contribute to children's body mass [32]. The rapid worldwide increase in obesity in the last three decades, particularly in Mexico, suggests that forces beyond the biology and behaviour of mothers are at play in shaping weight. Our ethnographic data showed how transformations in Mexico's food landscape made it easier than ever before for parents to provide children with cheap pleasurable processed foods and that at least 38 per cent of children's BMI is not linkable to heritable factors like mother's BMI. Attempts then at intervening in 'food' choices of mothers and families are less likely to be effective without interventions on the upstream drivers of diet and food availability, such as curtailing tax subsidies to transnational food and beverage corporations.

The bioethnographic findings of these two papers helped elucidate our first two principles for bioethnographic research described above: (1) eating and nutrition must not be understood through the lens of individual choice, and (2) biological conditions are inseparable from social processes. The effect of NAFTA on body mass over time makes it clear that metabolic processes are not separate from political economic processes, and trying to tease out the biological and social determinants of body mass may lead to missing the larger context producing the phenomena under question [33, 34]. In other words, the developmental origins of adult diseases such as obesity are not located solely, or even primarily, in the 'maternal environment'.

Additionally, our initial papers on eating and nutrition provided support for our third principle that ethnography can become a key driver for iteratively producing research questions, collecting data, and interpreting results, which then can generate hypotheses that are locally situated in the lived experiences of the study's participants. In 2017, we commenced a larger scale bioethnographic project – developed through initial ethnographic observations – that in working-class communities in Mexico City, water tends to arrive intermittently, with complex effects. Household members experienced water as unreliable and unhealthy even though state authorities declare that at least 85 per cent of the nation receives water that is safe to drink [35]. We also found that within the context of the advertising, ubiquity, reliability, and palatability of soda, drinking tap water made little sense.

These observations about the complex reality of water in working-class neighbourhoods have formed the basis for the bioethnographic study, 'Neighbourhood Environments as Socio-Techno-Bio Systems: Water Quality, Public Trust, and Health in Mexico City' (NESTSMX). NESTSMX combines ethnographic, environmental health, and environmental engineering methods to better understand the discrepancy between health messaging on the benefits and safety of water and residents' distrust in water. Over the course of three years, we carried out multiple visits in 60 ELEMENT households (a large 'n' by ethnographic standards), collecting water quality, real-time water sensors, biometrics, health biomarkers (epigenetic and cortisol), and ethnographic data pertaining to the household and neighbourhood water environment [36]. So far, our findings demonstrate that within these 60 households, water intermittency and low water pressure compel residents to install domestic water management infrastructure – that is storage units, tubing, and pumps – which can negatively impact water quality. When water stagnates at collection points, chlorine disperses, providing an excellent environment for bacterial growth. There are also indications that specific kinds of water intermittency might impact water quality: for example, receiving water a few days a week might encourage more harmful bacteria growth in storage units. Household residents, especially the adult women who manage water provisioning, are quite familiar with the signs of water quality deterioration, which contributes to their distrust of tap water. These complex biosocial findings point to how intermittency might contribute to making soda a more sensible choice than water and might contribute to the incidence of chronic diseases, like diabetes. Our team is currently collaborating with the Encuesta Nacional de Salud y Nutrición (ENSANUT) to examine the impact of water intermittency on health, gender, and economic dynamics at a national scale.

Our complex bioethnographic understanding of intermittency has been made possible through our open-ended ethnographic process. If we only carried out surveys about attitudes or beliefs about water, just collected biomarker data, or only conducted an ethnography of eating and drinking, we would have foreclosed the possibility of understanding the complex reasons people drink soda or bottled water. With NESTSMX, we can apprehend how food environments – now dominated by multinational corporations, as well as urban planning and domestic architecture – dramatically shape what and how people drink in Mexico City. NESTSMX's bioethnographic approach demonstrates that taking time to ascertain the *relevant* complex early life environments is a powerful means to understand health and disease over the lifecourse.

15.3 Bioethnography and Causal Mechanisms

The open-ended and iterative nature of bioethnography serves as a 'seed bed' for understanding and potentially measuring 'the how and the why'; in other words, what meaningfully shapes early life environments that contribute to later life disease [37, 359]. Most epidemiologically informed DOHaD studies deploy standard regression techniques that attempt to isolate the unidirectional effect of an exposure (e.g. maternal diet during pregnancy) on an outcome (e.g. offspring BMI) [38, 39]. Few pay attention to participants' bodies as dynamically situated in a specific time and space. By providing a means to examine how or why phenomena cause and are caused by more than one variable within a particular context, bioethnography enables the development and testing of context-specific theories behind these complex interrelationships.

Implementing an early open-ended ethnographic period can be used to develop theory-based hypotheses and to test causal mechanisms in specific contexts. For example, it is often assumed that proximity to supermarkets supports healthy diets. With this assumption in place, researchers have developed a suite of tools to measure the relationship of individual dietary intake to contextual factors like supermarket proximity. Ethnographic observations of ELEMENT participants revealed, however, that supermarket access might actually be detrimental to healthy eating patterns among people in working-class neighbourhoods in Mexico City. In these neighbourhoods, women procure fresh produce available from open-air mobile markets and procure sodas and processed food from supermarkets, where they are cheaper compared to their neighbourhood corner stores. In addition to measuring the proximity of supermarkets, which has become standard in food environment research, investigators could deploy ethnographic work early on to make more context-specific measures of food outlets and their role. By also including economic processes such as the displacement of mobile markets with supermarkets as part of the dynamic food environment, researchers can move beyond individual behaviour and develop a more accurate picture of the causal mechanisms behind nutritional intake that develop over time.

Open-ended bioethnographic research can identify more relevant, sensitive measures of behavioural mechanisms and improve upon a standard set of variables that are otherwise assumed to be universalisable from one context to another. After this open-ended stage, epidemiological methods can be implemented to test the generalisability of ethnographic observations in larger study populations. During survey question development and testing, bioethnographic research teams can test survey validity through cross-referencing responses to survey items with ethnographic observations of daily life on a sample of study participants. Such cross-referencing could also be used to further refine and extend survey instruments. Ultimately, the more comprehensive bioethnographically informed and highly granular data that are specific to the context and population under study can be used to statistically test causal mechanisms using traditional epidemiological methods. Validating and testing theories derived from ethnographic observations of mechanisms in the same population where they were observed can fill critical gaps in studies that associate environments with health and disease over the lifecourse.

15.4 Conclusion

As we have detailed elsewhere, there are enormous challenges to proposing, designing, and carrying out bioethnographic research [16, 37, 40]. Investigators in the life and social sciences are situated in radically different research ecologies with different obligations, incentive structures, epistemological assumptions, funding mechanisms, and research models and practices, all of which can pose challenges to interdisciplinary collaboration. Publishing can be difficult because of the specific disciplinary demands of journals around acceptable data sources and writing style. Perhaps the biggest challenge of all is how funding mechanisms are structured. For instance, in the United States, NIH funding requires researchers to narrow their research questions into specific aims and testable hypotheses in advance, which make it difficult to develop a comprehensive understanding of the complex environmental processes that shape the lifecourse. So far, our bioethnographic research within ELEMENT has been funded through the National Science Foundation and internal university sources. These sources, however, do not typically provide enough funds to carry out bioethnographic work with a large enough sample size for validity in life science research.

The challenges to bioethnographic research posed by structural issues like funding result in the exact reductionism and universalism that bioethnographic research seeks to overcome. Addressing these difficult issues is crucial, so that DOHaD researchers can adopt more open-ended and iterative approaches like bioethnography to ask better questions, produce better data, and arrive at more comprehensive knowledge about how environmental processes shape health and disease over the lifecourse.

References

1. Lock M. The Epigenome and Nature/Nurture Reunification: A Challenge for Anthropology. Medical Anthropology. 2013;32:291–308.

2. Landecker H, Panofsky A. From Social Structure to Gene Regulation, and Back: A Critical Introduction to Environmental Epigenetics for Sociology. Annual Review of Sociology. 2013;39:333–57.

3. Niewohner J. Epigenetics: Embedded Bodies and the Molecularisation of Biography and Milieu. BioSocieties. 2011;6:279–98.

4. Meloni M. How Biology Became Social, and What It Means for Social Theory. The Sociological Review. 2014;62 (3):593–614.

5. Jablonka E, Lamb MJ. Evolution in Four Dimensions : Genetic, Epigenetic,

Behavioral, and Symbolic Variation in the History of Life. Cambridge, MA: MIT Press; 2005.

6. Lamoreaux J. Reproducing Toxicity. Environmental History. 2021 Jul;26 (3):437–43.

7. Mansfield B. Race and the New Epigenetic Biopolitics of Environmental Health. BioSocieties. 2012;7(4):352–72.

8. Paxson H, Helmreich S. The Perils and Promises of Microbial Abundance: Novel Natures and Model Ecosystems, from Artisanal Cheese to Alien Seas. Social Studies of Science. 2014;44(2):165–93.

9. Pentecost M. The New Trial Communities: Challenges and Opportunities in Preconception Cohorts [Internet]. Somatosphere. 2021 [cited 9 Nov 2021]. Available from: http://somatosphere.net/2021/birth-cohort-studies-new-communites-pentecost.html/

10. Valdez N. Weighing the Future: Race, Science, and Pregnancy Trials in the Postgenomic Era. First ed. Oakland: University of California Press; 2021. 284 p.

11. Krieger N, Davey Smith G. The Tale Wagged by the DAG: Broadening the Scope of Causal Inference and Explanation for Epidemiology. International Journal of Epidemiology. 2016 1 Dec;45(6):1787–808.

12. Zamora AN, Arboleda-Merino L, Tellez-Rojo MM, O'Brien LM, Torres-Olascoaga LA, Peterson KE, et al. Sleep Difficulties among Mexican Adolescents: Subjective and Objective Assessments of Sleep. Behaviour Sleep Medicine. 2021 13 May;2:1–21.

13. Chung S, Wilson KE, Miller AL, Johnson D, Lumeng JC, Chervin RD. Home Sleeping Conditions and Sleep Quality in Low-Income Preschool Children. Sleeping Medical Research. 2014 30 Jun;5 (1):29–32.

14. Perng W, Tamayo-Ortiz M, Tang L, Sánchez BN, Cantoral A, Meeker JD, et al. Early Life Exposure in Mexico to ENvironmental Toxicants (ELEMENT) Project. BMJ Open. 2019 1 Aug;9(8): e030427.

15. Goodrich JM, Dolinoy D, Sanhez B, Zang ZZ, Mercado-Garcia A, Solano-Gonzalez M, et al. Adolescent Epigenetic Profiles and Environmental Exposures from Early Life through Peri-adolescence. Environmental Epigenetics. 2016;2(3). https://academic.oup.com/eep/article/2/3/dvw018/2415066

16. Roberts EFS, Sanz C. Bioethnography: A How To Guide for the Twenty-First Century. In: Meloni M, editor. A Handbook of Biology and Society. London: Palgrave Macmillan; 2017.

17. Diez-Roux AV. Multilevel Analysis in Public Health Research. Annual Review in Public Health. 2000;21:171–92.

18. Cantoral A, Téllez-Rojo MM, Ettinger AS, Hu H, Hernández-Ávila M, Peterson K. Early Introduction and Cumulative Consumption of Sugar-sweetened Beverages during the Pre-school Period and Risk of Obesity at 8–14 Years of Age. Pediatric Obesity. 2016 Feb;11 (1):68–74.

19. Jansen EC, Zhou L, Perng W, Song PX, Rojo MMT, Mercado A, et al. Vegetables and Lean Proteins-Based and Processed Meats and Refined Grains-Based Dietary Patterns in Early Childhood Are Associated with Pubertal Timing in a Sex-Specific Manner: A Prospective Study of Children from Mexico City. Nutritional Research. 2018 Aug;56:41–50.

20. Mulcahy MC, Tellez-Rojo MM, Cantoral A, Solano-González M, Baylin A, Bridges D, et al. Maternal Carbohydrate Intake during Pregnancy Is Associated with Child Peripubertal Markers of Metabolic Health But Not Adiposity. Public Health Nutrition. 2021 24 Nov;9:1–13.

21. Wu Y, Sánchez BN, Goodrich JM, Dolinoy DC, Cantoral A, Mercado-Garcia A, et al. Dietary Exposures, Epigenetics and Pubertal Tempo. Environmental Epigenetics. 2019 Jan;5(1):dvz002.

22. Carsten J. The Substance of Kinship and the Heat of the Hearth: Feeding, Personhood, and Relatedness among Malays in Pulau Langkawi. American Ethnologist. 1995;22(2):223–41.

23. Weismantel M. Making Kin: Kinship Theory and Zumbagua Adoptions. American Ethnologist. 1995;22(4):685–704.

24. Carney MA. The Unending Hunger: Tracing Women and Food Insecurity Across Borders. Oakland: University of California Press; 2015. 272 p.

25. Fielding-Singh P. How the Other Half Eats: The Untold Story of Food and Inequality in America. New York: Little, Brown Spark; 2021. 352 p.

26. Kulick D, Meneley A. Fat : The Anthropology of an Obsession. New York: Jeremy P. Tarcher/Penguin; 2005. p. 246 p.

27. Yates-Doerr E. The Weight of Obesity Hunger and Global Health in Postwar Guatemala. Oakland: University of California Press; 2015.

28. Roberts EFS. Food is Love: And So, What Then? BioSocieties. 2015;10:247–52.

29. Berrigan D, Arteaga SS, Colón-Ramos U, Rosas LG, Monge-Rojas R, O'Connor TM, et al. Measurement Challenges for Childhood Obesity Research Within and Between Latin America and the United States. Obesity Review. 2021 Jun;22(Suppl 3):e13242.

30. Delgado S. México, primer consumidor de refrescos en el mundo [Internet]. Gaceta UNAM. 2019 [cited 16 Dec 2022]. Available from: www.gaceta.unam.mx/mexico-primer-consumidor/

31. Jansen E, Marcovitch H, Wolfson J, Leighton M, Peterson K, Téllez-Rojo M, et al. An Analysis of Dietary Patterns in a Mexican Adolescent Population: A Mixed Methods Approach. Appetites. 2020;

32. Téllez-Rojo MM, Trejo-Valdivia B, Roberts E, Muñoz-Rocha TV, Bautista-Arredondo LF, Peterson KE, et al. Influence of Post-Partum BMI Change on Childhood Obesity and Energy Intake. PLOS ONE. 2019 Dec 12;14(12):e0224830.

33. Gálvez A. Eating NAFTA: Trade, Food Policies, and the Destruction of Mexico.

1st ed. Oakland: University of California Press; 2018. 288 p.

34. Vaughan M, Adjaye-Gbewonyo K, Mika M, editors. Epidemiological Change and Chronic Disease in Sub-Saharan Africa: Social and Historical Perspectives. London: UCL Press; 2021. 378 p.

35. Espinosa-Garcia AC, Diaz-Avalos C, Villarreal FG, Malvaez-Orozco RVS, Mazari-Hiriart M. Drinking Water Quality in a Mexico City University Community: Perception and Preferences. EcoHealth. 2015;12:88–97.

36. Martinez Paz EF, Tobias M, Escobar E, Raskin L, Roberts EFS, Wigginton KR, et al. Wireless Sensors for Measuring Drinking Water Quality in Building Plumbing: Deployments and Insights from Continuous and Intermittent Water Supply Systems. ACS EST Eng. 24 Oct 2021;acsestengg.1c00259.

37. Roberts EFS. Making Better Numbers Through Bioethnographic Collaboration. American Anthropologis. 2021;123(2):355–59.

38. Clark J, Martin E, Bulka CM, Smeester L, Santos HP, O'Shea TM, et al. Associations between Placental CpG Methylation of Metastable Epialleles and Childhood Body Mass Index Across Ages One, Two and Ten in the Extremely Low Gestational Age Newborns (ELGAN) Cohort. Epigenetics. 2019 Nov;14(11):1102–11.

39. Strohmaier S, Bogl LH, Eliassen AH, Massa J, Field AE, Chavarro JE, et al. Maternal Healthful Dietary Patterns During Peripregnancy and Long-Term Overweight Risk in Their Offspring. European Journal of Epidemiology. 2020;35(3):283–93.

40. Leighton M, Roberts E. Trust and Distrust in Multi-disciplinary Collaboration: Some Feminist Reflections. Catalyst: Catalyst: Feminism, Theory, Technoscience [Internet]. 2020;6(2):1–27. Available from: https://catalystjournal.org/index.php/catalyst/article/view/32956/26855

Chapter

Translating Evidence to Policy
The Challenge for DOHaD Advocacy

16

Felicia Low, Peter Gluckman, and Mark Hanson

16.1 Introduction: DOHaD over Two Decades

Maternal, newborn, child, and adolescent health (MNCAH) is clearly established to be a driver of health across the lifecourse and generations [1]. It is now 20 years since the founding of the International DOHaD Society, based on the research themes of the Fetal Origins of Adult Disease (FOAD) established by David Barker and others at the end of the last century. From its inception, Developmental Origins of Health and Disease (DOHaD) research largely focused initially on metabolic control and the major organ systems, such as cardiovascular, lung, and kidney; it also focused on pathophysiology rather than on normal development. It took some time for the incorporation of phenotypic variation in normal development to be recognised as part of the continuum of adaptive and maladaptive developmental plasticity [2, 3]. Similarly, the field has been slow to recognise that the same conceptual paradigm applied to the effects of developmental processes on brain development and socio-emotional health – with effects in the short term on infant and early childhood neurocognitive, emotional, and behavioural development – and then on school readiness, educational attainment, employment prospects, and wider contributions or costs to society [4, 5]. [See also Cohen in this volume.]

Research in DOHaD accords with other agendas that have developed in parallel over the last two decades, such as The First 1000 days and Best Start to Life [6, 7]. It is referred to in the 2011 UN Political Declaration on the Prevention and Control of NCDs [8], the 2015 Global Strategy for Women's, Children's and Adolescents' Health [9], and the 2016 report of the WHO Commission on Ending Childhood Obesity [10]. From this point of view, it could be argued that DOHaD has already been translated to inform policymaking at an international level. However, it has only been referred to in very general terms rather than indicating or identifying specific interventions, and so it has not influenced policymaking significantly. Even the lifecourse concept that underlies DOHaD has not been widely adopted within health policies, for example in Europe where a specific review was commissioned [11].

Although the epidemiological observations of Barker and other researchers in FOAD and DOHaD initially focused on high-income countries (HICs), it was clear from the outset that the insights into the impact of early development on later health and disease would be even greater in low-middle-income countries, especially as their societies passed through nutritional and economic transitions towards aspects of HIC lifestyles [12]. From this standpoint, much of DOHaD thinking was reflected in the Sustainable Development Goals (SDGs; e.g. Target 3.4 that aims to reduce by one-third premature mortality from NCDs by 2030). Again this was largely aspirational and not linked to specific actions. Since 2015, many additional challenges to health have arisen globally, in particular those stemming from the COVID-19 pandemic, continuing food insecurity, the accelerating impact of climate change and environmental degradation, and conflict and economic factors leading to large-scale migrations. The midterm evaluation of progress towards attaining the SDGs shows that insufficient progress has been made [5] and most areas of MNCAH have even deteriorated [13].

An aspect that is only now receiving significant attention concerns the ethical, moral, and social justice arguments for advocating greater policy focus on the application of DOHaD science. (See Chiapperino et al. and Kenney and Müller in this volume.) Many forms of disadvantage are passed across generations in multiple ways, and this raises questions about individual and societal responsibilities to protect the environment and the health prospects of future generations. DOHaD research has extended our understanding of intergenerational disadvantage, including the biological mechanisms by which environmental influences can project across generations to have significant implications for their future well-being. Examples of these mechanisms include having a shared nutritional environment [14], microbiota transfer [15], and the influences of maternal mental state on offspring brain development [16]. Epigenetic processes may play a role in embedding these intergenerational embodiments of disadvantage [17].

Maternal, newborn, child, and adolescent health is particularly vulnerable to the detrimental effects of challenges faced by societies, as is clear from the effects of COVID-19, climate change, and conflict, all of which are known to exacerbate pre-existing inequalities in MNCAH. Examples from COVID-19 include unplanned pregnancies resulting from lack of access to contraception, missed child vaccinations, teenage girls dropping out of school, and domestic violence [18]. DOHaD insights therefore provide an understanding of how the bedrock of social and economic resilience of societies to such challenges, now and in the future, can be undermined, and make a powerful argument for greater investment in MNCAH during socio-economic shocks [19].

The UN Global Strategy for Women's, Children's and Adolescents' Health (2016–2030) states that economic investment in this area will yield a tenfold return [9] (but see the chapter by Cohen in this volume). This argument is based on the long-standing work of the Nobel Laureate in Economics Professor James Heckman and his team; even so there are compelling reasons to think this may be an underestimate [20, 21].

For these reasons, DOHaD researchers need to equip themselves to argue that their research and concepts should inform health and wider policymaking. To a great extent, this has not happened. Here we discuss why.

16.2 Understanding the Role of Scientists in Policymaking

Translating scientific knowledge and evidence into policy is far from straightforward. Science alone rarely makes policy; there are always considerations that extend well beyond the ambit of science and that mostly lie with policymakers and society [22, 23]. While science itself is not value-free, many other value-based considerations influence decision-making. All policymaking involves making a choice (including whether to act or not), and in making such choices, decision-makers must assess which stakeholders benefit from a decision, and which do not. This is core to the political dimension of policymaking [24].

Science has its own distinct cultures, methods, and epistemologies and is not simply a matter of assimilating 'facts' universally agreed by researchers [25]. Even though it may be badged as objective, in reality science too involves value judgements, for example over what questions to investigate and how to do so, and especially over the sufficiency and quality of evidence from which to draw conclusions [26]. Such values – which may vary between disciplines, research teams, or institutions – shape the knowledge about which there is consensus. Policymakers also have their own cultures and values, which are likely to accord more closely with wider social values than with those of scientific researchers. Faced with this potential gap, there is increasing recognition of the need for boundary structures and processes to broker the interchange between science and policy [23].

Scientific data, however robust, do not equal information, or the knowledge and evidence that policymakers will accept as sufficiently important or compelling to necessitate a potential policy initiative. Moreover, policymakers have many sources of information in addition to that from scientists – tradition and beliefs, local knowledge, anecdotes, and the personal representations made to them all the time by a range of stakeholders or 'experts'. Science is but one source of such information, and when it is constantly contested, by scientists themselves as well as other constituencies and wider dissemination of misinformation, its impact is diminished. Scientists should not put the policymaker in the position of being a scientific referee as this will lead to uncertainty and inaction [23].

It is therefore more important than ever for scientists to understand how policy-making works, recognising that it is not a linear process and does not necessarily have clear or straightforward objectives. It is usually shaped by acute external factors, as well as by political and societal values. In addition, politicians increasingly must make decisions on a very short timescale, perhaps even a few days for major issues, with suboptimal information and little opportunity to consult experts. They are unlikely to be trained in scientific methodology. They will have to depend on input from civil servants, who may have considerable experience but who may also bring their own agendas and reflect departmental priorities.

Policymaking is thus essentially about making choices between different options that affect different stakeholders in different ways, and with different consequences, many of which are not certain. Virtually all policymaking involves complexity, uncertainty, and a degree of risk. But perceptions of complexity and risk vary, not only between scientists and policymakers but also between government departments too: a policy that seems to carry a low risk for the treasury may have an unacceptably high risk for a defence department.

The so-called 'policy cycle' almost never operates as is sometimes suggested in textbooks, and perhaps it never did except in the minds of theorists [22]. The cycle (awareness raising > problem definition > identification of options > policy selection > implementation > evaluation) is manifestly cumbersome and time-consuming and requires consensus and concerted action across government departments. Getting beyond the mindset of the policy cycle first requires recognition of the complex nature of policymaking and ensuring that awareness-raising by scientists addresses what policymakers need.

There are two distinct components to translating evidence to policymaking: evidence synthesis and evidence brokerage. Evidence synthesis must be much more than a narrow summary from a single field of science. It must be pluralistic and consider all the domains that might impact on achieving a policy goal and the questions that will matter to a policymaker (e.g. direct and indirect impact, effect size, and so forth). Evidence brokerage requires individuals who are skilled in the language and needs of both the policy and scientific communities and are able to translate between them. This requires what has often been called honest brokerage [27]. The basis of effective brokerage is being clear about what the science shows, what questions it does not answer, and what options emerge from it [23].

Problem definition by scientists does not help the policymaker. They expect the science community to present solutions they can enact. So when problems are presented they must be accompanied by solutions that are scalable, impactful, and supportable both ideologically and by a broad range of stakeholders [22]. In general, this favours attention to problems that have an identifiable single solution rather than a complex and complicated set of potential solutions. Yet, DOHaD science is unlikely to deliver simple single interventions with significant impact; rather it indicates the need for a broad shift in attitude and priorities within the policy and political community. A further complexity is that while interventions must be early in the lifecourse, the economic return accumulates over many subsequent decades [20, 28, 29]. Indeed, as has been suggested in areas such as climate change, issues where the return is in the distant future are unlikely to secure urgent political attention [30]. This is not helped by the use of discounting in economic forecasting [31], which argues against the deployment of funds to address long-term objectives, especially those affecting the beginning of life.

16.3 Translating DOHaD: What Do Policymakers Need from Scientists?

Any solution to a problem presented to policymakers must be based on a high degree of scientific consensus. This is seldom the case; scientific research by its nature competes for funding and recognition. Thus policymakers will be justifiably suspicious if the suggested solution is simply a disguised request for more funds for an area of research.

Even where there is consensus within the scientific community, it must still be presented to policymakers without hubris, condescension, or alarmist speculation. Wherever possible, economic and societal-value considerations of the proposed solutions need to be included, but again these should not stray beyond evidence. The gathering of such evidence may require participatory research, for example with a population or patient group, but this is time-consuming and raises its own methodological problems, especially where children and adolescents are concerned. (See Tu'akoi et al. in this volume.)

DOHaD science in many ways has not matured to the point where this participation has been achieved. Nor has the scale of the solution to the problem it encompasses been adequately defined. For example, while it is widely accepted that the risk of later NCDs has in part its origin in early life, and while there is no dispute that over 70 per cent of deaths globally every year result from NCDs [32], the contribution of DOHaD processes to the risk, *vis a vis* unhealthy lifestyles in adulthood and genetic variation, is not really known. This needs to be addressed if future advocacy is to be effective. At present, the strongest advocacy for DOHaD involves the counterfactual, based on untestable assumptions; that is the health and financial cost of inaction rather than the benefits of action.

DOHaD is a multidimensional issue, so interventions to address it will be complex. However, there is a lack of compelling research showing the benefit of such interventions. Rather, based on the evidence to date, a likely programme of intervention would involve a diffuse set of recommendations for preconception health for both parents, pregnancy management, nutrition, and nurturing care for the early years. Recommendations involve in part changing individual behaviour and in part structural issues concerning inequality and intergenerational disadvantage; these are holistic issues that challenge all governments and societies. There are no good precedents on which advocacy can be based.

DOHaD science will inevitably suffer from the fact that it advocates for preventive measures to address future burdens of ill health. Policymakers are not likely to act on prevention measures other than vaguely agreeing that 'prevention is better than cure' [33]. Because the benefits of an intervention based on DOHaD science will accrue at some point in the future well beyond the duration of an electoral cycle or two, it is unlikely to convey any sense of urgency. For this reason, DOHaD advocacy needs to encompass the short- (e.g. pregnancy outcomes and socio-emotional health in the pre-school years), medium- (educational attainment, adolescent health, and well-being), and longer-term (NCDs) implications of its evidence.

A first question policymakers will inevitably ask when presented with the evidence for a solution will be the following: given all the competing demands on resources and the interests of a range of stakeholders, do they need to do anything about it and, if so, when? As in other areas of advocacy for a cause, the evidence behind the message is only one aspect of the process; at least as important can be who is conveying the message and how it is framed. Clearly DOHaD needs to employ its most influential spokespersons, but it also needs to couch its messages in terms of other policy issues that are relevant, such as climate change, the impact of pandemics such as COVID-19, economic development, and ongoing conflicts and migration. Each of these has detrimental effects on population health and economic consequences, and each raises questions of equity and social justice [34–36]. There is a strong argument that each of these challenges has the most pronounced short- and longer-term effects on MNCAH, and therefore insights from DOHaD research could be highly relevant to mitigating such effects.

It has to be recognised that most advocacy-based approaches to policymakers fail. Persistence and reshaping the brief with relevant influential stakeholders therefore need to be the key aspects of the process, built in from the start. It can be helpful to ensure that a multiple streams theory approach is adopted, by which the domains or streams of problem, policy, and political components are included [37]. It may then be necessary to wait for a window of opportunity to open, for example as a result of external events, which makes a change in policy desirable, necessary, or appropriate, so making reception of an advocacy approach more likely to be positive. Successful approaches usually involve a collaboration between and consensus among a range of groups. Therefore, DOHaD advocates need to work with allies and form allegiances in ways that have not been undertaken to date. Even more important is to work towards providing advocacy for 'the right intervention at the right time'. In practice, this means considering how a particular policy initiative might align with other ongoing initiatives. Spillover benefits may be critical, for example plans to address childhood obesity may have benefits for educational attainment.

While DOHaD has a broad agenda and relevance globally, nonetheless from a practical point of view any advocacy initiatives must be relevant and deliverable at a local level. This may involve comparisons between populations or regions and perhaps include accountability for previous commitments. DOHaD advocacy needs to link to ongoing initiatives and be locally adaptable as well as globally relevant.

16.4 An Alternate and Complementary Approach: Devolved Solutions

DOHaD science effectively argues for a greater focus on the state of the parents before conception and on the support of the parent and infant in multiple ways through and after pregnancy, in the expectation that the offspring's potential through life will be protected or enhanced. Indeed, many of the later costs to that individual and to society are predictable from the age of about three [5, 38]. But the interventions needed are complex and context dependent. What might be appropriate in terms of nutritional advice for a family in a high-income country is not the same as that needed in a country where food insecurity is endemic. And even within a high-income country, there will be large foci of nutritional deficiencies within some components of the community. Further the very nature of the DOHaD challenge requires a multilateral approach that is both universal and targeted. For example, to focus on nutrition and not to consider emotional stress would be unlikely to improve outcomes significantly. That said, the DOHaD agenda aligns with wider issues of great concern, such as environmental despoliation and climate change, the impact of climate change, COVID-19, and the current cost of living crisis [39].

It is difficult in the current state of DOHaD knowledge to get beyond the conclusion that most progress will be made through local action. Certainly, this needs government support, but communities are in the position in many places to identify needs and to take action. However, this requires a new form of partnership with the science community, one that is meaningful and involves, codesign, respect for lay input, and a long-term commitment. This type of action-focused transdisciplinary research is neither easy to do nor easy to fund. It requires researchers to get out of their comfort zones, and it requires a commitment to long-term engagement, which in turn does not fit well with traditional academic incentives. Building trust with a community, adjusting scientific ideas to local knowledge and expertise, and through a local cultural lens can require sustained commitment before anything concrete can be planned. Many issues here outside the scope of this review are discussed in this handbook and elsewhere [40]. Yet if the DOHaD community is to see its knowledge turned into action, local engagement offers a productive and rewarding pathway. In turn, with a local focus, a broader form of advocacy for wider action is created.

16.5 Final Comments

Since the field first emerged, most DOHaD research has been premised and designed on the assumption that a singular developmental trigger would change biology with specific latter outcomes that manifest under particular conditions [41]. That model assumed that devising a singular intervention might be possible. But, 35 years on, it is clear that subsumed within the DOHaD 'space' are multiple and overlapping ways in which the developmental trajectory can be affected that in turn can have variable impacts later depending on genetic influences and later environmental exposures. With this understanding comes the need to think differently about how DOHaD knowledge enters the public domain. This requires partnership with others committed to the MNCAH field and translation of DOHaD knowledge and advocacy into a greater awareness of the importance of intergenerational health and circumstance. The solutions needed do not involve singular interventions and will require a reorientation of society and community values. An approach in part focused on the community, in part on the policymaker, is required. The DOHaD research community itself must now also evolve to meet these obligations.

References

1. Godfrey, K.M. et al. (eds.), Developmental Origins of Health and Disease, 2nd ed. 2022, Cambridge, UK: Cambridge University Press.

2. Bateson, P., et al., Developmental plasticity and human health. Nature, 2004. 430(6998): pp. 419–21.

3. Gluckman, P.D., M.A. Hanson, and T. Buklijas, A conceptual framework for the Developmental Origins of Health and Disease. Journal of Developmental Origins of Health and Disease, 2010. 1(1): pp. 6–18.

4. Low, F., P. Gluckman, and R. Poulton, Executive Functions: A Crucial But Overlooked Factor for Lifelong Wellbeing. 2021. Auckland: Koi Tū: The Centre for Informed Futures.

5. Moffitt, T., R. Poulton, and A. Caspi, Lifelong impact of early self-control. American Scientist, 2013. 101(5): pp. 352–59.

6. FHI Solutions. 1,000 days. [cited 12 January 2023]; Available from: https:// thousanddays.org/.

7. Early Years Healthy Development Review. The best start for life: A vision for the 1,001 critical days. The Early Years Healthy Development review report. 2021, London: Department of Health and Social Care.

8. United Nations General Assembly, Resolution adopted by the General Assembly on 19 September 2011. 66/2. Political Declaration of the High-level Meeting of the General Assembly on the Prevention and Control of Non-communicable Diseases. 2012.

9. Every Woman Every Child, The Global Strategy for Women's, Children's and Adolescents' Health (2016–2030). 2015, New York: Every Woman Every Child.

10. World Health Organization, Report of the Commission on Ending Childhood Obesity. 2016, Geneva: World Health Organization.

11. Jacob, C.M., et al., Health Evidence Network synthesis report 63: What quantitative and qualitative methods have been developed to measure the implementation of a life-course approach in public health policies at the national level? 2019, Copenhagen: WHO Regional Office for Europe.

12. Popkin, B.M., L.S. Adair, and S.W. Ng, Global nutrition transition and the pandemic of obesity in developing countries. Nutrition Reviews, 2012. 70(1): pp. 3–21.

13. World Health Organization and United Nations Children's Fund (UNICEF), Protect the promise: 2022 progress report on the Every Woman Every Child Global Strategy for Women's, Children's and Adolescents' Health (2016–2030). 2022, Geneva: World Health Organization and the United Nations Children's Fund (UNICEF).

14. Dalrymple, K.V., et al., Longitudinal dietary trajectories from preconception to mid-childhood in women and children in the Southampton Women's Survey and their relation to offspring adiposity: a group-based trajectory modelling approach. International Journal of Obesity, 2022. 46(4): pp. 758–66.

15. Calatayud, M., O. Koren, and M.C. Collado, Maternal microbiome and metabolic health program microbiome development and health of the offspring. Trends in Endocrinology & Metabolism, 2019. 30(10): pp. 735–44.

16. Meaney, M.J., Perinatal maternal depressive symptoms as an issue for population health. American Journal of Psychiatry, 2018. 175(11): pp. 1084–1093.

17. Scorza, P., et al., Research review: Intergenerational transmission of disadvantage: Epigenetics and parents' childhoods as the first exposure. Journal of Child Psychology and Psychiatry, 2019. 60(2): pp. 119–32.

18. Krubiner, C., et al., Working Paper 577. April 2021: Addressing the COVID-19 crisis's indirect health impacts for women and girls. 2021, Washington, DC: Centre for Global Development.

19. Jacob, C.M., et al., Building resilient societies after COVID-19: The case for investing in maternal, neonatal, and child health. Lancet Public Health, 2020. 5(11): pp. e624–e627.

20. Caspi, A., et al., Childhood forecasting of a small segment of the population with large economic burden. Nature Human Behaviour, 2016. 1(1): p. 0005.

21. Richmond-Rakerd, L.S., et al., Childhood self-control forecasts the pace of midlife aging and preparedness for old age. Proceedings of the National Academy of Sciences of the United States of America, 2021. 118(3): pp. e2010211118.

22. Cairney, P., The Politics of Evidence-based Policy Making. 2016, Basingstoke: Palgrave Macmillan. 137.

23. Gluckman, P.D., A. Bardsley, and M. Kaiser, Brokerage at the science–policy interface: From conceptual framework to practical guidance. Humanities and Social Sciences Communications, 2021. 8(1): p. 84.

24. Gluckman, P., The role of evidence and expertise in policy-making: The politics and practice of science advice. Journal and Proceedings of the Royal Society of New South Wales, 2018. 151(467/468): pp. 91–101.

25. Latour, B. and S. Woolgar, Laboratory Life: The Social Construction of Scientific Facts. 1979, Beverly Hills: SAGE Publications. 272.

26. Douglas, H.E., Science, Policy, and the Value-Free Ideal. 2009, Pittsburgh: University of Pittsburgh Press. 256.

27. Pielke, R., The Honest Broker. 2007, Cambridge: Cambridge University Press. 188.

28. Heckman, J., Pre-K researchers can't get past the third grade, in The Hechinger Report. 2015, New York: The Hechinger Report.

29. García, J.L., et al., Quantifying the life-cycle benefits of a prototypical early childhood program. NBER Working Paper No. 23479, in NBER Working paper series. 2019, Cambridge, MA: National Bureau of Economic Research.

30. Gluckman, P. and A. Bardsley, Policy and political perceptions of risk: The challenges to building resilient energy systems. Philosophical Transactions of the Royal Society A, 2022. 380: p. 20210146.

31. Hepburn, C., Valuing the far-off future: Discounting and its alternatives, in Handbook of Sustainable Development, ed. G. Atkinson, S. Dietz, and E. Neumayer, 2007, Cheltenham: Edward Elgar. 109–124.

32. World Health Organization. Noncommunicable diseases: Mortality. 2022 [cited 13 January 2023]; Available from: www.who.int/data/gho/data/themes/topics/topic-details/GHO/ncd-mortality.

33. Cairney, P. and E. St Denny, Why Isn't Government Policy More Preventive? 2020, Oxford, UK: Oxford University Press. 304.

34. Penkler, M., et al., Developmental Origins of Health and Disease, resilience and social justice in the COVID era. Journal of Developmental Origins of Health and Disease, 2022. 13(4): pp. 413–16.

35. Modi, N., G. Conti, and M. Hanson, Post-COVID economic recovery: Women and children first . . . or last? Archives of Disease in Childhood, 2022. 107(3): p. 214–15.

36. Campbell-Lendrum, D. and C. Corvalán, Climate change and developing-country cities: Implications for environmental health and equity. Journal of Urban Health, 2007. 84(1): p. 109–17.

37. Kingdon, J.W., Agendas, Alternatives, and Public Policies. 1984, Boston, MA: Little, Brown & Co. 240.

38. Moffitt, T.E., et al., A gradient of childhood self-control predicts health, wealth, and public safety. Proceedings of the National Academy of Sciences, 2011. 108(7): p. 2693–2698.

39. Mahase, E., UN warns of 'devastating' effect of Covid-19, conflict, and climate change on women's and children's health. BMJ, 2022. 379: p. o2497.

40. OECD, Addressing societal challenges using transdisciplinary research. OECD Science, Technology and Industry Policy Papers, No. 88. 2020, Paris: OECD Publishing.

41. Hanson, M.A. and P.D. Gluckman, Early developmental conditioning of later health and disease: Physiology or pathophysiology? Physiological Reviews, 2014. 94: pp. 1027–1076.

Chapter

17

Framing DOHaD for Policy and Society

Chandni Maria Jacob, Michael Penkler, Ruth Müller, and Mark Hanson

17.1 Introduction

Developmental Origins of Health and Disease (DOHaD) research has shown that social, economic, and environmental experiences and exposures in early life greatly affect an individual's ability to develop, grow, and experience long-term health and well-being. Recently, the focus has moved from animal and biomedical studies on DOHaD mechanisms [1] to the translation of research findings into wider public health intervention and policy. The DOHaD concept has gained some international attention in the last 10 years, for example figuring prominently in reports from the World Health Organization (WHO), including the Commission on Ending Childhood Obesity [2]. At the same time, a lack of clear strategies to implement the concept has led to only partial translation into policies, public health interventions, and clinical practice [3].

When communicating with policy and other audiences, researchers usually engage in a practice known as 'framing'. Framing is a concept from communication studies, social psychology, and sociology that is based on the premise *'that an issue can be viewed from a variety of perspectives and be construed as having implications for multiple values or considerations'* [4, p. 104]. Framing is an act of communication that presents a specific view and thereby *'enables individuals to organize experience, to simplify and make sense of the world around them, and to justify and facilitate collective action'* [5, p. 183]. Frames can highlight specific aspects of an issue or solution and implicate particular moral judgements [6]. Frames are collectively shared and persistent, often developing over time, but can also be used strategically to champion specific interpretations of facts and to promote specific avenues for collective or policy action. The concept can be used as a tool to understand how scientific facts are ordered and presented, thus imbuing them with meaning and values when communicating findings to policy and society (see also Kenney and Müller in this volume).

In this chapter, we investigate how DOHaD researchers and interdisciplinary networks rooted in the DOHaD paradigm frame their research in attempts to translate it into policy, and we discuss the potential and challenges of these frames. We first provide a brief overview of prevalent forms of framing in DOHaD more generally before we discuss two empirical examples in which some of the authors have been involved.

CMJ is supported by the European Union's Horizon 2020 LifeCycle Project under grant agreement No. 733206. MH is supported by the British Heart Foundation and the National Institute for Health Research, UK, through the Southampton Biomedical Research Centre. RM and MP were supported by the DFG German Research Foundation through the project 'Situating Environmental Epigenetics' (403161875). Both CMJ and MH are members of the Preconception Partnership and the Venice Forum.

We conclude by highlighting opportunities to frame DOHaD messages in a social justice framework, and we propose directions for future research and advocacy.

17.2 Overview of Common DOHaD Frames

Other contributions to this handbook discuss at length how DOHaD science has been and continues to frame its findings. Hanson and Buklijas show how a social medicine frame was prominent in the formation of the early DOHaD field. David Barker's work, for instance, had a strong focus on how social and health inequalities are linked and perpetuated, and Barker was centrally involved in efforts to promote social policies aimed at reducing inequities in health. This frame, with its strong focus on social determinants of health, was increasingly replaced by a biomedical frame that foregrounded individual and somatic factors, particularly the maternal body. According to Hanson and Buklijas, this 'telescoping' [7], from social conditions to dietary components and molecular pathways, has been the result of broader socio-political contexts and a related restructuring of DOHaD as a firmly biomedical field.

The foregrounding of different causal factors within a DOHaD frame is tied to how responsibilities are distributed and to who is regarded as the most pertinent agent for action. Chiapperino et al., also in this handbook, highlight the 'paradox' that DOHaD research communication, while often rhetorically acknowledging social determinants, still in practice often focuses on individual responsibility for action, especially targeting women's dietary and other health behaviours [8, 9]. The frames used for communication to the general public about preventing non-communicable diseases (NCDs), for instance, through the media, largely emphasise individual behaviour change (particularly mothers' lifestyles, weight loss, and diet modification) and diminish the role of other agencies (e.g. food industries and marketing) [10]. Framing DOHaD findings in a way that emphasises women as primarily responsible for their offspring's healthy development has been criticised as promoting maternal blame and stigma. Richardson et al. (2014) in a critical article wrote that 'exaggerations and over-simplifications are making scapegoats of mothers, and could even increase surveillance and regulation of pregnant women' [11].

Many DOHaD researchers welcome this critique, and prominent figures have co-authored articles that call for a wider framing that moves away from maternal blame and individual attributions of responsibility. Such a *social justice framing* [12] instead empha-sises the social, political, and economic dimensions that shape developmental outcomes and calls for policy translations of DOHaD that emphasise the need for action through social policy and health equity [9]. Yet, based on reviews of interventions using a DOHaD model [13] and a recent ethnographic study of researchers working in DOHaD-focused institutes [14], it is evident that the DOHaD and lifecourse fields largely still use a biomedical frame. More recently, some DOHaD scholars have begun to promote the formation of wider multidisciplinary coalitions and advocacy networks to improve messaging, framing, and ultimately policy impact. In the following, we explore two such coalitions and if and how their framing activities depart from and improve on the status quo in DOHaD.

17.3 Case Studies of Two Multidisciplinary Coalitions and Advocacy Networks

As Low and colleagues describe in this volume, there is a serious effort to translate DOHaD knowledge into policy and society through advocacy by collaborative networks.

These have been based on a 'facilitational' model of advocacy [15] that emphasises the joint and participatory production and communication of knowledge by collaborations between scientists, civil society organisations, and policymakers, as seen for instance with climate change-related policies [16]. Several such multi-sectoral alliances have been formed in the last decade to advocate for collective action to translate DOHaD and lifecourse research into policy at national and international levels. Below, we discuss two such networks – the Venice Forum [17] and the UK Preconception Partnership [18].

In order to explore how DOHaD messages have been framed by these two networks, we consider two aspects proposed by global health policy experts [5]: problem definition (internal framing) and positioning (external framing). Problem definition is concerned with how actors internal to the network view or conceptualise the issue and its solutions. Within a network, there may be a common understanding of or disagreement on the primary rationale for why an issue is important. Positioning on the other hand deals with how the messages are communicated to an audience external to the network, with the goal of inspiring them to act. While an internal consensus on framing increases credibility when presented to external audiences (such as policymakers), the success of a frame can also depend on the legitimacy of the experts endorsing it. Positioning is often tailored to resonate with the target external actors such as policymakers or funding bodies [5].

As both the Venice Forum and the UK Preconception Partnership broadly focus on the translation of messages from DOHaD research, with common actors in membership for both groups, there has been overlap in frames used by them. We first present an overview of each network (Table 17.1)[1] and the frames they use in their collective advocacy before discussing the implications of the employed frames.

17.3.1 The Venice Forum (Global)

The Venice Forum was established in 2019 by a group of independent academics and healthcare professionals to explore the impact of economic and other crises (e.g. war and famine) on DOHaD outcomes globally. Based on evidence that crises such as the 2008 economic downturn have a disproportionate impact on women and children, the main goal of the Venice Forum is to advocate for an ethical imperative of supporting early childhood development, thus preventing the intergenerational passage of risk.

This agenda gained new urgency by the COVID-19 pandemic, which further exposed inequalities in health and well-being [14], but also inequalities in responses to the pandemic. For example, research during the early stages of the pandemic (for example on vaccine safety) often excluded children and pregnant or breastfeeding women [20]. Post-pandemic, the focus of the Venice Forum shifted from the impact of economic crises and natural disasters on MNCH to understanding factors that build resilient

---

[1] Both networks have partly overlapping membership. For example, the first and last authors of this chapter have been actively involved in both networks. The Partnership and the Forum have also collaborated to write joint statements, for example, providing input into the call for evidence for the UK Women's Health Strategy in 2021. This written input has focused on building a robust case for MNCH through measurement, monitoring, and better-quality data and implementation through a multi-sectoral approach, developing practical messages for the public and addressing ethnic and socio-economic disparities in women's health.

Table 17.1 Overview of the two advocacy networks

	Venice Forum	Preconception Partnership
Aim/Key agenda	To make the case for increased investment in maternal, newborn, and child health (MNCH) for long-term benefits to the population and for inter-generational impact	To 'normalise' the concept of pregnancy preparation and improve population health through intervention in the preconception period
Focus	DOHaD-related outcomes, transgenerational health, and engagement with policymakers for advocacy	DOHaD-related outcomes, translation of evidence into policy, and co-production with public health authorities in the UK. Key target groups have been future parents, policymakers, and practitioners.
Origin	Established in 2019 as an informal think tank	Established in 2018 with the publication of the landmark *Lancet* series [19] on preconception health
Governance and membership	Led by a core team of six board members with a clinical and academic background in DOHaD. The annual international forums include an informal network of health-oriented professionals, academic and scientific societies (from obstetrics and gynaecology, neonatology and paediatrics, public health, health economics, social science, and education), clinical organisations, patients' rights groups, and NGOs predominantly from high-income and European contexts.	Led by two academic chairs with well-defined subgroups and roles. The remit of the group has expanded with membership predominantly from UK-based academics (from fields of nutrition, sexual reproductive health, public health, psychology, mental health, epidemiology, etc.), public health entities, NGOs, charities, and healthcare professionals (obstetrics and gynaecology, community health workers, and general practitioners).
Target audience	Global policymakers	Predominantly UK focused policymakers, the general public, and clinical organisations

societies, making an argument for embedding MNCH as core to research and policy-making aimed at developing healthier societies [21].

The Forum has often framed its policy messages in economic terms. It has developed key arguments from early-life interventions such as the Perry Preschool and Abecedarian programmes that show how such interventions can have long-term economic benefits, higher school completion rates, college attendance, lower rates of teenage pregnancy, dependency, and welfare [22, 23]. The rationale for employing an economic frame that emphasises long-term cost reductions and returns on investment has been the assumption that non-health outcomes are important issues from a policymaker's perspective. Ongoing projects by the Forum include specific recommendations for policy, for example introducing parental leave for the first six months of life. The assumption is that the economic frame is more likely to elicit a response from finance ministers and other governmental departments outside healthcare. In this context, the Forum has strategically tried to promote a 'technification'[24] of the issue – in this case conveying the economic costs of a lack of investment in early years and in parenthood and portraying the issue as one that can – and should – be addressed primarily through science and economics, and not necessarily on the individual level, thus developing an 'investment case' for MNCH.

At the same time, the Forum has also adopted a contrary approach, emphasising the need to reframe the way 'value' is conceptualised in policymaking and financing. While supporting the development of an investment case described above, the Venice forum has also challenged the dominant view that economic growth measured by GDP is an adequate measure of success, when it does not include unremunerated contributions to society such as childbearing, domestic work, and care – largely conducted by women in most societies [17]; see also Cohen in this volume. The Venice Forum has explored and promoted newer frames of a 'caring economy' [25] that include well-being as an indicator of economic success over GDP and employ alternative measures to include unremunerated work, such as the Human Capital Index or the Genuine Progress Indicator. The goal of these new frames is to shift the approach from mainstream economics that focuses predominantly on market relations towards feminist economics that values women's contributions. However, framing issues of health in terms of economic benefits always carries the risk of contributing to rather than resisting approaches in which health only matters in terms of its economic impact, rather than emphasising health and access to healthcare as human rights and values in themselves.

The Forum has also strategically engaged in linking MNCH to the climate crisis, recommending inter-sectoral actions required to address climate change – such as reducing air pollution and low-environmental impact diets – that are also beneficial for health. Such focus on policy framed in terms of human and planetary well-being might benefit from the existing momentum for the climate crisis agenda. The Forum perceives that climate is of high importance to younger people, thus providing an opportunity to disseminate messages by highlighting their concurrent benefits for health and the environment.

The Venice Forum has also strategically decided to emphasise the benefits of inter-generational health to prioritise investments in MNCH. While a focus on child/newborn health might have greater political traction, such a focus potentially competes with the maternal health agenda when the health of the fetus is emphasised at the expense of women's health for their own benefit [26]. A framing of MNCH in terms of long-term investments used by the forum can thus compete with an ethical frame that positions MNCH as a matter of women's rights and equity – a frame that was also utilised by the Forum, which called for urgent action in this area due to slow progress.

Overall, the Venice Forum has targeted policymakers and international health organisations using a variety of different framings – a social justice framing, economic framings, frames related to intergenerational health benefits, synergies with climate change, and ethical frames for women's rights.

17.3.2 The UK Preconception Partnership (United Kingdom)

The 2018 landmark *Lancet* series on preconception health [19] made a strong case that 'preconception' forms a key period for health interventions that have long-term benefits for subsequent maternal and child health. The Partnership that formed after this series meets regularly and has worked extensively with local authorities in the UK and stakeholders such as the Office for Health Inequalities and Disparities (OHID) (under the Department of Health and Social Care, UK). Targeted engagement, particularly in the local/national context, has been an advantage for the Partnership, facilitated by the inclusion of knowledge brokers (stakeholders facilitating knowledge transfer from research to policy) in the network.

While the Partnership is interdisciplinary in its membership, there is a higher representation from healthcare organisations and the biomedical sciences (see Table 17.1). The Partnership's stated goal is to 'normalise' the concept of preparation for pregnancy and parenthood, thus framing adolescence and early adulthood as a 'pre-conception period' where young people should be encouraged and empowered to engage in healthy activities both for the sake of their own health and also to prepare for (potential) pregnancies.

The Preconception Partnership has overall adopted a lifecourse approach to preconception care, focusing on adolescent health, inter-pregnancy health, and post-partum care as key periods to include in the definition of preconception health. The Partnership has positioned this approach within a reproductive justice framework that considers 'the human right to maintain personal bodily autonomy, have children, not have children, and parent the children we have in safe and sustainable communities' [27]. In supporting women's rights to make decisions related to fertility and contraception, the Preconception Partnership (among other global networks) has endorsed universal screening for pregnancy intention with clinical tools to discuss the desire to be pregnant or avoid pregnancy [28, 29]. This also relates to the reproductive justice framework that includes equitable access to a range of health services such as contraception, sexual health, and abortion (which women of colour and marginalised groups often have barriers accessing as a core component). However, an overemphasis on reproductive health could propagate a view of women as 'vessels of reproduction' [30], in which young women are primarily viewed and addressed as future mothers [31]. Ongoing work by members also has focused on the extension of health behaviours to adolescence, for example through school-based interventions to promote scientific and health literacy [32].

A recent study by Jacob [33] has shown different and partly competing ways of framing the internal discussions and external communications of the Partnership. On the one hand, the Partnership has framed preconception health as a systemic issue and promoted policies and public health campaigns aimed at addressing socio-economic inequalities in women's health. One prominent Partnership initiative has been to improve the evidence base for health policy focused on the preconception period and to hold policymakers accountable for issues in preconception care that show links with deprivation. To this end, the Partnership has focused on using routine data from maternity care programmes to develop a report card on preconception health status in the UK [34]. The analysis of national maternity services data (England) highlighted inequalities based on age (e.g. younger women were less likely to take folic acid supplements preconception), ethnicity, and deprivation and in turn provided outcomes and indicators for accountability. Members' publications have also emphasised the impact of wider determinants of health [35] and called on governments as key actors to address preconception health at the policy level.

At the same time, framings of risk factors like obesity as being linked to systemic problems influenced by the environment and deprivation contrasted with recommendations to change lifestyles with support from clinicians. The clinical setting, where clinicians often meet women with or without their partners, was often framed as an effective and easily accessible platform for the dissemination of preconception health messages. In this view, postnatal care presents a 'window of opportunity' for both the next pregnancy and early childhood development [29, 36]. However, such recommendations were also critically discussed within the Partnership, as it was argued that they could lead to individual attributions of responsibility and a stigmatised framing of behaviours deemed unhealthy, particularly among low-income populations. It was argued that focusing on influencing behaviours through the dissemination of health messages also assigns a set of values and moral implications, falling disproportionately on women and addressing them primarily as reproductive agents [33].

In order to address these issues, the Partnership has recently conducted several public engagement activities to investigate appropriate ways for developing and framing health messages that avoid unintended and harmful consequences. Unsurprisingly, using the term 'preconception' was not preferred by participants (women living in the UK) [37]. Additionally, participants also recommended gender-inclusive terms that could capture the interest of men, who often felt excluded from the conversation on health for their children [38]. While the area of male preconception health and its impact on long-term health has been increasingly discussed within the Partnership, messages related to men's health before pregnancy were often lacking in their outputs. Framing preconception health mainly around women's health and bodies could further alienate men and non-binary individuals from engaging in health messages and conversations around preconception care [38]. Studies from low- and middle-income settings have, however, shown that men were keen to be involved in engaging in such conversations [39]. The need to represent health findings without causing alarm is key for the public's engagement with preconception health messages, considering the probabilistic nature of the associations in DOHaD studies [9]. Framings related to 'unplanned pregnancies' as a risk factor for a negative outcome were often used by the Partnership. This may also need to be revisited as studies have shown that people may not perceive unplanned pregnancies to be a negative outcome, nor is pregnancy intentionality a straightforward idea [40, 41].

Another question that proved internally contentious within the Partnership was how to frame obesity. Though publications have acknowledged the wider determinants of obesity and the need to reduce stigma in clinical conversations, obesity is also framed as a condition in need of medical treatment or intervention [29, 36, 42], in accordance with recent World Obesity Federation campaigns (2018–19). However, internally members of both the Partnership and the Venice Forum have contested this medical framing, as over-medicalising the issue presents challenges in policy translation. One such challenge is that an increased focus on addressing obesity through healthcare and weight management services might lead to reduced investments in preventive policies that target systemic drivers of obesity, such as the marketing of foods or food composition. Framings of obesity as a medical condition also potentially conflict with a social justice framework. Feminist scholars and fat activists have argued that framing obesity in medical terms may contribute to weight stigma in which individuals are blamed for their body shape and ill health. Such frames in particular target women and minorities and lead to localising structural problems within individual bodies, thus potentially deflecting policy attention away from the systemic conditions that drive inequities in health. (See Lappé and Valdez in this handbook.) Additionally, conversations focusing only on weight can also lead to unintended consequences such as repeated cycles of weight gain and loss, eating disorders, weight stigmatisation, and mental health issues, thus calling for a person-centred approach [43].

From a social justice perspective, health interventions and policies based on individual behaviour change appear as particularly problematic. Such interventions were also debated internally within the Partnership, with one point of debate being how health messages related to preconception health should be framed. Preconception health interventions that target individual behaviour change predominantly focus on rational aspects of decision-making (e.g. providing information on food-based dietary guidelines and Eatwell plates), and overall DOHaD health messaging tends to focus on risks and potential negative outcomes. In contrast, the Preconception Partnership has recommended appealing to emotional aspects of the benefits of healthy growth and development [8]. This is especially relevant as health messages compete with framings by the private sector, which focus on selling comfort and happiness – for example with the use of infant formula. Framing preconception health messages in more positive terms has the goal of improving the public and policy uptake of these messages.

Thus the Preconception Partnership has used framings similar to the Venice Forum on intergenerational benefits and health across the lifecourse, social justice, and the reproductive justice framework. However, medicalised framings of obesity are still evident along with a focus on women's fertility and pregnancy planning.

17.3.2.1 Competing Framings in DOHaD Health Advocacy

Research findings from DOHaD can be framed in different ways, imbuing them with different meanings to link to different types of policy recommendations. Such frames may not incorporate all aspects of the issue in question and present a risk of oversimplification of a complex field, as seen in the above examples. Figure 17.1 is a conceptual figure summarising examples of framings used by the networks in publications and other

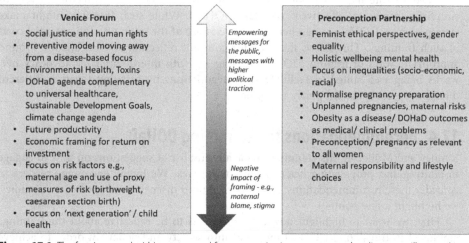

Figure 17.1 The framings used within groups and for communicating to an external audience are illustrated in the figure. Certain framings may have potentially negative consequences, while others have more positive effects as shown by the arrow.

media, which we have listed by the potential impact it could have if applied in healthcare, policy, and interventions.

DOHaD frames may emerge in multiple ways, not limited to evidence generated from research but also as a response to the evidence demand from governments/policy-makers, major societal events, and public opinion. Efforts to bring DOHaD insights into policy and health interventions are often driven by a sense of urgency and an under-standing that it is an ethical imperative to act now to improve MNCH and to address persistent inequalities in health. This sense of urgency often translates into efforts to influence policy and the public 'effectively', for example through strategically framing DOHaD messages in ways that make them more palatable to policymakers and the public, and thus more likely to influence policies and health behaviours.

Such efforts and emphasis on urgency can also lead to unintended consequences that may be at odds with the goal of promoting health equity and social justice – especially when the potential negative impacts of employed framings are not given adequate consideration. For example, alarmist language – obesity as 'a ticking time bomb', or the 'war on obesity' – might be an adequate way to garner policy and media attention, but it also has the potential to increase weight stigma when fat people are implicitly framed as a threat to society, economic prosperity, and the welfare state's future [44]. This becomes particularly problematic when public health campaigns are aimed at marginalised parts of the population.

Similarly, an economic frame of 'returns on investment' might be well suited to attract policymakers' interests – but it carries the danger of propagating eugenic logics when women are targeted primarily in the name of the offspring's health, as discussed by Cohen in her contribution to this volume. And a framing that highlights individual agency in relation to factors that influence the development of health and disease may be well suited to inform individual action – but runs the risk of also increasing blame and of reinforcing health inequalities as not everybody has the necessary resources to act.

The analysis of our two case studies has shown contestations around how to frame DOHaD for policy and society. Individualising and potentially stigmatising frames were critiqued in internal discussions. At the same time, there are strong incentives for simplistic frames to 'effectively' translate DOHaD. While such framings might make strategic sense, DOHaD researchers should be aware of the trade-offs and potential costs of such framings. This shows the need for constant reflection and negotiation around appropriate ways of framing DOHaD messages – with interdisciplinary advocacy net-works being well suited to facilitate such negotiations by bringing together different disciplinary, societal, and policy viewpoints.

17.4 Recommendations for Reframing DOHaD

Kenney and Müller in this volume provide a useful list of suggestions on how to engage in crafting and propagating health-related narratives. We highly encourage readers to consider these recommendations. Here, based on our discussion of our two case studies, we highlight a few points.

First, we want to highlight how important it is to be reflective about the framings employed in translating DOHaD messages into society and policy. In order to achieve societal and policy impact, there is a need to strategically employ specific framings. At the same time, scholars and practitioners should also be conscious of the potential negative impacts of the framings employed and about what trade-offs are involved when employing specific frames. However, this demand for 'targeted messaging' could also have led to competing or conflicting frames within the same network, as seen in the case studies. We advise DOHaD researchers to be particularly cautious when employing economic framings when talking about the value of health, when employing alarmist language, and when promoting interventions that target predominantly individual health behaviours.

Second, our discussion of the two case studies shows that finding and employing appropriate framings is a continuous process. As Chiapperino et al. in this volume discuss, DOHaD researchers often in principle subscribe to and are motivated by a social justice framing of DOHaD, which highlights the need to address inequities in health through social policy. Such a social justice framing is also fundamental to the Forum's and Partnership's work, but at the same time there are powerful institutional and policy incentives to frame health messages in ways that are antithetical to such a social justice framing (see also Penkler 2022). There are competing interests and factors at work that encourage perhaps more reductionist framings of DOHaD findings that imply more individual translations. Finding the adequate balance and engaging in DOHaD messaging that is both effective and avoids negative outcomes is a continuous process that DOHaD researchers should be reflective about. Such ongoing reflection can also help tackle the challenge of developing messages that account for both the individual-level and population-level actions required to address the health issues in consideration. An example of work towards this is the Preconception Partnership's multidisciplinary representation and ongoing study with the public on the appropriate inclusive language to be used in public health messaging related to preconception health [38]. We recommend a continued need for engagement and reflection on the frames used by both networks due to the conflicting frames discussed.

Thirdly, advocacy networks such as the case studies included here are particularly well suited for such negotiations. They offer ways of breaking the siloes of academic research groups and allow researchers to engage with the public, wider disciplines, and policymakers. They allow the inclusion of different disciplinary, societal, and policy viewpoints and a forum to engage and negotiate about appropriate framings. Diversity within networks (disciplinary and geographic) and links with a wider range of actors outside research (policy, communities, private sector, healthcare sector, charities, and activists) are needed to develop solutions that are sensitive to the available resources and environmental and socio-economic factors influencing health behaviours, cultural practices, and differences in behaviours based on ethnicity/income groups. Our recommendation in this context is to further broaden advocacy coalitions to also include more non-scientific, non-health, and non-policy actors, such as activists and community members. Co-creating frames is a way of making them more socially robust and aligned with values of social justice and equality, as work in the Preconception Partnership has shown when including civic society. In order to pursue co-creation effectively, it is important to include a wider range of stakeholders (including civic society) proactively and early on, including them in upstream discussions about what appropriate frames and goals are, and not only downstream. Such engagement can help ensure that the very goals of advocacy networks (such as 'improving health') should not be taken as given, but up for negotiation when engaging collectively in finding appropriate frames for translating DOHaD into policy and society.

In conclusion, we argue that a return to 'business as usual' by adopting medical and individual framings for DOHaD translation would be inadequate to address the increasing disparities in MNCH, obesity, and NCD-related issues. Such a global outlook, which includes justice and addressing inequalities, will help in translating the DOHaD and lifecourse models into policy that integrates not only life stages from preconception but also all wider societal factors that shape human well-being.

References

1. Hanson MA, Gluckman P. Early developmental conditioning of later health and disease: Physiology or pathophysiology? Physiological Reviews. 2014;94(4):1027–76.

2. World Health Organization. Consideration of the evidence on childhood obesity for the Commission on Ending Childhood Obesity: Report of the ad hoc working group on science and evidence for ending childhood obesity, Geneva, Switzerland. 2016. Available from: https://apps.who.int/iris/handle/10665/206549 [Accessed 1st March 2022]

3. Hanson MA, Poston L, Gluckman PD. DOHaD: The challenge of translating the science to policy. Journal of Developmental Origins of Health and Disease. 2019;10(3):263–67.

4. Chong D, Druckman JN. Framing theory. Annual Review in Political Science. 2007;10:103–26.

5. Shiffman J. Four challenges that global health networks face. International Journal of Health Policy and Management. 2017;6(4):183–89.

6. Scheufele B. Framing-effects approach: A theoretical and methodological critique. Communications. 2004:29 (4):401–28.

7. Warin M, Moore V, Zivkovic T, Davies M. Telescoping the origins of obesity to women's bodies: How gender inequalities are being squeezed out of Barker's hypothesis. Annals of Human Biology. 2011;38(4):453–60.

8. McKerracher L, Moffat T, Barker M, Williams D, Sloboda D. Translating the Developmental Origins of Health and Disease concept to improve the nutritional environment for our next generations: A call for a reflexive, positive, multi-level approach. Journal of Developmental Origins of Health and Disease. 2019;10(4):420–28.

9. Müller R, Hanson C, Hanson MA, Penkler M, Samaras G, Chiapperino L, et al. The biosocial genome? Interdisciplinary perspectives on environmental epigenetics, health and society. EMBO Reports. 2017;18 (10):1677–82.

10. Penkler M, Hanson MA, Biesma R, Müller R. DOHaD in science and society: Emergent opportunities and novel responsibilities. Journal of Developmental Origins of Health and Disease. 2019;10 (3):268–73.

11. Richardson SS, Daniels CR, Gillman MW, Golden J, Kukla R, Kuzawa C, et al. Society: Don't blame the mothers. Nature. 2014;512(7513):131–32.

12. Policy UNDfS. Social Justice in an Open World: The Role of the United Nations: United Nations Publications; 2006.

13. Jacob CM, Newell ML, Hanson MA. Narrative review of reviews of preconception interventions to prevent an increased risk of obesity and non-communicable diseases in children. Obesity Reviews. 2019;20:5–17.

14. Penkler M. Caring for biosocial complexity. Articulations of the environment in research on the Developmental Origins of Health and Disease. Studies in History and Philosophy of Science. 2022;93:1–10.

15. Oliver K, Cairney P. The dos and don'ts of influencing policy: A systematic review of advice to academics. Palgrave Communications. 2019;5(1):1–11.

16. Gluckman PD, Bardsley A, Kaiser M. Brokerage at the science–policy interface: From conceptual framework to practical guidance. Humanities and Social Sciences Communications. 2021;8 (1):1–10.

17. Meka K, Jacob CM, Modi N, Bustreo F, Di Renzo GC, Malamitsi-Puchner A, et al. Valuing maternal, newborn, child and adolescent health for societal progress– Going beyond the economic orthodoxy of gross domestic product. Acta Paediatrica. 2023;112(4):630–34.

18. UK Preconception Partnership. About the partnership. 2022. Available from: www.ukpreconceptionpartnership.co.uk/ [Accessed 1 April 2023]

19. Stephenson J, Heslehurst N, Hall J, Schoenaker DA, Hutchinson J, Cade JE, et al. Before the beginning: Nutrition and lifestyle in the preconception period and its importance for future health. The Lancet. 2018;391(10132):1830–41.

20. Vassallo A, Womersley K, Norton R, Sheel M. Pregnant women's appetite for risk. The Lancet Global Health. 2021;9(5): e593.

21. Jacob CM, Briana DD, Di Renzo GC, Modi N, Bustreo F, Conti G, et al. Building resilient societies after COVID-19: The case for investing in maternal, neonatal, and child health. The Lancet Public Health. 2020;5(11):e624–e7.

22. Heckman JJ. Skill formation and the economics of investing in disadvantaged children. Science. 2006;312(5782):1900–2.

23. Heckman JJ, Moon SH, Pinto R, Savelyev PA, Yavitz A. The rate of return to the HighScope Perry Preschool Program. Journal of Public Economics. 2010;94 (1–2):114–28.

24. Shiffman J, Shawar YR. Framing and the formation of global health priorities. The Lancet. 2022;399(10399):1977–90.

25. Group WsB. Creating a Caring Economy: A Call to Action. 2020 [cited 20 April 2023]. Available from: https://wbg.org .uk/analysis/creating-a-caring-economy- a-call-to-action-2/.

26. Shiffman J, Smith S. Generation of political priority for global health initiatives: A framework and case study of maternal mortality. The Lancet. 2007;370 (9595):1370–79.

27. Song S. Reproductive Justice. 1997. Available from: www.sistersong.net/ reproductive-justice [Accessed 1 April 2023]

28. Hall JA, Barrett G, Stephenson JM, Edelman NL, Rocca C. Desire to Avoid Pregnancy scale: Clinical considerations and comparison with other questions about pregnancy preferences. BMJ Sexual & Reproductive Health. 2023;0:1–9. doi:10.1136/bmjsrh-2022-201750.

29. Stephenson J, Schoenaker DA, Hinton W, Poston L, Barker M, Alwan NA, et al. A wake-up call for preconception health: A clinical review. British Journal of General Practice. 2021;71(706):233–36.

30. Verbiest S, Shawe J, Steegers EA. Advancing Preconception Health Globally: A Way Forward. Preconception Health and Care: A Life Course Approach. Springer; 2020. p. 299–308.

31. Waggoner MR. Motherhood preconceived: The emergence of the preconception health and health care initiative. Journal of Health Politics, Policy and Law. 2013;38(2):345–71.

32. Woods-Townsend K, Hardy-Johnson P, Bagust L, Barker M, Davey H, Griffiths J, et al. A cluster-randomised controlled trial of the LifeLab education intervention to improve health literacy in adolescents. PLoS One. 2021;16(5):e0250545.

33. Jacob CM. Preconception Health and the Life Course Approach to Prevention of Non-Communicable Diseases: Implications for Informing Policy and Practice [PhD]. United Kingdom: University of Southampton; 2022.

34. Schoenaker DA, Stephenson J, Smith H, Thurland K, Duncan H, Godfrey KM, et al. Women's preconception health in England: A report card based on cross-sectional analysis of national maternity services data 2018/19. BJOG:

An International Journal of Obstetrics & Gynaecology. 2023;130:1187–1195.

35. Hall J, Chawla M, Watson D, Jacob CM, Schoenaker D, Connolly A, et al. Addressing reproductive health needs across the life course: An integrated, community-based model combining contraception and preconception care. The Lancet Public Health. 2023;8(1):e76-e84.

36. Jacob C, Killeen S, McAuliffe F, Stephenson J, Hod M, Diaz Yamal I, et al. Prevention of noncommunicable diseases by interventions in the preconception period: A FIGO position paper for action by healthcare practitioners. International Journal of Gynecology & Obstetrics. 2020;151 (Suppl. 1): 6–15.

37. UK Preconception Partnership. Survey by Tommy's charity and the preconception partnership. 2022 [cited April 2023]. Available from: www .ukpreconceptionpartnership.co.uk/ projects/survey-by-tommys-charity-and-the-preconception-partnership.

38. Schoenaker DA, Gafari O, Taylor E, Hall J, Barker C, Jones B, et al. Informing public health messages and strategies to raise awareness of pre-conception health: A public consultation. The Lancet. 2021;398:S77.

39. Watson D, Chatio ST, Barker M, Boua PR, Compaoré A, Dalaba M, et al. Men's motivations, barriers to and aspirations for their families' health in the first 1000 days in sub-Saharan Africa: A secondary qualitative analysis. BMJ Nutrition, Prevention & Health. 2023.

40. Grace B, Shawe J, Barrett G, Usman NO, Stephenson J. What does family building mean? A qualitative exploration and a new definition: A UK-based study. Reproductive Health. 2022;19(1):203.

41. Johnson-Hanks J. When the future decides: Uncertainty and intentional action in contemporary Cameroon. Current Anthropology. 2005;46 (3):363–85.

42. Barker M, Dombrowski SU, Colbourn T, Fall CH, Kriznik NM, Lawrence WT, et al. Intervention strategies to improve nutrition and health behaviours before conception. The Lancet. 2018;391 (10132):1853–64.

43. Bacon L, Aphramor L. Weight science: Evaluating the evidence for a paradigm shift. Nutrition Journal. 2011;10(1):1–13.

44. Penkler M, Felder K, Felt U. Diagnostic narratives: Creating visions of Austrian society in print media accounts of obesity. Science Communication. 2015;37 (3):314–39.

Chapter

18 The Impact of Community-Based Participatory DOHaD Research

Siobhan Tu'akoi, Mark H. Vickers, Celeste Barrett-Watson, Kura Samuel-Ioane, Teaukura Puna, Drollet Joseph, and Jacquie L. Bay

18.1 Introduction

As outlined in the preceding chapters, the Developmental Origins of Health and Disease (DOHaD) concept is a lifecourse approach that describes how environmental exposures in the early-life stages can impact later-life health outcomes. This paradigm has developed considerably since Barker's early findings, solidifying links between adverse early-life events in childhood, pregnancy, and preconception and later risk for non-communicable diseases (NCDs) [1, 2]. Such risk events are not experienced equally, with structural and social determinants such as economic stability, housing, access to health-care, and the wider built environment influencing the ability of individuals and communities to experience good health. Within the DOHaD field, there is increasing support for the integration of social justice and participatory lenses in research, acknowledging that all people deserve equal opportunities to be healthy [3–5]. Such approaches require partnerships that empower and collaborate with the communities who participate in research in order to reduce the power imbalance and better understand the contexts in which health challenges are situated [4]. This encourages the normalisation and inclusion of different types of evidence that are all valuable for addressing health issues, including scientific evidence, sociological factors, and local community knowledge. This chapter describes how a community-based participatory research (CBPR) approach used within the DOHaD field could significantly benefit researchers, communities, and health outcomes. It outlines what CBPR involves and current participatory DOHaD work being undertaken and draws on examples of our own CBPR in the Cook Islands.

18.2 Community-Based Participatory Research in DOHaD

18.2.1 What Is Community-Based Participatory Research?

Community-based participatory research is a collaborative approach to research that aims to engage researchers and community members in equal partnership throughout all stages of the research process [6]. It is widely understood that CBPR developed from action research, an approach proposed in the 1940s by social scientist Kurt Lewis as a way of addressing social problems by undertaking research with or by the study population [7]. Although referred to by a variety of terms, such as action research, participatory research, action science, co-operative inquiry, and community-based research, the shared idea between these concepts is participatory knowledge production that involves the study population [7]. A critical aspect of the CBPR approach is acknowledging that both researchers and community members hold essential knowledge that is equally valuable for conducting rigorous and impactful research. Western research approaches have traditionally assumed that research phenomena can and should be separated from their broader context to conduct valid and reliable studies [7]. CBPR rejects this assertion and recognises the value of different types of knowledge and contextual evidence. In his work exploring the power of professionals and local communities working together, Corburn describes expertise not as an objective truth but as something that can be collaboratively produced to enable better research and policy solutions [8]. Researchers are trained in experimental, epidemiologic, and systematic data collection practices, validated by statistical significance and other professional standards [8]. This knowledge is typically tested via forums such as peer review processes and media. On the other hand, communities hold important local knowledge that has been acquired through experiences, cultural and social traditions, and intergenerational storytelling. This knowledge can be tested via forums such as public narratives, community stories, and media [8]. CBPR approaches emphasise that both forms of evidence are critical for improving research validity and driving social change within communities.

Table 18.1 outlines nine general principles of CBPR proposed by Israel and colleagues that reflect multiple approaches and lessons learned from previous participatory research structures [9].

Empowering communities to be actively involved in conceptualising and leading research is important from a social justice perspective. Criticisms of non-participatory research studies often include a lack of understanding of local socio-cultural factors, leading to limited acceptability of findings by the communities themselves [10]. In particular, research on Indigenous and marginalised communities has historically been conducted without community input, leading to uninformed conclusions that may not address community priorities and contributing to a general mistrust of research by those communities [11]. Fitzpatrick and colleagues acknowledge that 'researchers have often been perceived as doing research *on*, and not *with* Indigenous people, with little regard to local cultural protocols and languages and without seeking consent from communities' [11]. Social justice and empowerment are the foundations of CBPR, ensuring that communities are equal partners in setting research questions, conducting the research, and interpreting what the data mean. This approach not only values the community's expertise but also addresses their moral right to data ownership and leading research that affects their own community.

Key benefits of CBPR include the potential for research findings to be more acceptable and impactful, leading to community-led action and, in turn, increased potential for long-term benefits [12]. Salimi and colleagues systematically reviewed CBPR health projects and found that they enhanced skills and capabilities within the community, resulting in community-level action [13]. CBPR approaches can also be valuable in ensuring the participation and retention of historically marginalised ethnic groups who are traditionally underrepresented in health research [14]. A review by Cook found reciprocal benefits of working together, stating:

> Academic researchers reported that community collaboration had been valuable in making the studies possible and valid and in generating credible data. Community partners helped academic researchers to recruit and retain study participants ... (and) to render research more culturally sensitive and acceptable to the participants and relevant to the local context. [12, p. 669]

Table 18.1 General principles of CBPR [9]

Principles	Explanation
1. Acknowledges the community as a unit of identity.	Identifying and working with groups that share a common membership or identity, such as a social network, ethnic group, or geographical neighbourhood.
2. Builds on the strengths and resources within the community.	Developing the strengths, expertise, and assets that already exist within a community.
3. Facilitates a collaborative, equitable partnership across all research phases.	Requires a foundation of mutual respect and trust to ensure all partners share decision-making and control throughout the research.
4. Fosters reciprocal exchange and capacity building among all partners.	Recognising that all parties bring diverse and valuable knowledge and experiences.
5. Integrates knowledge generation and translation of research findings for the mutual benefit of all partners.	Making a commitment to ensuring research findings are translated into action.
6. Focuses on public health concerns that are relevant to the community using an ecological perspective that recognises the multiple determinants of health.	Recognising the individual, community, and societal contexts and considering broader determinants of health and disease.
7. Involves systems development using a cyclical and iterative process.	Within the system or partnership, this involves a cycle of feedback to develop and improve each stage of the research.
8. Disseminates findings to all partners and engages them in wider dissemination.	Ensuring the research is disseminated in ways that are useful and appropriate for all partners.
9. Prioritises a long-term process and commitment to sustainability.	Making a long-term commitment to ensuring the sustainability of projects or action outcomes beyond a single funding period is critical.

To create better and more robust DOHaD knowledge for action and social change, particularly for Indigenous and disadvantaged groups, partnerships between researchers and the communities that contend with the real-world challenges are essential.

18.2.2 CBPR in the DOHaD Field

Penkler and colleagues argue that better understandings of the health contexts where communities engage are critical to equitably improving intergenerational health and well-being [4]. Utilising CBPR and actively engaging communities in co-developing research projects can provide major benefits for DOHaD research, local community capabilities, and health outcomes [4]. While CBPR approaches remain limited in the DOHaD field, there are key examples where partnerships and participatory frameworks have enhanced the research and knowledge translation processes. Presented below is a snapshot of three participatory approaches grounded in DOHaD theory. Each carries out important work to contribute to the health and well-being of their communities.

In recognition of the inequitable health outcomes faced by Australia's Aboriginal population, for example the increased likelihood of premature birth and poorer infant outcomes compared to the rest of the population, the Gomeroi Gaaynggal programme was established [15]. Initially designed by reproductive scientists, the study underwent an extensive two-year community consultation phase with Aboriginal organisations and health services, Elders, young mum's groups, men's and women's groups, prison staff, and wider community members that revealed key community priorities [15, 16]. As a result, Gomeroi gaaynggal became a two-pronged approach, including a research study and a community-focused arts health programme. Working in partnership with Aboriginal communities in New South Wales, the programme's research focuses on understanding the drivers of adverse health outcomes during pregnancy among Indigenous women and how that affects long-term health and infant health. One study on the prospective cohort of Aboriginal women and infants showed that less than 50 per cent of breastfeeding women were meeting nutrient requirements for folate, iodine, and calcium. Although breastfeeding initiation was high at 85.9 per cent, the median duration of breastfeeding was only approximately 42 days, in contrast to the recommended six months [17]. The research identified the need for promoting sustained breastfeeding practices and improving education on optimal nutrition for mothers and infants.

The arts health portion of the programme was initiated after Aboriginal partners identified a widely held view among the community that existing antenatal education classes were not culturally appropriate for their community [15]. Acknowledging that antenatal class attendance can have benefits not only for improving education and access to healthcare but also for increasing social connectedness and support networks, Gomeroi Gaaynggal established a culturally appropriate arts health centre [15, 16]. A range of topics are covered in the education programme, including antenatal care, mental health, and dietetics [18]. The centre also facilitates cooking classes, cultural art activities, baby health checks, and spaces for local artists and Elders to share stories. The programme continues to evolve in line with what is needed and relevant as decided by the community themselves. By fostering strong relationships with Aboriginal families, Elders, and community members, the Gomeroi gaaynggal research team recognised the positive impact this had on building an Aboriginal research cohort, study retention, and improvements in health literacy and antenatal outcomes from the arts health programme. While acknowledging that this participatory approach can be a costly and lengthy process, the benefits for research, translation of research findings, and, importantly, for the health and social outcomes of the local Aboriginal community are clear [15].

In Alberta, Canada, the ENRICH research team has developed similar CBPR approaches. In particular, their collaborative work with a large Cree First Nations community aims to address the disproportionate health burden experienced by Indigenous women by exploring better ways of supporting women and families in pregnancy and post-partum [19]. After an initial year and a half of strong engagement with the community, a research partnership was formalised via a Community Advisory Committee, which included Elders, health and social service professionals, and wider community members [20]. This committee collaborated with researchers to jointly design research protocols, interpret data, and contribute to dissemination. This resulted in several research and knowledge translation pathways, including exploring Cree men's experiences of their partner's pregnancy, implementing cultural sensitivity interventions for primary care staff, and understanding effective prenatal care for Cree women

[19, 20]. The latter involved an ethnographic CBPR study investigating views and perceptions of prenatal healthcare providers in the Cree community of Maskwacis, Alberta [20]. Interview findings showed that strong relationships, cultural understanding, and a sense of trust and non-judgement were key for First Nations women to receive effective prenatal care, while a lack of cultural appropriateness could lead to poorer outcomes and sustain health inequities. The study emphasised that time invested in such healthcare interactions to build relationships and trust should be standard and not viewed as extra [20]. The authors encouraged healthcare providers to actively engage with local Indigenous communities, stressing that reviewing literature or completing cultural competency courses is not enough to gain meaningful understandings of Indigenous experiences. By using a CBPR approach, the ENRICH team and the Cree First Nations community have built a strong research–community partnership that can investigate and address important health issues to improve the overall well-being of the Indigenous community.

Another example of research–community collaboration is the Abuela, Mamá y Yo (AMY) project. The AMY project was established by a partnership between the Oregon Health and Science University and Familias en Acción, a non-governmental community organisation focused on the health of Latino families in Oregon, the United States. The research-based programme partners with Latinx families and Latinx-serving organisations and is centred on DOHaD and intergenerational well-being, recognising the high rates of obesity and type 2 diabetes in the local Latino community [21]. Abuela, Mamá y Yo provides a culturally specific food equity nutrition education programme that addresses the root causes of health inequities and builds participants' knowledge around upstream determinants [21]. Community leaders have been trained to facilitate the AMY curriculum in community classes with core topics including the first 1000 days, breastfeeding, and decolonising food systems [22, 23]. Although evaluation is ongoing, initial mixed methods research, including pre- and post-surveys, has reported an increase in participant knowledge across all topics, particularly in relation to the first 1000 days concept. Similarly to other CBPR approaches in the DOHaD field, AMY researchers acknowledge the benefits of close community partnership, including the ability to constantly adapt and tailor to the community's needs, ensuring their work is relevant and impactful for the population of interest [22].

These research–community partnerships emphasise the importance of strong and sustained relationships in DOHaD research. This process can be particularly impactful for Indigenous and/or low- and middle-income communities where there may be mistrust due to past experiences of exploitative, one-sided research. Simply presenting to a community and requesting permission to undertake a research proposal is inadequate [24]. Community engagement and collaboration before a proposal is created and throughout each stage of research can ensure respect and integrity. Such collaborations build a greater level of trust and can strengthen 'buy-in' or willingness to participate in studies. When communities are actively leading research, there can also be a better understanding of where research needs to be targeted. The participatory DOHaD projects above describe how continuous feedback loops enable communities to contribute perspective and guidance regarding research directions and issues of local relevance and ultimately lead to the translation of evidence into action. CBPR approaches that co-construct research priorities and co-design studies ensure that the dignity of communities is upheld and can result in more relevant and impactful interventions. This is particularly important for Indigenous, historically marginalised, and low-income communities that are often disproportionately impacted by risk factors and, as a result, can experience poorer health outcomes.

18.3 A Case Study in the Cook Islands

We have previously published a systematic review that found a lack of DOHaD research occurring in low- and middle-income countries, particularly within the Pacific region [5]. The Cook Islands, with a resident population of 14,802, is one such Pacific nation that lacks research into DOHaD and early-life causes, despite experiencing some of the highest rates of NCDs and related-risk factors worldwide. Through a CBPR partnership focused on addressing these health challenges, researchers and the Cook Islands community co-developed research questions, data collection methods, and ways of knowledge translation. This section outlines the background of our Cook Islands partnership and the importance of using local models in research and explores a selection of research studies that have been carried out under this collaboration.

18.3.1 The Cook Islands

The Cook Islands is a self-governing state in free association with New Zealand. Its current health status is greatly influenced by a history of colonisation, Westernisation, and changing trade policies. Food imports have increased considerably since the late twentieth century, influencing a nutrition transition from traditional diets sourced from the land and ocean to more processed foods high in fat and sugar [25]. Approximately, 88.5 per cent of adults aged 18–64 years old are overweight and 61.4 per cent are obese [26]. Insufficient physical activity is reported among 33 per cent of adults, raised blood pressure affects 28.5 per cent, and raised blood glucose levels impact 23.5 per cent of adults [26]. Non-communicable diseases affect approximately 30 per cent of the population and contribute to 80 per cent of all deaths in the country, 36 per cent of which occur before 60 years old [27]. Risk factors among younger age groups are also of concern, with a 2015 global school health survey reporting 63.7 per cent of Cook Islands students aged 13–17 years were overweight/obese [28]. Although biannual school health checks are conducted in the Cook Islands to assess body mass index, lice, and skin conditions, there was a lack of in-depth data on metabolic health and, concurrently, no data on how this might be influenced by the early-life environment. This gap was identified, and action was taken to begin to address it within the work of The Pacific Science for Health Literacy Project (PSHLP) [29], a CBPR partnership between researchers, health professionals, educators, and community members.

The Pacific Science for Health Literacy Project is a multi-sectoral community-based participatory research project established initially across partners in the Cook Islands, Tonga, and New Zealand, and currently in action via an ongoing partnership between the Cook Islands Ministry of Education, Te Marae Ora Cook Islands Ministry of Health, and the Liggins Institute, University of Auckland. The partnership was established in 2012 via a pre-feasibility grant from the New Zealand Ministry of Foreign Affairs and Trade, which identified perceived commonalities in goals between potential partners, those being the Ministries of Education and Health in Tonga and the Cook Islands, and the University of Auckland's Liggins Institute in New Zealand. Staff from the Ministry of Foreign Affairs and Trade in New Zealand, Tonga, and the Cook Islands facilitated partner introductions over a period of four months, resulting in an agreement to enter into a six-month pre-feasibility study. The purpose of this study was to build relationships by enabling potential partners to meet, share, and listen, examine the potential of a partnership, and, importantly, co-write a grant application for pilot funding [30].

The PSHLP phase I pilot was funded from 2013 to 2016 and extended through to 2017, examining the potential of the school curriculum for developing scientific, sociological, and health literacies and facilitating adolescent-led actions [31]. Learning programmes were established that facilitated this development via the exploration of local community health challenges such as diabetes, obesity, and nutrition. This included examining the science of DOHaD using local and international evidence. By involving teachers from science, health and physical education, and social sciences, the programme encouraged the examination of issues from a systems perspective while also promoting educational goals associated with assessing multiple perspectives in relation to complex issues [32–34]. Engagement in the programme encouraged further locally led questions and provided opportunities for research capability development. In 2016, the funder and community representatives decided that a deliberation process should be undertaken to identify whether and how the programme should be developed. Stakeholders including community leaders, health and education experts, parents, diplomats, and representees from nongovernmental organisations and government agencies such as sport, child development, and agriculture met over a period of two days. This resulted in a plan to again work in partnership to propose the next phase of this CBPR and seek funding. Achieving funding to scale up took a further two years, during which time all partner schools from the pilot continued to use and grow the programmes. Resourcing partnership building and acknowledging the importance of local evidence guided by local frameworks that can inform community interventions and policies is key to effective CBPR.

18.3.2 Local Models and Methodologies

Research conducted using mainstream research frameworks and resulting programmes often have limited transferability for Indigenous and historically marginalised communities [35]. Framing research using local customs, traditions, and ways of knowing is one way to ensure it is contextualised and culturally relevant to the community of interest. Cook Islands collaborators within the PSHLP discussed the importance of utilising local frameworks and methodologies to ensure the research had a strong foundation in local knowledge. *Oraanga pitoenua*, or health and well-being, is a holistic concept in the Cook Islands that refers to what makes people healthy, happy, and well [34]. The five dimensions include *kopapa* (physical well-being), *tu manako* (mental and emotional well-being), *vaerua* (spiritual well-being), *kopu tangata* (social well-being), and *aorangi* (total environment) [34]. Like other holistic health models, *oraanga pitoenua* includes considerations for the health of one's body, thoughts and feelings, values, and beliefs, and for social and family relationships. It also incorporates *aorangi* and the recognition that one's connections with the land, the sky, and the ocean are important aspects of holistic health and wellbeing. This concept of *oraanga pitoenua* was central to the adolescent health research conducted in the Cook Islands, acknowledging that well-being is not simply an individual issue but related to our community relationships and connections to the environment.

Another key framework used in this research was the Tivaevae model, a Cook Islands research methodology first established by Teremoana Maua-Hodges in 1999 [36]. The framework uses the traditional tivaevae quilt-making process as a metaphor for a collaborative approach to research [37]. In the Cook Islands, tivaevae are colourful, hand-sewn patchwork quilts commonly created by a group of women and led by one *ta'unga* (expert). The three key stages of tivaevae-making are 1. *Koikoi* (picking), the preparation stage where patterns for the quilt are discussed and selected, 2. *Tuitui* (stitching), whereby patterns are stitched together and sewn onto the blank canvas, and 3. *Akairianga* (reviewing), where the completed tivaevae are gifted or displayed at birthdays, graduations, and other special occasions [38]. Five key principles underpin this tivaevae-making process: *taokotai* (collaboration), *akairi kite* (shared vision), *tu inangaro* (relationships), *uriuri kite* (reciprocity), and *tu akangateitei* (respect). The Tivaevae model applies this same process and key principles to research. *Koikoi* represents the initial stages of a research project where collaborations, ideas, and knowledge sharing occur to conceptualise research questions and plan a project. *Tuitui* is the 'making' stage of research where data are collected, analysed, and interpreted to create a story. *Akairianga* refers to disseminating research findings and determining how the evidence can be translated into real outcomes for the community. The Tivaevae model ensured PSHLP research was grounded in local Cook Island ways of knowing and emphasised the importance of having a shared vision and reciprocal relationships between researchers and the community.

18.3.3 Partnerships for DOHaD Research

The PSHLP partnership between researchers and the Cook Islands community embedded the Tivaevae model and local concepts of *oraanga pitoenua* from the beginning of the research process. As discussed previously, the PSHLP was formed to support health and science literacies within Cook Islands schools. Over time, knowledge sharing and collaborative discussions of DOHaD resulted in local partners questioning why there was no local evidence, given the high rates of NCDs and related risk factors. Cook Islands students participating in the PSHLP learning programme at school also began to consider the lack of local evidence and became increasingly interested in having access to and understanding their own health data. These discussions from Cook Islands students, educators, and health professionals within the PSHLP led to a research project aimed at extending local adolescent health measurements, linking these back to birth records to explore potential DOHaD associations and considering how to translate this evidence into positive outcomes for students themselves and the wider community.

We have previously published a short report on the process and key results from this initial study [39]. Educators, health professionals, and researchers worked together to facilitate and measure a range of health indicators among Year 9 adolescents (approximately 13 years old) in Cook Islands high schools from 2016 to 2018. Measures included height, weight, waist circumference, blood pressure, blood glucose, and total cholesterol levels. To support participating adolescents in understanding and having access to their own data, the PSHLP team co-created a resource named 'My Health Profile' where students could record and chart their measurements, alongside simple, informative health facts [40]. Teachers supported the development of these understandings during class time. Of the 195 students included in the study, our findings showed that approximately 68 per cent were overweight/obese, 46 per cent were affected by central obesity, and 43 per cent had raised blood pressure [39]. When linked with birth data, this study found a significant inverse association between birthweight and central obesity in Rarotongan adolescents. Data sense-making workshops with collaborators and community members emphasised the potential for DOHaD and investment into the early-life environment in the Cook Islands in order to optimise *oraanga pitoenua* later in life and across generations. They also recognised key areas of improvement for future research, including larger sample sizes, increasing the accuracy of measures, and further exploring the influence of school, home, and community contexts.

A key part of the Tivaevae model is *akairianga*, referring to the appropriate dissemination and knowledge translation of the evidence collected. Collaborators discussed how the local early-life data collected in addition to international evidence could be translated into positive outcomes for the community. A key discussion point was the need to increase community awareness of early-life concepts and provide an easily accessible, localised resource for new mothers, fathers, and families. We have previously published a paper that reports the CBPR process we undertook with a range of professional and lay groups in Rarotonga, Cook Islands, in order to co-design a local early-life resource [41]. With recruitment led by our Cook Islands collaborators, we conducted a series of collaborative focus group workshops with the House of Ariki and Koutu Nui (traditional chiefs and leaders in the Cook Islands), health professionals, pregnant women, current mothers of young children, Takamoa Theological College students, the Cook Islands National Youth Council, Internal Affairs, and the Child Welfare Association. After a series of co-designing workshops and draft reviews, a finalised resource titled 'Lifelong health: Our Tamariki' was created. Participants discussed the lack of physical resources available to expecting mothers and fathers, particularly emphasising the lack of locally relevant, contextualised information. They expressed that Cook Islanders would be able to relate to and form an attachment with the finalised resource and that it would help to start the conversation of nutrition, early-life health, and intergenerational impacts [41]. Although initially delayed by COVID-19, research is underway to assess the understanding of DOHaD and early-life concepts in the community both before and after the booklet is released. Local collaborators are also planning the initial launch of the resource in the community and its distribution to antenatal clinics, workplaces, and high schools across the islands.

The research described above is just a portion of the ongoing PSHLP work in the Cook Islands with other studies including investigations into adolescent physical activity levels, mental health, and the co-development of other health literacy resources as requested by the community. The CBPR approach has enabled strong relationships and reciprocal exchanges of knowledge between researchers and community members. Local partners set research directions that they feel are important and relevant for their community. Side-by-side collaboration throughout data collection and interpretation phases not only enabled 'buy-in' but also allowed for insight into relevant contextual factors that may explain specific data trends. Taking a CBPR approach has also proved beneficial for research translation. Ensuring the community was involved from the beginning helped to increase the acceptability of findings and strengthen community-led action. The views held among communities are not always homogenous, and thus it is important that this process of building and maintaining relationships is given the necessary time and breadth. CBPR is an approach that respects the dignity of local communities, prioritises shared power and reciprocal knowledge, and can ensure research evidence is translated to be impactful.

18.4 Future for CBPR in DOHaD

Although there is increasing recognition from researchers in the DOHaD field about the need to conduct research alongside community partners, projects where this has occurred remain limited. This may be due to the challenges of developing strong community engagement. First and foremost, building relationships and trust with a community can be a lengthy and sometimes difficult process. Many communities already harbour a mistrust of science and research due to historical experiences of exploitation. Developing strong, trusting relationships should therefore be a long-term commitment and is not typically acknowledged under the traditional role of a researcher [7]. Additionally, as funding structures require a research proposal to be set out before funding is allocated, this can lead to many hours of unpaid work to develop strong collaborations with communities that can then together put forward a project proposal. However, ensuring a 'cyclical and iterative process' where research projects are able to be sustainable and fully owned by the community to ensure continuation beyond research funding limits is important and achievable via CBPR [7]. Regardless of the challenges, there is a need for more DOHaD research to adopt CBPR moving forward. The current examples in the DOHaD field typically relate to community awareness or education programmes within Indigenous and historically marginalised communities. While this is important and needed, researchers outside these spaces should also consider adopting CBPR principles and local cultural models for both quantitative and qualitative DOHaD research to ensure relevancy and contextually appropriate outcomes. CBPR can ensure the reciprocal sharing of different forms of knowledge, develop capabilities, and contribute to improving overall health and well-being.

18.5 Conclusion

Community-based participatory research aims for equal partnership and sharing of knowledge between researchers and communities. It has its foundations in social justice and empowerment and can be used to build trust and capabilities in underprivileged communities. There are examples in the DOHaD field of how CBPR positively guides how research is conducted. Our own work in the Cook Islands shows that CBPR relationships may develop slowly and over a long time. However, what can result is a community that is empowered to learn, ask questions, and make positive social changes, and researchers that can also learn and adapt research contextually. Institutions and funding bodies should acknowledge and promote such forms of collaborative partnerships to ensure that research can be appropriately conducted and sustainably embedded with the goal of improving long-term and intergenerational well-being.

References

1. Hanson MA, Gluckman PD. Early developmental conditioning of later health and disease: Physiology or pathophysiology? Physiol Rev. 2014; 94(4):1027–76.

2. Barker DJ, Osmond C. Infant mortality, childhood nutrition, and ischaemic heart disease in England and Wales. Lancet. 1986; 327(8489):1077–81.

3. M'hamdi HI, de Beaufort I, Jack B, Steegers E. Responsibility in the age of Developmental Origins of Health and Disease (DOHaD) and epigenetics. JDOHaD. 2018; 9(1):58–62.

4. Penkler M, Jacob CM, Müller R, Kenney M, Norris SA, da Costa CP, et al. Developmental Origins of Health and Disease, resilience and social justice in the COVID era. JDOHaD. 2021;13(4):1–4.

5. Tu'akoi S, Vickers MH, Bay JL. DOHaD in low-and middle-income countries: A systematic review exploring gaps in DOHaD population studies. JDOHaD. 2020; 11(6):557–63.

6. Tremblay M, Martin DH, McComber AM, McGregor A, Macaulay AC. Understanding community-based participatory research through a social movement framework: A case study of the Kahnawake Schools Diabetes Prevention Project. BMC Public Health. 2018; 18(1):1–17.

7. Holkup PA, Tripp-Reimer T, Salois EM, Weinert C. Community-based participatory research: An approach to intervention research with a Native American community. ANS Adv Nurs Sci. 2004; 27(3):162.

8. Corburn J. Street science: Community knowledge and environmental health justice. Cambridge, MA: MIT Press; 2005. 271 p.

9. Israel BA, Eng E, Schulz AJ, Parker EA. Introduction to methods for community-based participatory research for health. Methods for community-based participatory research for health. 2nd ed. San Francisco: John Wiley & Sons, Incorporated; 2012. pp. 1–38.

10. De las Nueces D, Hacker K, DiGirolamo A, Hicks LS. A systematic review of community-based participatory research to enhance clinical trials in racial and ethnic minority groups. Health Services Res. 2012, 47(3pt2):1363–386.

11. Fitzpatrick EF, Martiniuk AL, D'Antoine H, Oscar J, Carter M, Elliott EJ. Seeking consent for research with indigenous communities: A systematic review. BMC Med Ethics. 2016; 17(1):1–18.

12. Cook WK. Integrating research and action: A systematic review of community-based participatory research to address health disparities in environmental and occupational health in the USA. JECH. 2008; 62(8):668–76.

13. Salimi Y, Shahandeh K, Malekafzali H, Loori N, Kheiltash A, Jamshidi E, et al. Is community-based participatory research

(CBPR) useful? A systematic review on papers in a decade. Int J Prev Med. 2012; 3(6):386.

14. De las Nueces D, Hacker K, DiGirolamo A, Hicks LS. A systematic review of community-based participatory research to enhance clinical trials in racial and ethnic minority groups. Health Serv Res. 2012; 47(3pt2):1363–86.

15. Rae K, Weatherall L, Clausen D, Maxwell C, Bowman M, Milgate P, et al. Gomeroi gaaynggal: Empowerment of Aboriginal communities through ArtsHealth to understand health implications of research in pregnancy. 2013.

16. Rae K, Weatherall L, Hollebone K, Apen K, McLean M, Blackwell C, et al. Developing research in partnership with Aboriginal communities: Strategies for improving recruitment and retention. Rural Remote Health. 2013;13(2):1–8.

17. Ashman A, Collins C, Weatherall L, Keogh L, Brown L, Rollo M, et al. Dietary intakes and anthropometric measures of Indigenous Australian women and their infants in the Gomeroi gaaynggal cohort. JDOHaD. 2016; 7(5):481–97.

18. Rae K, Weatherall L, Blackwell C, Pringle K, Smith R, Lumbers E. Long conversations: Gomeroi gaaynggal tackles renal disease in the Indigenous community. Australas Epidemiol. 2014; 21(1):44–48.

19. ENRICH. Working with a First Nations community Alberta: University of Alberta (no date). Available from: https://enrich.ualberta.ca/our-research/working-with-a-first-nations-community/.

20. Oster RT, Bruno G, Montour M, Roasting M, Lightning R, Rain P, et al. Kikiskawâwasow-prenatal healthcare provider perceptions of effective care for First Nations women: An ethnographic community-based participatory research study. BMC Pregnancy Childbirth. 2016;16(1):1–9.

21. Familias en Acción. Abuela, Mamá y Yo! Oregon. 2021. Available from: www.familiasenaccion.org/abuela-mama-y-yo/.

22. Arnold B, Márquez R, Gurrola A, Ventura Meda I. Abuela, Mamá y Yo;

Nutritional resiliency for the Latinx community. OSHU-PSU School of Public Health Annual Conference; Oregon: Oregon Health & Science University; 2020.

23. Gautom P, Richardson DM. Evaluation of Abuela, Mamá y Yo: Informing programmatic level change. OSHU-PSU School of Public Health Annual Conference; Oregon: Oregon Health & Science University; 2021.

24. O'Donahoo FJ, Ross KE. Principles relevant to health research among Indigenous communities. IJERPH. 2015; 12(5):5304–9.

25. Ulijaszek SJ. Trends in body size, diet and food availability in the Cook Islands in the second half of the twentieth century. Econ Hum Biol. 2003; 1(1):123–37.

26. Cook Islands Ministry of Health. Cook Islands NCD risk factors STEPS report 2013–2015. Suva, Fiji; 2016.

27. World Health Organization. Western Pacific region health information and intelligence platform (HIIP): Noncommunicable disease mortality, data by country. Geneva: World Health Organization; 2008. Available from: http://hiip.wpro.who.int/data.

28. World Health Organization. Global school-based student health survey: Cook Islands 2015 fact sheet. Geneva: World Health Organization; 2015.

29. LENScience. Pacific science for health literacy project Auckland. Auckland: University of Auckland; 2013. Available from: www.lenscience.auckland.ac.nz/en/about/partnership-programmes/pacific-science-for-health-literacy-project.html.

30. Bay JL, MacIntyre B. Pacific science for health literacy pre-feasibility study report. Auckland: University of Auckland; 2013.

31. Bay JL, Yaqona D, Oyamada M. DOHaD interventions: Opportunities during adolescence and the periconceptional period. In: Sata F, Fukuoka H, Hanson M, editors. Pre-emptive medicine: Public health aspects of developmental origins of health and disease. Singapore: Springer; 2019. pp. 37–51.

32. Barrett-Watson C, Bay JL. Two hundred years of lifestyle change on Rarotonga. Auckland: Read Pacific Publishers Limited; 2017. 58 p.

33. Bay JL, Mora HA, Tairea K, Yaqona D, Sloboda DM, Vickers MH. Te maki toto vene (T2): E manamanata no toku iti tangata. Teacher resource. Auckland: Read Pacific Publishers Ltd; 2016.

34. Bay JL, Yaqona D. Ko au te toku aorangi: Kai no te oraanga meitaki. Student book. Cook Islands edition. Auckland: Read Pacific Publishing Ltd; 2015.

35. Chino M, DeBruyn L. Building true capacity: Indigenous models for Indigenous communities. AJPH. 2006; 96 (4):596–99.

36. Maua-Hodges T. Ako Pai ki Aitutaki: Transporting or weaving cultures: What effects and influences do the visits of Ako Pai to Aitutaki, Cook Islands, have on principals, teachers, island council and community? Wellington; 1999.

37. Futter-Puati D, Maua-Hodges T. Stitching tivaevae: A Cook Islands research method. AlterNative. 2019; 15 (2):140–49.

38. Te Ava A, Page A. How the Tivaevae Model can be used as an Indigenous methodology in Cook Islands education settings. Aust J Indig Educ. 2018; 49 (1):70–76.

39. Tu'akoi S, Bay JL, Aung YYM, Tamarua-Herman N, Barrett-Watson C, Tairea K, et al. Birth weight and adolescent health indicators in Rarotonga, Cook Islands. APJPH. 2022; 34(1):118–22.

40. Herman H, Tairea K, Bay J. My health profile. Auckland: Liggins Institute; 2016.

41. Tu'akoi S, Tamarua-Herman N, Tairea K, Vickers MH, Aung YYM, Bay JL. Supporting Cook Island communities to access DOHaD evidence. JDOHaD. 2020; 11(6):564–72.

Chapter

19 The First 1000 Days and Clinical Practice in Infant Mental Health

Anusha Lachman, Astrid Berg, Fiona C. Ross, and Simone M. Peters

19.1 Introduction

The chapter begins with two premises. First, infancy is a crucial time in human develop-ment, both physically and cognitive-affectively. During the first three years of life, the infant develops from being helpless and absolutely dependent to being able to move independently and make its needs known through language. In this time, the foundations are laid for socio-emotional and cognitive development. These premises are confirmed in DOHaD research, where the earliest period of life has clearly been demonstrated to be significant in shaping individual health over the life cycle and intergenerationally, and thence shaping population health over time. The second premise arises from the recogni-tion by the World Health Organization (WHO) that mental health is a right. It is included in the United Nations Sustainable Development Goals (SDGs), where Goal 3 makes explicit its significance for the accomplishment of other goals [1]. The latest State of the World's Children Report [2] specifically focuses on children's mental health.

A large body of research suggests that some aspects of mental health and illness may be heritable. There is also clear evidence that environmental factors in the perinatal period can have durable effects on cognitive and emotional development and function and that infancy and the perinatal period offer opportunities to identify and ameliorate such effects [3]. The DOHaD-inspired 'first 1000 days of life' campaigns, for example, indicate the potential to alter developmental trajectories and protect children against environmental risk factors through early intervention. There is also growing recognition that supportive social relations in the early period promote adaptive cognitive and emotional functioning over time and potentially through the generations. The WHO et al.'s [4] endorsement of 'nurturing care' is a recognition of how material and emotional care produce improved long-term individual and social outcomes. These include better social relationships and psychological stability and improved schooling outcomes. In the longer term, they are assumed to result in greater work productivity and economic stability. So compelling are the findings that the Lancet Commission on Mental Health identifies child and youth mental health as 'a moral imperative' (1 p1578). This gives impetus to work that seeks to support caring relations and ameliorate the conditions under which human development takes place.

19.2 Why Infants? Infant Mental Health and Well-Being

Infant mental health refers to the 'young child's capacity to experience, regulate, and express emotions, form close and secure relationships, and explore the environment and learn' [5, p. 6].

Like DOHaD, infant mental health (IMH) is a convergent field of study, informed by multiple disciplines, including paediatrics, allied medical disciplines, developmental psychology, psychiatry, neuroscience, clinical practice, and public mental health advocacy. As such, it cuts across disciplines, giving it a broad and inclusive foundation for research and implementation. Its aim is to identify and enable positive developmental trajectories for children [5]. Its central tenet is that the human infant is born with a capacity to explore the environment, learn, experience, and express emotions. While learning is lifelong, the plasticity of the developing brain makes early childhood critical. From the start, in utero, the infant takes in and absorbs the stimuli from its environment and gradually forms internal images and representations in its mind of what it means and what it requires to be a member of a particular community. Far from being a blank slate or *tabula rasa*, the infant comes into this world with a 'story' and sensory experience [6].

Cognitive well-being and affective stability are critical to adaptive responses to the world and, in addition to their individual effects, are seen by developmental practitioners as central to the making of stable societies and productive workforces. For these capacities to unfold, the baby requires human relationships. Infant mental health thus takes as its central concern the relationship between infants and caregivers. The emphasis on *relations* is vital, marking an important shift away from the focus on individual psychological disturbance to a concern with the promotion of infant well-being and flourishing within the networks of relations that comprise their lives. To theorise this, IMH draws on developmental psychology, particularly attachment theory, in explaining well-being and promoting secure relationships that form the basis of social and intellectual functioning.

While it is not always thought of as DOHAD research, there is considerable evidence from multiple fields that demonstrates that the early social environment is an important shaper, sometimes determinant, of early child psychological development, which in turn influences long-term child health outcomes [7, 8]. A robust body of scholarship shows that stressors during early development (including prenatally) can affect cognitive and emotional development and generate mental health problems that endure into or may only fully materialise in adulthood [9]. Stressors produce neuro-biological effects that have lasting, potentially heritable effects on mental health [10]. Different kinds of stressors at different times in development may have different effects and different outcomes [11]. Specific biological and chemical pathways are disputed [12] and are still under investigation [13]. Some of these findings are also attributable to the broader socio-economic circumstances under which children are raised. In addition to these influences, there is growing attention to the possibilities of transgenerational transmission of mental health risks and illness. This may be a result of genetic inheritance, epigenetic processes [14], and/or because affected adults may be less able to provide secure environments for raising children, particularly where social-political-economic circumstances are inhospitable.

The interplay between genetic predispositions and the physical and psycho-social environment thus lays the foundations for mental and physical health [15]. Infant mental health understands that these are mediated by *relations in context*. The emphasis on relations is critical. Relationships are embedded in context, and we suggest that more attention needs to be paid to the latter. In the remainder of the chapter, we explore contextual factors significant for infant mental health before turning to our work on localising the model of IMH, a process we characterise as *attunement* to context. The latter seeks to enable a picture of well-being that has resonance and efficacy in the contexts in which we work in southern Africa and that has the potential to shift the gamut of social relations to enable better support of infants and their relational worlds.

19.3 Exposure and Resilience

While the epigenetic and neurobiological processes that shape outcomes are still under investigation, knowledge of the effects of psycho-social stressors in infancy on child and adult mental health has a history that predates DOHaD. Socio-economic factors are particularly significant. There is a substantially higher prevalence of common perinatal mental health disorders in low- and middle-income countries (LMICs) than in higher income countries, particularly in poorer peri-urban and rural areas [16, 17]. Mother–infant dyads in LMICs may be exposed to multiple cumulative environmental factors that may confer risk on infant outcomes. Parental capacity to provide the kind of care that promotes security in infancy and good developmental outcomes can be severely compromised in adverse conditions such as poverty, particularly when mothers are themselves at risk for mental health disorders [18]. Concern has been raised about the links between maternal stress and later mental health disorders in children, including, among others, attention deficit hyperactivity disorders (ADHD), depression, and poor development of linguistic, cognitive, and socio-emotional skills [9].

In South Africa, for example, poverty, inequality, insecurity, and gender-based violence produce and compound very high rates of perinatal depression and anxiety and mental illness [19, 20]. Risks appear to be cumulative: for example, shocks in early childhood are correlated with a greater risk of mental illness in adulthood [2, 21]. Research on Adverse Childhood Experiences suggests that there is a 'graded relationship' between early exposure to emotional, physical, and sexual abuse and later disease and risk behaviours [22]. More recent cohort studies in South Africa have suggested that there is a graded relationship between ACEs, adult ill health, and adult risk behaviours including antisocial behaviours.

Longitudinal studies are increasingly showing the effects of early life experiences, particularly toxic stress, on development [23, 24]. There is robust evidence pointing to the transmission of maternal (and some paternal) factors in mental ill health, especially regarding the links between maternal depression and stress and child development. However, the precise mechanisms remain complex. In a review, Wan and Green [25] highlighted that most children of mothers with mental health problems do not inevitably develop lasting attachment difficulties. While children in settings of vulnerability (social adversity and caregiver mental illness) may be at higher risk of developing relational difficulties, many go on to develop positive developmental outcomes and secure attachments, indicating that childhood resilience may be facilitated by the efforts of mothers and others to mitigate the immediate and potential impact of maternal mental illness [26].

Indeed, evidence from the cognate fields of psychiatry, psychology, and child development [5] clearly demonstrates that the kinds of insults described above can be partially offset by attentive care practices. These are presumed to provide the grounds for secure relating that in turn sets in motion processes of resilient adaptation shown to be critical in long-term health. A large body of evidence demonstrates that attachment relations between the infant and the caregiver are critical for physical survival, optimal development of the brain, and resilience through the lifecourse. Interventions in this early sensitive phase of life have been shown to promote well-being in a more effective way than interventions later in the life cycle.

This is a critical concern for international organisations such as UNICEF, Save the Children, and the WHO, among others, which have become increasingly focused on 'parenting' to ameliorate or offset social shocks and promote resilience and social competence. It is important that 'parenting' be understood as a component of the infant's environment and not as the solution for factors that lie well beyond parental control. This suggests that we need to pay critical attention to how to theorise the contexts and environments that shape exposures and resilience. Given the emphasis on 'environment' in DOHAD research, this should not come as a surprise.

19.4 Universalist Models and Local Contexts

As Zeanah and Zeanah note, 'One of the most distinctive features of the early years is the clear importance of multiple interrelated contexts (e.g. caregiver–infant relationship, family, cultural, social, and historical) within which infants develop' [5, p. 19]. How we theorise those relationships and their 'multiple, interrelated contexts' matters, as do the assumptions we make about their role in well-being. Much of what has been written on human development has been drawn from populations from Western, educated, industrialised, rich and democratic (WEIRD) societies [27]. This leaves out or ignores the majority of the world's infants and young children. It also means that much of what has been 'evidence-based' comes from a biased and limited sample. Work from South Africa, particularly from the Parent-Infant Mental Health Service in Cape Town [28] and the *Ububele Umdlezane* Parent-Infant Project in Johannesburg [29], and from ongoing practical work in parenting centres, child support services, and perinatal healthcare projects, suggests that care needs to be taken in how we understand the formative influences on babies of the specific social worlds around them. Contextual factors, including ongoing legacies of racism and social inequalities, combined with cultural variations in ideas about parenting, childrearing, and diverse family structures, make it difficult to apply a 'one-size-fits-all' approach to understanding IMH and the interventions needed to support and protect it. This is an important consideration for DOHaD scholarship, especially as questions about how to understand and investigate the 'environment' and its press on partly permeable bodies become more critical [30].

Take, for example, the assumptions about kinship embedded in theoretical models animating IMH. Attachment theory anticipates that a child learns the security from which to explore the world with confidence from its primary caregiver's arms. This caregiver is frequently posited to be the mother – as is often the case. But it is also the case that many people are involved in childcare, especially after an early period of seclusion. Some are recognised in the literature: female relatives such as aunts and grandmothers; people employed to offer care, such as nannies and workers in early childhood development centres [31, 32]. Much less recognised are the informal networks of adults and older children whose supportive care generates a wide social net for children – as Keller and Chaudhary [33] call it, 'cradles of care' – that can be endangered if it is not recognised as part of social and emotional well-being. While the responsibility of infant care rests mainly with adult caregivers, in many places, younger generations share in childcare roles. These in turn are dependent on the immediate and distal social environment in which they live. Economic hardship or ease, disadvantages, cultural norms and values, and political circumstances impact the parent and other caregivers and the relationship with the infant. As a common African proverb has it, 'It takes a village to raise a child'. Indeed, it was precisely this proverb that was used in South Africa to launch a Provincial First Thousand Days Campaign in 2016 that seeks to undo historical legacies of ill health, particularly stunting, through close attention to infant well-being.

The impact of historical factors on structures supporting infant well-being is particularly significant in the southern African context. For example, the migrant labour system that long characterised family life for many Black South Africans and those in neighbouring states has produced complex familial arrangements across the region. The HIV pandemic that, until relatively recently, produced mass illness and death in the absence of antiretro viral drugs, shifted caring practices to a wider range of kin and other networks, some of which became tightly stretched in impoverished contexts. Ongoing political instabilities and economic insecurities in the subregion generate considerable mobility in family life, including ongoing separations of mothers and babies. The resultant social forms are not the simple 'nuclear family' long presumed to be desirable and normative, but complex and shifting adaptations to changing circumstances. And indeed, there is growing evidence that the nuclear family itself, on which much developmental theory rests, makes caring effectively for children much more difficult than is the case in more complex households – the same households that have long been stigmatised for their deviation from the nuclear model [34]. There is therefore a need to factor into our models of well-being the diverse sources from which children receive nurturing care while still recognising and supporting the primary (dyadic) caregivers. Doing so presents a more accurate perspective on the environments that support children and complicates an overly simplistic equation of relations as solely dyadic and the 'woman as environment model' that has, until recently, beset DOHaD research [35, 36].

While DOHaD research has largely focused on the effects of maternal factors on epigenetics and neuropsychological development, there is growing interest in the paternal factors [37]. Similarly, in psychiatry, there is a small but growing body of research that explores paternal factors on infant well-being [38]. This suggests that a father(-figure)'s mental state affects infants directly (through inheritance and parenting practices) and indirectly (through the effects of mental illness on family stability and emotional tenor) and contributes to infants' internalising and externalising behaviours. Lasting consequences include the risk of child psychopathology [ibid.].

In psychology, although there was early recognition that infants attach to their fathers as well, most research has also focused on the mother–child dyad. More recent scholarship on paternity demonstrates that fathers affect the infant's well-being both indirectly and directly [39] and that positive infant–father relationships result in healthy emotional and social outcomes for the infant [40] and over the lifecourse [41, 42]. The father's relationship with the infant's mother indirectly affects the infant's well-being. Indeed, research conducted in Soweto, South Africa [43], concluded that father involvement may reduce postnatal maternal depression and improve maternal mental health, with important implications for infant well-being.

Well-being needs to be broadly understood. In many parts of southern Africa, it is the father's responsibility to ensure the incorporation of the child into meaningful social worlds and secure wider sets of relationships. Andile Mayekiso describes this as 'social attachment': the work of enabling cultural identifications and securing social well-being through the rituals that identification enjoins [44]. In contexts where historical processes have shattered family life, the absence of a paternal figure whose kin can be relied on to structure belonging may have severe mental health consequences. And yet, despite the significance of the paternal role in an infant's life, men are still marginalised in both practices of parent–infant psychotherapy and psychoanalytic and IMH theory [45].

19.5 Translation to the Clinical Setting: Increasing Awareness and Increasing Knowledge

The reality for many South African infants and young children, and indeed children in much of the world – including in some of the world's richest countries – remains one of significant deprivation. Beyond the drivers of socio-economic disadvantage, access to quality healthcare and mental health services – in particular, for caregivers – remains neglected and under-resourced. Limited mental health resources (including both physical structures and human resources) impact clinicians' abilities to screen and offer support, referrals, and appropriate early interventions.

In South African public health, there has been tragically poor investment in mental health services and support at both community and district levels [46, 47]. While our IMH training programme (described below) responds to the need for awareness and upskilling of local care providers at a grassroots level, the ability to integrate screening and support of infants at risk remains out of reach. Health and family support network providers are faced with a difficult choice: to identify problematic or at-risk dyads early but be limited in what they can be offered or to continue to focus on purely physical and social risks that can be addressed within a resource-constrained system. With task shifting/sharing[1] being one of the key focus areas of the SDGs, we believe the answer may lie in innovative approaches that attempt to upskill existing allied and support workers to identify mental health risks in their standard practices of care and to adapt treatment models to this and similar settings. This has the potential to bring mental health into the mainstream of everyday clinical practice. So, if infants are routinely weighed, immunised, and assessed for physical health conditions at local clinics, an IMH-friendly approach would then include additional questioning around the relationship and interactions of the infant and caregiver. Caregiver mental health screening is then included as part of the infant health screening, true to IMH's relational underpinnings. Where health practitioners are attuned to cultural values, practices, and historical circumstances, this can also contribute to aligning scientific knowledge about infant well-being to specific contexts, helping to create the localised 'nurturing care' imagined in global health discourse.

To bring awareness of IMH into everyday clinical practice, we needed a simple screening tool that would blend in with existing local conditions and practices. Drawing from European work on caregiver and infant screening at the primary healthcare level, Puura, Berg, and Malek developed the Basic IMH Screen (BIMHS) [48], a five-

---

[1] Task shifting or task sharing refers to the re-allocation of healthcare tasks to non-traditional healthcare workers (HCWs) such as community HCWs and allied professionals. This is particularly important in low-resource settings.

item tool that can be readily identified by a primary HCW. Items are 'basic' in the sense of being universally present or valid for infants and their caregivers. They are embedded in and form an implicit *sine qua non* in the World Association of Infant Mental Health Position Paper on the Rights of Infants [49].

The items consist of two simple questions for the mother/primary caregiver: *Are you worried about your infant/child? How have you been feeling?* The third item is the weight of the infant that is routinely plotted on a growth chart. The fourth and fifth items are simple observations of the infant's eye contact with the caregiver or health worker, and moments of shared pleasure between the infant and caregiver. The last item is the intuitive sense of the HCW about the dyad: is the relationship between the two of concern or not?

If there is concern about any of these items, the caregiver may be given an earlier appointment to determine whether the concern persists or not. Only after several such checks, should the infant be followed up at a more specialised clinic or service. The BIMHS is thus meant to 'flag' vulnerable dyads and to provide them with additional support, which, if given early enough, may prevent a less-than-optimal trajectory.

The BIMHS has been incorporated by the Western Cape Provincial Department of Health into existing maternal and infant screening tools as part of a DOHaD-inspired focus on the first thousand days of life.

In environments characterised by inequality, support in this respect can be significant, although it does not outweigh the importance of structural reform for population-level effects. This is particularly true where mental health challenges in the perinatal period continue to be overshadowed by complex systemic issues in health systems. These include a lack of resourcing, limited collaborative care between obstetric antenatal and psychiatric services, stigma, cultural misconceptions, and a lack of accessible and sustainable service delivery models. They can be partly addressed by general and mental healthcare professionals encouraging an awareness of the impact of perinatal mental health on early IMH, as well as early dyadic screening and intervention, and careful attention to cultural and social factors shaping infant potential and well-being.

19.6 Developing Comprehensive Approaches to IMH

In stark contrast to international standards of care espoused by high-income countries (HICs) and international organisations such as the WHO and UNICEF, the African continent offered no professional postgraduate degrees focusing on IMH until the development of a structured master's degree programme at Stellenbosch University to attempt to address this need [50]. This programme applies social medicine principles to train interdisciplinary practitioners to enter a diverse workspace, with the intention of integrating IMH-specific approaches into existing clinical offerings. Its diverse curriculum addresses human development, social and mental health influences on parenting practices, and accommodates both professional diversity and cultural diversity. It aims to develop interdisciplinary practitioners skilled in clinical observation and screening while also contributing to the critical local research agenda in the IMH field.

The ways that care, attachment, and relationships form and are understood in everyday practices are not universal. This raises the challenge of developing teaching models and course content to reflect local practice while remaining true to the core principles of the field of IMH. The ambitious degree programme has navigated pedagogic and logistical challenges in training and assessment methods, content applicability, and competency evaluation. Legacies of economic, social, and political disadvantage in South Africa continue to impact higher education and training, especially in multiculturally diverse classrooms such as ours. Teaching faculty has to navigate sensitively, with awareness of an underlying English language and Eurocentric bias on pedagogy and outcome assessments. A critical stance is required when evaluating students within the field of their own training background (such as allied health and humanities) while integrating a new field of IMH (relying on psychological and biological health origins). The programme integrates alternative blended teaching methods with traditional coursework to accommodate students' academic and professionally diverse backgrounds. The result has been a rich and evolving offering of a complex and diverse learning environment that speaks to the true cultural and ethnic diversity of South African students and the health-seeking population of its children.

Graduates of the MPhil programme integrate their learnings in context-specific health and psychological settings, including infant feeding clinics, well-baby immunisation visits, and mothers attending routine antenatal or assisted fertility services. This demonstrates the relative ease with which IMH can be included in standard packages of care, without requiring greater specialisation. This speaks to the true nature of IMH and its influence across sectors. Such findings can be applied to DOHaD interventions also.

There has been resistance. One of the main challenges in approaching an established subject field in Africa is the ability to share and contribute to the existing international literature. 'Publish or perish' has never been more relevant than in the current climate. Yet there is resistance from peer-reviewed publication avenues to specific contextual offerings that are not considered favourably by or as being of interest to 'global' (i.e. American-Eurocentric) audiences [51]. The field of IMH disproportionately favours a Eurocentric approach [52]. This is a contentious issue for researchers in LMIC settings who struggle to balance the desire to produce locally relevant and culturally sensitive research with the need to accommodate Euro-American expectations and HIC contexts. Infant mental health work in Africa challenges that norm, desiring to develop a field and produce academic offerings originating in Africa and for Africa; offerings that are sensitive to the manifold ways people produce well-being in different contexts. In localising the model of health, then, we seek to enable a picture of well-being that has resonance and efficacy in the contexts in which we work and may shift the gamut of social relations to enable better support of infants and their relational worlds. The model we have described here may be useful to DOHaD practitioners seeking to do the same.

19.7 Conclusion

Broad environmental factors – poverty, malnourishment, racism, interpersonal and structural violence, and inequality – are critical factors shaping mental well-being. Such environmental insults have lasting, possibly heritable effects. Research on brain development and plasticity suggests that early experience of positive dyadic and broader relational ties is critical in supporting infant well-being, promoting resilience, and potentially reducing rates of mental illness later in life. Relationships are not only outer social connections but are also evident as inner neural brain circuitry in every individual. The context and relationships that each infant is born into give meaning and voice to this complex matrix of inner and outer and bind the subjective with the objective. There is here an important project in bridging the divide between the sciences of the brain and heredity and those of the psyche and relationship. Drawing from the literature and southern African experience, we suggest that approaches to human well-being that centre relationality both enable optimal outcomes and may map onto ontologies in much of the non-Western world. This in turn enables knowledge to be localised to specific conditions, something that is critical in DOHaD research. In southern Africa, understanding and supporting infant well-being requires attunement to the damaging effects of colonialism and postcolonial economic formations on family life and an effective training infrastructure. Southern scholarships, concerned with the interplay of power, history, and everyday life, can help to illuminate some of the more problematic assumptions about social environments and generate interventions that are reflective and responsive to local conditions. The result will be the culturally and socially adaptive approaches called for in the WHO's Nurturing Care Framework, with particular emphasis on promoting secure relationships that are essential for future social and cognitive functioning.

References

1. Patel, V. S., Saxena, C., Lundt†, G., Thornicroft, F., Bainga, P. et al. The Lancet Commission on global mental health and sustainable development. The Lancet, 2018. 392:1553–1598.

2. UNICEF. The state of the world's children: On my mind – Promoting, protecting and caring for children's mental health. 2021. New York: UNICEF.

3. Monk, C., Spicer, J., Champagne, F. Linking prenatal maternal adversity to developmental outcomes in infants: The role of epigenetic pathways. Development and Psychopathology, 2012. 24: 1361–1376.

4. World Health Organization, United Nations Children's Fund, World Bank Group. Nurturing care for early childhood development: A framework for helping children survive and thrive to transform health and human potential. 2018. Geneva: World Health Organization. https://apps.who.int/iris/handle/10665/272603

5. Zeanah, C. H. Jr. and Zeanah, P. D. Infant mental health: The science of early experience' pp. 16–35 in C. Zeanah (ed.) The handbook of infant mental health. 2019. New York: Guildford Press.

6. Marx, V.,and Nagy, E. F.. Behavioural responses to maternal voice and touch. PLoS ONE. 2015. 10(6): e0129118. doi:10.1371/journal.pone.0129118

7. Maggi, S., Irwin, L. J., Siddiqi, A., and Hertzman, C. The social determinants of early child development: An overview. Journal of Paediatrics and Child Health, 2010. 46(11), 627–635.

8. Richter, L. M., Orkin, F. M., Adair, L. S., Kroker-Lobos, M. F., Mayol, N. L., Menezes, A. M. B., . . . and Victora, C. Differential influences of early growth and social factors on young children's cognitive performance in four low-and-middle-income birth cohorts (Brazil, Guatemala, Philippines, and South Africa). SSM-Population Health. 2020. 12: 100648.

9. Shonkoff, J. and Garner, A. The lifelong effects of early childhood adversity and toxic stress. Pediatrics. 2012. 29(1): e232–46. doi: 10.1542/peds.2011-2663.

10. Schmidt, L., Burack, J., and Van Lieshout, R. Themed Issue on Developmental Origins of Adult Mental Health and Illness. Journal of Developmental Origins of Health and Disease, 2016. 7(6): 564–564. doi:10.1017/S204017441600060X

11. Cameron, J. L., Eagleson, K. L., Fox, N. A., Hensch, T. K., and Levitt, P. Social origins of developmental risk for mental and physical illness. The Journal of

Neuroscience, 2017. 37(45): 10783–10791.

12. O'Donnell, K. J., Meaney, M. l. J.. Origins of mental health: The developmental origins of health and disease hypothesis. American Journal of Psychiatry, 2017. 174: 319–328; doi: 10.1176/appi.ajp.2016.16020138.

13. Huizink, A. and De Rooij, S. Prenatal stress and models explaining risk for psychopathology revisited: Generic vulnerability and divergent pathways. Development and Psychopathology, 2018. 30(3): 1041–1062. doi: 10.1017/S095457941800034

14. Taouk, L. and Schulkin, J. Transgenerational transmission of pregestational and prenatal experience: Maternal adversity, enrichment, and underlying epigenetic and environmental mechanisms. Journal of Developmental Origins of Health and Disease, 2016. 7(6): 588–601. doi:10.1017/S2040174416000416

15. Shonkoff, J., Slopen, N., and Williams, D. R. Early childhood adversity, toxic stress, and the impacts of racism on the foundations of health. Annual Review of Public Health, 2021. 42(1): 115–134.

16. Fisher, J., Mello, M. C. D., Patel, V., Rahman, A., Tran, T., Holton, S., and Holmes, W. Prevalence and determinants of common perinatal mental disorders in women in low- and lower-middle-income countries: A systematic review. Bulletin of the World Health Organization, 2012. 90: 139–149.

17. Brittain, K., Myer, L., Koen, N., Koopowitz, S., Donald, K. A., Barnett, W et al. Risk factors for antenatal depression and associations with infant birth outcomes: Results from a South African birth cohort study. Paediatric and Perinatal Epidemiology, 2015. 29(6): 505–514.

18. Patel, V., Flisher, A. J., Nikapota, A., and Malhotra, S. Promoting child and adolescent mental health in low and middle income countries. Journal of Child Psychology and Psychiatry, 2008. 49(3): 313–334.

19. Redinger, S., Pearson, R. M., Houle, B., Norris, S. A., and Rochat, T. J. Antenatal depression and anxiety across pregnancy in urban South Africa. Journal of Affective Disorders, 2020. 277: 296–305. https://doi.org/10.1016/j.jad.2020.08.010.

20. Honikman, S., Sigwebela, S., Schneider, M., and Field, S. Perinatal depression and anxiety in resource-constrained settings: Interventions and health systems strengthening. South African Health Review, 2020. 1: 30-40.

21. Tomlinson, M., Kleintjes, S., and Lake, L. South African Child Gauge 2021/22: Child and Adolescent Mental Health. 2022. Cape Town: Children's Institute, University of Cape Town.

22. Feletti, V. J., Anda, R. F., Nordenberg, D., Williamson, D. F., Spitz, A. M., Edwards, V. et al. Relationship of childhood abuse and household dysfunction to many of the leading causes of death in adults: The Adverse Childhood Experiences (ACE) Study. American Journal of Preventive Medicine, 1998. 14(4): 245–258.

23. Lyons-Ruth, K., Bureau, J-F., Easterbrooks, M. A., Obsuth, I., Hennighausen, K., and Vulliez-Coady, L. Parsing the construct of maternal insensitivity: Distinct longitudinal pathways associated with early maternal withdrawal. Mental & Human Development. 2013. 15(5–6): 562–582

24. Beebe, B. and Lachmann, F. The Origins of Attachment – Infant Research and Adult Treatment. 2014. New York and London: Routledge.

25. Wan, M. W. and Green, J. The impact of maternal psychopathology on child–mother attachment. Archives of Women's Mental Health, 2009. 12(3): 123–134.

26. Cooper, P. J., Tomlinson, M., Swartz, L., Landman, M., Molteno, C., Stein, A. et al. Improving quality of mother-infant relationship and infant attachment in socioeconomically deprived community in South Africa: Randomised controlled trial. BMJ, 2009. 338:b974. doi: https://doi.org/10.1136/bmj.b974

27. Henrich, J., Heine, S., and Norenzayan, A. The weirdest people in the world? Behavioral and Brain Sciences, 2010. 33

(2–3): 61–83. doi:10.1017/S0140525X0999152X

28. Berg, A. Infant-parent psychotherapy at primary care level: Establishment of a service. South African Medical Journal, 2012;102(6): 582–584. www.samj.org.za/index.php/samj/article/view/5772

29. Frost, K. The Ububele Baby Mat Project: A community-based parent-infant intervention at primary health care clinics in Alexandra Township, Johannesburg. South African Journal of Psychology. 2012. 42(4): 608–616. https://doi.org/10.1177/008124631204200414

30. Lock, M. Permeable bodies and environmental delineation pp. 15–43 in Jens Seeberg, Andreas Roepstorff, Lotte Meinert (eds) Biosocial worlds: Anthropology of health environments beyond determinism. 2020. UCL Press. Open Access. www.jstor.org/stable/j.ctv13xpsqt.6

31. Dugmore, N. The presence of a 'nanny' in South African infant observations: Learning opportunities and challenges for student observers and their teachers. Infant Observation, 2019. 22(1): 42–56. doi: 10.1080/13698036.2019.1571934

32. Armstrong, K. Nannies or creche? Exploring child carers' knowledge of the first 1000 days and their perception of the significance of their role as carers. 2022. Unpublished M Phil dissertation, University of Stellenbosch, South Africa.

33. Keller, H. and Chaudhary, N. Is the mother essential for attachment? Models of care in different cultures pp. 109–138 in H. Keller and K. A. Bard (eds) The cultural nature of attachment: Contextualising relationships and development. 2017. Cambridge, MA: MIT Press.

34. Voges, J., Berg, A., and Niehaus, D. J. H. Revisiting the African origins of attachment research – Fifty years on from Ainsworth: A descriptive review. Infant Mental Health Journal, 2019. 40: 799–816.

35. Richardson, S. Maternal bodies in the postgenomic order: Gender and the explanatory landscape of epigenetics pp. 210–231 in S. S. Richardson and H. Stevens (eds.) Postgenomics: Perspectives on biology and the genome. 2015. Durham, NC: Duke University Press.

36. Pentecost, M. and Ross, F. C. The first thousand days: Motherhood, scientific knowledge, and local histories. Medical Anthropology, 2019. 38(8): 747–761. https://doi.org/10.1080/01459740.2019.1590825

37. Soubry, A. POHaD: Why we should study future fathers. Environmental Epigenetics. 2018. 4(2): 1–7. doi: 10.1093/eep/dvy007.

38. Fisher, S. Paternal mental health: Why is it relevant? American Journal of Lifestyle Medicine. 2016. 11(3): 200–211. doi: 10.1177/1559827616629895.

39. Bingham, C. R., Loukas, A., Fitzgerald, H. E., and Zucker, R. A. Parental ratings of son's behavior problems in high-risk families: Convergent and structural validity, and interparental agreement. Journal of Personality Assessment, 2003. 80: 237–251.

40. Henry, J. B., Julion, W. A., Bounds, D. T., and Sumo, J. Fatherhood matters: An integrative review of fatherhood intervention research. The Journal of School Nursing, 2020. 36(1): 19–32. doi: 10.1177/1059840519873380

41. Jackson, D. B. The interplay between early father involvement and neonatal medical risk in the prediction of infant neurodevelopment. Prevention Science, 2017. 18: 106–115. https://doi.org/10.1007/s11121-016-0734-4

42. McKee, C. L., Stapleton, P. B., and Pidgeon, A. M. History of pre and perinatal (PPN) parenting education: A literature review. Journal of Prenatal & Perinatal Psychology & Health, 2018. 32: 191–219.

43. Drysdale, R. E., Slemming, W., Makusha, T., and Richter, L. M. Father involvement, maternal depression and child nutritional outcomes in Soweto, South Africa. Maternal Child Nutrition, 2021. 17(S1): 1–12. doi: https://doi.org/10.1111/mcn.13177-

44. Mayekiso, A. 'Ukuba yindoda kwelixesha' ('To be a man in these times'): Fatherhood, marginality and forms of life among young men in Gugulethu, Cape Town. 2017. Unpub. PhD diss, University of Cape Town. https://open.uct.ac.za/handle/11427/24447

45. Baradon, T. The bodies and minds of babies in relationship: Dialogues in a multidisciplinary context. Conference 30–31 October 2022. Johannesburg.

46. Lund, C., Petersen, I., Kleintjes, S., and Bhana A. Mental health services in South Africa: Taking stock. African Journal of Psychiatry 2012. 15(6): 402–405. https://doi.org/10.4314/ajpsy.v15i6.48

47. Bain, K. The challenge to prioritise infant mental health in South Africa. South African Journal of Psychology, 2019. 50(2): 1–11.

48. Puura, K., Malek, E., and Berg, A. Integrating infant mental health at primary care level. Perspectives in Infant Mental Health, 2018. 26(2–3): 4–6.

49. World Association of Infant Mental Health. WAIMH Position Paper on the Rights of Infants. 2016. https://perspectives.waimh.org/2016/06/15/waimh-position-paper-on-the-rights-of-infants/positionpaperrightsinfants_-may_13_2016_1–2_perspectives_imh_corr/

50. Berg, A. and Lachman, A. Infant mental health in Africa: Developing a Master's programme that addresses the need for Afrocentric training. International Journal of Birth and Parent Education, 2019. 6(3): 19–21

51. Lachman, A., Berg, A., Ross, F. C., and Pentecost, M. Infant mental health in southern Africa: Nurturing a field. Lancet. 2021. 398(10303): 835–836. doi: 10.1016/s0140-6736(21)00998-3. PMID: 34058135.

52. Tomlinson, M., Bornstein, M. H., Marlow, M., and Swartz, L. Imbalances in the knowledge about infant mental health in rich and poor countries: Too little progress in bridging the gap. Infant Mental Health Journal, 2014. 35(6): 624–629.

Chapter 20

Understanding Child Development: A Biosocial Anthropological Approach to Early Life

Emily H. Emmott and Sahra Gibbon

20.1 Introduction

A biosocial understanding of child development frames development as a dynamic process that influences, and is influenced by, childrearing environments [1]. This encourages a complex understanding of the determinants of development by considering both biological and socio-cultural factors, which in turn encourages cross/interdisciplinary approaches. There is strong evidence that the Developmental Origins of Health and Disease (DOHaD) is best understood from a biosocial perspective that acknowledges and seeks to better understand the dynamic interactions between the biological and social [1]; however, cross/interdisciplinary research often encounters barriers and challenges such as epistemological differences and misunderstandings [2]. Understanding how research around child development has been conducted may help inform and facilitate effective biosocial collaborations.

Anthropology, being a diverse discipline spanning biological and social-cultural studies, is well positioned to examine and inform biosocial approaches. There has been long-standing interest in the biosocial within and beyond anthropology [3] as well as established traditions such as biocultural approaches in US-based anthropology that have long sought to better align social and biological sciences [4]. Recently, there is an emerging biosocial agenda in anthropology, in particular, medical anthropology (cf. Singer et al. on 'syndemics' [5], Lock on 'local and situated biologies' [6], Roberts on 'bioethnography' [7], and Gibbon et al. on 'biosocial medical anthropology' [8]; see also Alvergne on 'evolutionary medicine' [9]). Anthropology is as a result particularly well placed to contribute to work within DOHaD to foster better biosocial frameworks of understanding child development.

Building on this previous work, in this chapter we reflect on how different disciplines have conceptualised 'early life' with particular insights from evolutionary, social, and medical anthropology to challenge and further expand the narrow framing of DOHaD focus and to show the scope of a biosocial perspective. First, we introduce how childhood and early life have been studied in anthropology, followed by a discussion on how early life has been conceptualised in public health, lifecourse, and development research. We then discuss how concepts of early life may impact caregiving practice and childhood environments, which in turn impacts research on early life itself, with longitudinal birth cohort studies as an example. While recognising that there are points of difference in approach and analysis in the disciplinary reflections brought together in this chapter, and also that our discussion and analysis are far from comprehensive, we nonetheless highlight the need for critical and reflective thinking about the ways in which we do biosocial research, and the impact it has on our understanding of DOHaD. Overall, we suggest that a more reflexively engaged biosocial anthropological dialogue around research on early life helps to broaden the scope of cross-disciplinary work that can more fully engage with the complex and dynamic process of childhood development and present a more nuanced framework of early life for DOHaD informed research and health practice.

20.2 'Early Life' in Anthropology

Children, childhood, and child development have long been a focus of interest in anthropology, with some considering it as central to its foundation and disciplinary development [10]. By studying children across cultures, anthropologists in the early twentieth century directly challenged the notion of 'childhood' as universal or that child development is shaped solely by physiology, biology, or hormones, instead showing how early life is a period of both intense socialisation and cultural transmission [11–13]. Anthropologists continue to engage with early life by describing the variety of child-hoods across cultures, examining how ecology and culture impact development, and testing processes of cultural transmission, to name a few [14–16].

At the same time, there is a great deal of heterogeneity in the way that children and childhood have been studied [17, 18], and how this period of the lifecourse is approached; a diversity that provides a particular resource for widening the lens of DOHaD research and perspectives on early life. This is reflected in a more psychologic-ally informed focus on child development in US-based anthropology that draws from lifecourse theory [19]. A focus on childhood in anthropology is also informed by what is called 'four field' approaches that include physical and cultural anthropology as well as archaeology and linguistics [14, 16], as demonstrated, for example, in the classic work of Margaret Mead [12]. While European anthropology also attended to children's lives, this was by contrast more as part of an evolving ethnographic tradition that aimed to examine wider social structures rather than child development per se (cf. Malinowski [20] and Richards [21]). A more explicit focus on childhood, however, emerged within a constructivist-situated paradigm that highlights personhood and agency in examining early socialisation [18, 22, 23]. While there are differences in the historical evolution of research in anthropology on children and childhood development, it is true to say that diverse traditions of anthropology (including those beyond a Euro-American context – see, for instance, work in South Africa such as Reynolds [24] and Ross and Pentecost [25]) have collectively helped to show how child socialisation is variably influenced by both culture and ecology, while also recognising that there are some shared mechanisms and processes.

Notably this broad landscape of anthropological work has led to directly challenging Eurocentric ideas in developmental psychology and beyond, including Bowlby and Ainsworth's 'attachment theory', which not only fails to consider non-Western caregiving approaches [26] but sees intensive caregiving by a primary caregiver as biologically adaptive [27]. An evolutionary anthropological perspective highlights the importance of a wide range of caregivers beyond the mother, with humans evolving a cooperative childrearing system [28]. Cross-cultural, comparative research highlights how attachment to a single individual is not always observed nor optimal [26]. In summary, diverse histories of engagement with early life across different traditions of anthropology provide an important basis and resource in widening biosocial dialogue. This enables us to consider how DOHaD-informed research, policies, and practices might be expanded to encompass a broader range of factors and contexts in childhood development.

20.3 Concepts of 'Early Life' and Optimal Developmental Environments

In contemporary public health research and practice, child development is typically viewed as a *process of growth* where individuals gain socio-emotional, physical, and cognitive traits until they reach their 'final state' in adulthood [29]. Development is often represented in terms of trajectories, where there is an expected and optimal path of growth, or in terms of milestones, where development is sequential and additive. Taking physical development as an example, anthropometric measures are commonly mapped onto the WHO's child growth standards, which describe 'normal child growth [trajectories] from birth to 5 years under optimal environmental conditions' [30]. Here, average development is often perceived as 'good development', and being under- or overdeveloped may potentially be problematic with an increased risk of negative health outcomes. Similarly, motor skills may be mapped onto expected milestones using the Ages and Stages Questionnaire, a threshold-based, age-specific global screening tool assessing developmental progress [31]. Here, development is conceptualised as hierarchical where later stages of development are 'more advanced' and often perceived as 'good development'. For both trajectories and milestones, development is underpinned by biology, interacts with the environment, and builds through time. What children experience and how they develop in early life act as foundations for later life, framing the lifecourse approach as critical for developmental research. Combined with this is the idea of sensitive and critical periods, particularly in the first few years of life where 'the brain is "tuned" by the input from the environment' [32].

This view of early life, by default, places children as immature beings on their journeys to adulthood, with implications for how we research and engage with children and caregivers, and what we consider as optimal childrearing practices and environments. For example, in 'Western' countries such as the United Kingdom, United States, and Australia where such views are normative, children are typically viewed as being different to adults, and as highly sensitive to caregiver input and external environments [33–35]. Research findings recommend sensitive parenting practices that focus on understanding and responding to the child's needs without frightening the child, and such parenting practices are argued to be crucial in constructing secure attachments to the caregiver, and a foundation for 'good development' across a range of socio-emotional and behavioural outcomes [33]. Consequently, there are social expectations to create child-centred, developmentally appropriate, and stimulating environments that are typically age specific and separated from the adult world, allowing 'children to be children' [33–36]. For instance, caregivers in England are encouraged to 'read and look at books together' because 'it will help [children] with their future learning ... allows you to bond with them and is good for emotional wellbeing' [37], informed by evidence that 'books serve as inputs to influence an infant's visual, social and linguistic development' [32]. Here, the act of reading books together is framed as a scientifically recommended extra activity caregivers can carry out for the infant, independent of their day-to-day 'adult activities', which serves as a developmentally appropriate stimulus to encourage 'good development'.

However, not all cultures share the view that childhood is foundationally a time of growth, conflicting with the dominant notions of 'early life' in contemporary public health, lifecourse, and development literature [38]. For example, Helen Kavapalu [39] describes how concepts of childhood in Tonga stemmed from how 'children are perceived as inherently *vale* (foolish, ignorant, "crazy")' where socially undesirable characteristics such as laziness, aggression, and disobedience were viewed as 'natural'. Punishment, including corporal, was commonly used by caregivers to remove such traits and instil socially desirable traits – a form of caregiving practice viewed as harmful, outdated, and often outlawed in high-income nations. In Tonga, however, 'good development' is dependent on *removing* traits, contrasting with the idea that development is necessarily a process of cumulative growth, with caregiver punishment being an effective tool to guide children away from socially undesirable characteristics.

Broadly, the belief that development requires removal of traits is not necessarily an incorrect one, from what might be seen as a traditional science perspective. Removal of traits occurs throughout childhood, with processes such as synaptic pruning (a process of development in the nervous system that eliminates synapses) being a core aspect of brain development and possibly later health [40]. Humans also possess a range of ontogenetic adaptations that are traits with specific functions for specific timepoints in development, to address the challenges associated with childhood and adolescence [41]. These traits may disappear before adulthood and are not immature versions of adult traits. A simple example is the newborn rooting reflex, where neonates turn their heads with an open mouth when touched around their cheek or mouth; a trait that disappears during infancy. High self-efficacy in early childhood, where young children aged 3–4 years tend to overestimate their abilities, has also been argued to be an ontogenetic adaptation to facilitate exploration and engagement with the external environment [42]. If focusing on these characteristics of development, children could be conceptualised as 'full beings' who are perfectly adapted to their socio-ecological niche of childhood.

The view that children are 'full beings' has been documented across cultural contexts outside of the Western world, reported by many anthropologists including Margaret Mead who described Samoans as viewing 'children as little adults' [12]. Reframing children as 'full beings' somewhat conflicts with the Western focus on early life as an immature period of growth – with potential implications for what might be considered as an optimal developmental environment. In contrast to the child-centred approach frequently championed in the West, Samoan children were not provided with tailored age-specific, developmentally appropriate environments: when describing their play, Mead states, 'For dolls they have real babies; at six they are expected to sweep up the real house and pick all the scraps off the floor' [12]. In Samoa, therefore, 'children being children' did not require children to be removed from the adult world; they were assumed to be competent in carrying out specific tasks, and play was incorporated into everyday life. Full societal participation was seen as key for children to develop the skills and knowledge they required for the future, meaning the child-centred approach promoted in the West may be seen as a poor caregiving practice.

Overall, the concept of early life as a period of growth, dominant in Western contexts, influences how we construct optimal childrearing practices and environments. The focus on growth frames children as immature and sensitive, reflected in the promotion of child-centred sensitive parenting practices. However, in cultural contexts where early life is not strongly equated to be a period of growth and immaturity, there may be fundamental schematic conflicts, particularly around removing children from the adult world. While evidence shows sensitive parenting leads to 'good development' in the West [33], it does not come without cost: assuming children are immature and vulnerable can encourage containment of children within developmentally appropriate and safe environments, which may limit their freedoms, agency, and social participation, which in itself impacts their learning and development [34, 35]. The presumed significance of caregiver input for 'good development' may lead to excessive and intrusive caregiving, or helicopter parenting, which has been associated with poorer mental and physical health outcomes for adolescents and young adults [42]. It may also overburden common caregivers such as mothers, with the emergence of intensive mothering cultures that have implications for their health and well-being [36].

20.4 How Concepts of Early Life Impact Research

We have seen above how concepts of childhood and development impact how caregivers interact with and construct environments around children and how in turn these conceptual framings themselves impact practices of child development. We suggest that concepts of early life also inform research and subsequently the understanding of the DOHaD. Here, we examine this hypothesis by using longitudinal birth cohort studies as a paradigmatic broad terrain of research on early childhood and the lifecourse. Analysis of how early life research is framed and situated theoretically and methodologically in birth cohort studies further illuminates how cultural framings of early development shape research practices. We suggest that critical reflection on how this terrain of research on early life is culturally constituted within birth cohort studies may also help to inform future directions for biosocial research.

Longitudinal birth cohort studies that follow the social and biological aspects of people's lives have been an important methodological tool for different research communities, mainly epidemiological, for over 60 years [43]. These studies have been particularly useful for understanding developmental patterns and causal pathways [44], contributing to the DOHaD knowledge/evidence base. In this sense, birth cohort studies serve as a resource for and are also a 'technology of' biosocial research [45]. Recently, there has been an explosion of interest in birth cohort studies, with renewed efforts to maintain existing cohorts and new birth cohorts being established in many national contexts [46]). Detailed historical records that track the social context of intergenerational lives, while not always necessarily formulated as birth cohort studies as such, have been equally important. With public health and child development often underpinned by DOHaD frameworks, birth cohorts and other longitudinal studies have fuelled and facilitated an intense research focus on the 'early life stage' of pregnancy, infancy, and childhood and now also encompass the preconception period [47]. In turn, a range of 'life stages' have become 'critical windows' for public and global health interventions, with early interventions championed for their preventative approach and effectiveness [32, 48]. As Lappé and Landecker [49] point out, specific environments have become foregrounded in postgenomic and biosocial research, with consequences for how different stages of the lifecourse, including childhood and parenting, are temporally situated as being relevant to health. In this way, birth cohort research contributes not only to new temporal framings of the lifecourse but also to its explicit periodisation, suggesting discrete and definable life stages.

While there is today an intensive contemporary research focus on early life, its environment, and its consequences, this is arguably far from comprehensive. Birth cohort studies do allow researchers to better understand the biological and social determinants of development, including in childhood development and also across the lifecourse of participants [44]. Nevertheless, these studies have traditionally focused on limited aspects of the childrearing environment, almost exclusively focusing on the 'microsystem' within the ecological system (i.e. the immediate environment experienced by the child) [50], and in particular relying on the concept of the nuclear family household. For example, the Avon Longitudinal Study of Parents and Children [51] reveals an impressively detailed account of parenting and the household environment, including the pets that were owned by the families of birth cohort participants, how much toothpaste was put on the toothbrush, and when children first ate a raw carrot. However, there is surprisingly little information from beyond the household, such as who children see outside of this social context and what activities they do with them. This household focus persists in recent British birth cohorts such as the Millennium Cohort Study [52], which continue to hold limited information on how families and children interact with potentially important caregivers such as grandparents and even siblings of cohort participants, who are not always included in such studies.

The prioritisation of the microsystem and the household arguably stems from biases in what is valued as important aspects of the childrearing environment, including by the DOHaD and birth cohort research community, with research focus (and funding) directed towards these topics. To date, researching 'early life' has been heavily influenced by norms such as intensive mothering and the perception that two-parent nuclear families are the 'default' family structure [36, 53]. However, it has long been established that the environments beyond the household matter [52], including non-parental caregivers who are essential in the human childrearing system [2, 53]. Disciplinary silos, with their own traditions and theories, not only limit the understanding of DOHaD but may also introduce monocultural biases [53] and perpetuate an ongoing tendency for dyadic thinking in foregrounding parent (mostly mother) and child relations [54]. We suggest therefore that biosocial collaborations require critical reflection on how early life and childhood environments are culturally framed and examined in research contexts such as longitudinal birth cohorts, including how this may vary depending on histories and genealogies that shape systems of public health, concepts of the biosocial, and the emergence and evolution of birth cohorts in diverse national contexts. Understanding how norms and assumptions are built into research on early life is the first step in both challenging these normative parameters and evolving new approaches that can more fully address both diversity and variability in childhood development.

20.5 Conclusion

The examples above evidence how societal views of childhood and development have implications for childrearing practices, and in turn, understanding children's developmental outcomes in DOHaD research, outlining how biology and society may interact to shape the DOHaD. Further, our cross-disciplinary and cross-cultural examinations show how our understanding of DOHaD is influenced by the meaning of childhood and development. This also has consequences for the staging and framing of the current intense focus on early life and childhood in birth cohort studies, raising many questions about what 'good' development in childhood looks like and challenging the idea of this process as necessarily linear and additive.

Cross-disciplinary research initiatives such as the Biosocial Birth Cohort Research (BBCR) network (https://bbcrnetwork.com) provide an important infrastructure for widening the frame of research in DOHaD on child development. They also help create contexts for collaboration, such as that between our own sub-disciplinary expertise of biological and medical anthropology. Such collaborations while nascent and in dynamic formation also lead to new research questions and challenges. This includes other dimensions of a biosocial approach that we have not been able to fully address in this chapter and that also need further elaboration through more detailed, reflexive, and engaged cross-disciplinary dialogue. Exactly how the cultural politics of childhood are variously invoked and contested in the intense focus on this stage of the lifecourse in birth cohort studies and in the way that DOHaD is implemented in public and global health are just some of the areas for future investigation. Similarly how the figure of the child and childhood continues to symbolically represent future promise in these contexts is, as yet, relatively underexamined. Integrating analysis of the wider institutional contexts of research cultures (including funding priorities) that are manifest in and help sustain the infrastructure for DOHaD-focused and birth cohort studies would also further expand the scope of critical reflexive engagement. DOHaD research has much to gain from viewing developmental processes that shape childhood and health outcomes in highly context-specific ways; an understanding that is both underlined and strengthened through cross-disciplinary dialogues, such as those with biosocial anthropology outlined here.

References

1. Harris KM, McDade TW. The Biosocial Approach to Human Development, Behavior, and Health Across the Life Course. RSF. 2018 Apr;4(4):2–26.

2. Emmott EH, Myers S, Page AE. Who Cares for Women with Children? Crossing the Bridge between Disciplines. Philosophical Transactions on Royal Society London B Biological Science. 2021/05/03 ed. 2021 21 Jun;376 (1827):20200019–20200019.

3. Fuentes A. The Extended Evolutionary Synthesis, Ethnography, and the Human Niche. Current Anthropology. 2016 1 Jun;57(S13):S13–26.

4. Goodman AH, Leatherman TL. Building a New Biocultural Synthesis: Political-Economic Perspectives on Human Biology. Ann Arbor: University of Michigan Press; 1998.

5. Singer M, Bulled N, Ostrach B, Mendenhall E. Syndemics and the Biosocial Conception of Health. The Lancet. 2017 Mar;389 (10072):941–50.

6. Lock M. Mutable Environments and Permeable Human Bodies. Journal of the Royal Anthropological Institute. 2018 20 Jun;24(3):449–74.

7. Roberts EFS. Bio-Ethnography: A Collaborative, Methodological Experiment in Mexico City. Somatosphere. 2015 26 Feb. Available from: http://somatosphere.net/2015/bio-ethnography.html/

8. Gibbon S, Daly L, Parkhurst A, Ryan C, Salali GD, Tasker A. Biosocial Medical Anthropology in the Time of Covid-19: New Challenge and Opportunities. London: UCL; 2020. Available from: https://medanthucl.com/2020/04/29/biosocial-medical-anthropology-in-the-

time-of-covid-19-new-challenges-and-opportunities/

9. Alvergne A, Jenkinson C, Faurie C. Evolutionary Thinking in Medicine: From Research to Policy and Practice. New York: Springer; 2016.

10. La Fontaine J. An Anthropological Perspective on Children in Social Worlds. In: Richards M, Light P, editors. Children of Social Worlds: Development in a Social Context. Cambridge: Polity; 1986. pp. 10–30.

11. Boas, F. Instability of Human Types. In: Spiller G, editor. Papers on Interracial Problems. Boston, MA: Ginn and Company; 1912. p. 99–103.

12. Mead, M. Coming of Age in Samoa. A Psychological Study of Primitive Youth for Western Civilisation. New York: William Morrow Paperback; 1971 [1928].

13. Benedict R. Continuities and Discontinuities in Cultural Conditioning. Psychiatry. 1938 May;1(2):161–7.

14. LeVine RA, New RS. Anthropology and Child Development: A Cross-Cultural Reader. Oxford: Wiley-Blackwell; 2008.

15. Lancy DF, Bock J, Gaskins S. The Anthropology of Learning in Childhood. Walnut Creek: AltaMira Press; 2010.

16. Lancy DF. Why Anthropology of Childhood? A short history of an emerging discipline. AnthropoChildren: French Studies in the Anthropology of Childhood. 2012 Jan; 1(1). Available from: http://popups.ulg.ac.be/AnthropoChildren/document.php?id=918

17. Levine RA. Ethnographic Studies of Childhood: A Historical Overview. American Anthropologist. 2007 Jun;109(2):247–60.

18. Montgomery H. An Introduction to Childhood: Anthropological Perspectives on Children's Lives. Malden: Wiley-Blackwell; 2009.

19. Giele J, Elder G. Methods of Life Course Research: Qualitative and Quantitative Approaches. 1998; Available from: http://dx.doi.org/10.4135/9781483348919

20. Malinowski B. Argonauts of the Western Pacific: An Account of Native Enterprise and Adventure in the Archipelagoes of Melanesian New Guinea, Enhanced Edition. Oxford: Routledge and Kegan Paul; 1922.

21. Richards A. Chisungu, a Girls' Initiation Ceremony among the Bemba of Northern Rhodesia. London: Faber & Faber; 1956.

22. Bluebond-Langer M. The Private Worlds of Dying Children. Princeton: Princeton University Press; 1978.

23. Hardman C. Can There Be an Anthropology of Children? Childhood. 2001 Nov;8(4):501–17.

24. Reynolds P. 'Not Known Because Not Looked for': Ethnographers Listening to the Young in Southern Africa. Ethnos. 1995 Jan;60(3–4):193–221.

25. Ross FC, Pentecost M. Still Unknown and Overlooked? Anthropologies of Childhood and Infancy in Southern Africa, 1995–2020. Ethnos. 2021 1 Nov;1–22. 10.1080/00141844.2021.1994622

26. Keller H. Universality Claim of Attachment Theory: Children's Socioemotional Development across Cultures. Proceedings of the National Academy Science USA. 2018 6 Nov;115(45):11414–19.

27. LeVine RA. Attachment Theory as Cultural Ideology. In: Otto H, Keller H, eds. Different Faces of Attachment: Cultural Variations on a Universal Human Need. Cambridge, UK: Cambridge University Press; 2014. pp. 50-65.

28. Emmott EH, Page AE. Alloparenting. In: Shackelford TK, Weekes-Shackelford VA, editors. Encyclopedia of Evolutionary Psychological Science [Internet]. Cham: Springer International Publishing; 2019 [cited 9 Jun 2023]. pp. 1–14. Available from: https://doi.org/10.1007/978-3-319-16999-6_2253–1

29. Larcher V. Children Are Not Small Adults: Significance of Biological and Cognitive Development in Medical Practice. In: Schramme T, Edwards S,

editors. Handbook of the Philosophy of Medicine [Internet]. Dordrecht: Springer Netherlands; 2015 [cited 9 Jun 2023]. pp. 1–23. Available from: https://doi.org/10.1007/978-94-017-8706-2_16–1

30. Child Growth Standards [Internet]. WHO. 2005 [cited 9 Jun 2023]. Available from: www.who.int/news-room/questions-and-answers/item/child-growth-standards

31. Singh A, Yeh CJ, Boone Blanchard S. Ages and Stages Questionnaire: A Global Screening Scale. Boletín Médico del Hospital Infantil de México (English Edition). 2017 Jan;74(1):5–12.

32. Krishnan S, Johnson MH. A Review of Behavioural and Brain Development in the Early Years: The "Toolkit" for Later Book-related Skills [Internet]. Booktrust. 2014. [cited 11 Apr 2022]. Available from: www.booktrust.org.uk/globalassets/resources/research/krishnan–johnson-2014-full-report-a-review-of-behavioural-and-brain-development-in-the-early-years-the-toolkit-for-later-book-related-skills-.pdf

33. Van der Voort A, Juffer FJ, Bakermans-Kranenburg M. Sensitive Parenting Is the Foundation for Secure Attachment Relationships and Positive Social-Emotional Development of Children. Journal of Children's Services. 2014 10 Jun;9(2):165–76.

34. Christensen PH. Childhood and the cultural constitution of vulnerable bodies. In The Body, Childhood and Society. London: Palgrave Macmillan UK. 2000;38–59.

35. Garlen JC. Interrogating Innocence: 'Childhood' as Exclusionary Social Practice. Childhood. 2018 22 Nov;26 (1):54–67.

36. Budds K. Validating Social Support and Prioritizing Maternal Wellbeing: Beyond Intensive Mothering and Maternal Responsibility. Philosophical Transactions on Royal Society London B Biological Science. 2021/05/03 ed. 2021 21 Jun;376(1827):20200029–20200029.

37. Baby and Toddler Play Ideas [Internet]. nhs.uk. 2020 [cited 9 Jun 2023]. Available from: www.nhs.uk/conditions/baby/babys-development/play-and-learning/baby-and-toddler-play-ideas/

38. Lachman et al., this volume.

39. Kavapalu H. Dealing with the Dark Side in the Ethnography of Childhood: Child Punishment in Tonga. Oceania. 1993 Jun;63(4):313–29.

40. Sakai J. Core Concept: How Synaptic Pruning Shapes Neural Wiring during Development and, Possibly, in Disease. Proceedings of the National Academy of Science U S A. 2020/06/24 ed. 2020 14 Jul;117(28):16096–9.

41. Bjorklund DF. Ontogenetic Adaptations. In: Weekes-Shackelford V, Shackelford TK, Weekes-Shackelford VA, editors. Encyclopedia of Evolutionary Psychological Science [Internet]. Cham: Springer International Publishing; 2016 [cited 9 Jun 2023]. pp. 1–3. Available from: https://doi.org/10.1007/978-3-319-16999-6_2388–1

42. Reed K, Duncan JM, Lucier-Greer M, Fixelle C, Ferraro AJ. Helicopter Parenting and Emerging Adult Self-Efficacy: Implications for Mental and Physical Health. Journal of Child and Family Studies. 2016 6 Jun;25 (10):3136–49.

43. Lawlor DA, Andersen AMN, Batty GD. Birth Cohort Studies: Past, Present and Future. International Journal of Epidemiology. 2009 26 Jun;38(4):897–902.

44. Bynner J, Joshi H. Building the Evidence Base from Longitudinal Data. Innovation: The European Journal of Social Science Research. 2007 Jun;20(2):159–79.

45. Gibbon S, Pentecost M. Excavating and (Re)creating the Biosocial: Birth Cohorts as Ethnographic Objects of Inquiry and Sites of Intervention. Somatosphere. 2019 14 Nov. Available from: http://somatosphere.net/2019/introduction-excavating-and-recreating-the-biosocial-birth-cohorts-as-ethnographic-object-of-inquiry-and-site-of-intervention.html/ [Accessed 01/01/22]

46. Wijmenga C, Zhernakova A. The Importance of Cohort Studies in the Post-GWAS Era. Nature Genetics. 2018 Mar;50(3):322–8.

47. Pentecost M, Meloni M. "It's Never Too Early": Preconception Care and Postgenomic Models of Life. Frontiers in Sociology. 2020 21 Apr;5:21–21:322–8.

48. Bruder MB. Early Childhood Intervention: A Promise to Children and Families for Their Future. Exceptional Children. 2010 Apr;76(3):339–55.

49. Lappé M, Hein RJ, Landecker H. Environmental Politics of Reproduction. Annu Rev Anthropol. 2019 Oct;48:133–50.

50. Bronfenbrenner U. Ecological Systems Theory (1992). In: Making Human Beings Human: Bioecological Perspectives on Human Development. Thousand Oaks, CA: Sage Publications Ltd; 2005. pp. 106–73. 10.1093/ije/dys064

51. Boyd A, Golding J, Macleod J, Lawlor DA, Fraser A, Henderson J, et al. Cohort Profile: The 'Children of the 90s' – The Index Offspring of the Avon Longitudinal Study of Parents and Children. International Journal of Epidemiology 2013 Feb;42(1):111–27.

52. Connelly R, Platt L. Cohort Profile: UK Millennium Cohort Study (MCS). International Journal of Epidemiology. 2014 17 Feb;43(6):1719–25.

53. Emmott EH, Myers S, Page AE. Who Cares for Women with Children? Crossing the Bridge between Disciplines. Philosophical Transactions on Royal Society London B Biological Science. 2021 21 Jun;376 (1827):20200019–20200019.

54. Pentecost M, Ross FC, Macnab A. Beyond the Dyad: Making Developmental Origins of Health and Disease (DOHaD) Interventions More Inclusive. Journal of Developmental Origins of Health and Disease. 2018 Feb;9(1):10–14.

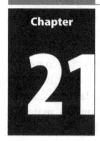

Chapter 21

Building Biosocial Collaboration in the HeLTI–South Africa Trial

Michelle Pentecost, Catherine E. Draper, Khuthala Mabetha, Larske M. Soepnel, and Shane A. Norris

21.1 Introduction

While the Developmental Origins of Health and Disease (DOHaD) as a field has been built on extensive physiological and epidemiological observational studies, there is recognition that the evidence base requires a shift to human intervention trials if it is to have any policy traction [1]. As intervention studies become more commonplace in the field of DOHaD, it is also essential to integrate a multidisciplinary perspective and social science approaches. Indeed, DOHaD is proving to be a productive and creative ground for biosocial collaboration between scientists and social scientists (including psychologists, anthropologists, sociologists, and science studies scholars), with recognition that integrating social science in interventions ensures that there is ongoing attention to assumptions embedded in research frameworks; maintenance of complexity in the face of the temptation to reach for the silver bullet; a retained sensitivity to socio-political and historical context; and active brokerage of new experimental forms of engagement with the communities of actors involved [2–4]. Such contributions are especially important given that DOHaD intervention studies will most frequently use complex public health interventions, where traditional methods are unable to capture the complexity of how context impacts intervention (and vice versa). New methods are required for understanding non-linear relationships and explaining results [5].

This chapter summarises lessons from the established literature on biosocial collaboration in trial contexts and considers their application in DOHaD intervention trials. Using the case study of the Healthy Life Trajectories Initiative (HeLTI), we illustrate the dynamics of a biosocial approach in action and discuss the benefits of building research infrastructures in DOHaD such that diverse disciplinary perspectives are given equal standing.

21.2 From Observation to Intervention: Time for Pragmatism?

As discussed in the introduction to this volume, DOHaD was formalised as a field with the consolidation of both physiological and observational studies of developmental programming that showed consistent associations between early life factors and adult health and disease outcomes, for example the relationship between birth size (lower birth weights) and adult non-communicable disease outcomes [6]. At the time the DOHaD Society celebrated its 10th World Congress in 2019, the field had expanded significantly to study a much wider range of associations, including the effects of early-life factors on mental health outcomes. However, both past and present DOHaD Society presidents highlight that DOHaD's translation to policy has been hindered by the kinds of evidence that DOHaD science has produced, citing the 'much needed transition from observational to interventional studies' [1, p. 265] alongside developing knowledge of the pathways to policymaking.

While interventions during pregnancy were an obvious first step, outcomes of behavioural interventions demonstrated limited evidence of efficacy in what is a very narrow time period. The LIMIT trial demonstrated that antenatal lifestyle interventions did not decrease the risk of infants born large for gestational age or impact maternal outcomes, but did reduce the risk of birthweight exceeding 4kg [7]. The UPBEAT trial similarly showed that antenatal lifestyle interventions for obesity in pregnancy are insufficient to affect rates of large-for gestational-age births and gestational diabetes [8]. A narrative systematic review of 27 studies of the effects of weight management via dietary counselling and dietary interventions in overweight or obese pregnant women showed little effect of these on childhood obesity outcomes [9].

There is thus a significant swing to assess interventions *before conception* to shape intergenerational health. Preconception care is an explicit focus of the World Health Organization's (WHO) 2017 report of the Commission on Ending Childhood Obesity and the subject of a 2018 *Lancet* Series [10]. A systematic review and meta-analysis of the association between pre-pregnancy body mass index and child obesity confirmed the significantly increased odds of child obesity with increased maternal BMI, to the order of 264 per cent [11], with those authors recommending preconception interventions as a logical course of action in the light of these findings.

Testing the preconception intervention hypothesis requires large-scale trials of complex public health interventions that commence before pregnancy and track individuals and their potential offspring for long periods to assess intergenerational health impacts. In partnership with WHO, HeLTI is the first consortium of randomised controlled trials of this kind in China, Canada, India, and South Africa. HeLTI aims to evaluate the efficacy of interventions initiated prior to conception and for those that become pregnant, continued during pregnancy, infancy, and early childhood to address offspring obesity and development. As the test case for starting interventions in the preconception period, HeLTI is thus of huge significance to DOHaD science. Building on long-standing efforts towards interdisciplinary collaboration in trial contexts, HeLTI is also an important test case for what this volume terms 'biosocial collaboration'. Biosocial collaboration here refers both to methodologically innovative ways of working and conceptual collaborations between disciplines (see Béhague et al., 2008 [12]), which should work in tandem to produce new models of understanding health and disease.

Lifecourse approaches encounter significant challenges around the best research practices and techniques in studies that include both long-term observational and interventional components [13]. Public health research thus increasingly works to understand not only whether a particular intervention will improve health or not but also how that intervention works to do so [14]. To achieve this, trial design, especially for behavioural and other complex public health interventions, increasingly employs 'complex', 'pragmatic', or 'realist' frameworks. As aims have shifted to encompass not only 'what' works (or not) but also 'how' it works (or not), trial design and process evaluation have incorporated interdisciplinary collaboration between epidemiologists, implementation scientists, evaluation specialists, and qualitative health researchers [15]. There is an expanding literature on the integration of qualitative methods into randomised controlled trials, especially of complex public health interventions [5]. Historically there have been epistemological limitations placed on the kinds of qualitative methods deemed applicable in the biomedical framework of trials, which has constrained the use of approaches from disciplines such as anthropology, sociology, or psychology [16]. However, the 'turn to the complex' in public health research acknowledges a broader set of social factors that influence health [14] and obliges pragmatic and adaptive trial designs that encompass more innovative and iterative qualitative methods.

21.3 Bukhali: The HeLTI–SA Trial

For HeLTI–South Africa, the *Bukhali* individual randomised controlled two-arm trial has recruited between 6000 and 7000 women aged 18–28 in Soweto for a complex public health intervention, which statistically should lead to a pregnancy and birth cohort of about 1530 mother–child pairs. All women aged 18–28 years are eligible except for those with a prior diagnosis of type 1 diabetes mellitus or epilepsy and those who are unable to provide informed consent. The primary trial outcome is to assess the effect of a four-phase intervention (preconception, pregnancy, infancy, and early childhood) on the index child's adiposity at five years of age (fat mass index [fat mass/height]2 derived from dual-energy X-ray absorptiometry). The trial also assesses a range of secondary child outcomes (anthropometric, metabolic, developmental, and behavioural); secondary maternal outcomes (anthropometric, nutritional, physical health, mental health, and behavioural); and phase-specific outcomes in the 4-phase trial [17]. The intervention is community healthcare worker-driven and comprises a programme of nutritional and health screening and support interventions, including micronutrient supplements, health information booklets, and monthly informational interventions in-person or by telephone that use healthy conversation skills, a motivational interviewing technique that focuses on empowering participants to explore opportunities for and obstacles to behaviour change [18]. These sessions cover themes, including diet, exercise, sleep, contraception, safe sex, and emotional well-being, as well as health checks and measurements at in-person visits. The control group receives 'standard of care plus', comprising access to standard community primary healthcare provisions, as well as additional services provided by the control team at the trial site, including free HIV and pregnancy tests, and general non-health-related advice, for example finances, insurance, and accessing child support. Women in the intervention arm who become pregnant receive additional interventions including an ultrasound scan and health promotion materials on diet and physical activity in pregnancy, child developmental milestones, and accessing state child support. In the postnatal period, interventions will focus on current messaging about breastfeeding, nutrition, care, and developmental stimulation outlined in the South African 'Road to Health' booklet received by each birthing parent at the child's birth, and women will be encouraged to return to preconception healthy behaviours. For the full trial protocol, see Norris et al. 2022 [17].

21.4 A Pragmatic DOHaD Trial

HeLTI–SA exemplifies the 'pragmatic' trial model. There is an explicit framework of trial as a process, where ongoing learning and adaptation to new knowledge as it arises are expected and desirable, such that the trial becomes a dynamic platform that does not just test the primary hypothesis – that preconception interventions might improve childhood metabolic and developmental outcomes – but also undertakes process evaluation analyses, as well as generating new hypotheses as situations arise, that can then also be tested in the course of the trial.

From the outset, the HeLTI team have needed to adapt the framework to a complex context of urban poverty. Pilot trial implementation of Bukhali led to significant changes to both the trial design and implementation approaches [19]. While the trial was initially conceptualised as a cluster randomised trial with 30 random geographical units in Soweto, the pilot demonstrated significant cluster contamination due to participants' movement between households and parts of Soweto as part of a strategy of resource-sharing between different households [19]. This accords with the 'domestic fluidity' that anthropologists have noted as common for southern African households [20, 21]. HeLTI–SA was consequently converted to an individual randomised model. Pilot qualitative work was also able to capture the key priorities and key challenges for women in Soweto. Women are focused on obtaining further education and securing employment, while navigating difficult socio-economic circumstances [19]. As a result of the pilot, other key changes to Bukhali design and implementation included modifications to the intervention delivery, from group to individual sessions and to mostly telephonic rather than in-person delivery (a requirement further amplified by the onset of the COVID-19 pandemic and lockdowns in South Africa); the inclusion of additional incentives that respond to some of the priorities women discussed (such as making provision for the printing of their CVs at the research unit); and the implementation of a system for the delivery of supplements to participants' homes.

The focused approach to adapt to the contextual complexities of the trial goes beyond the pilot. The pragmatic trial model means that the research team is highly responsive to new challenges or concerns as they arise [18]. The pilot findings that women preferred telephonic engagements meant a switch to delivering interventions telephonically. South Africa ranks third in Africa with regard to mobile phone penetration and therefore provides a robust platform for mHealth prospects [22]. The widespread availability of mobile phones has enhanced healthcare communication [23] as they are cost-effective and facilitate health professionals in clinical trials to stay in contact with participants and, where possible, deliver intervention components telephonically [23, 24]. Crucially, this adaptation preceded the COVID-19 pandemic and meant that the trial continued even during periods of lockdown in South Africa.

However, for the duration of the trial thus far, this has also meant a reliance on mobile coverage and continuity of mobile phone numbers for participants, raising concerns over participant accessibility in clinical trials that have been previously recognised within telemedicine and medical informatics [25]. Although a large proportion of individuals who are enrolled in the HeLTI trial own mobile phones, lower retention rates were observed among some participants who were hard to reach by mobile phone. The lack of accessibility and reachability of these participants was largely attributed to changes in their mobile phone numbers. Losing contact with some participants prompted further qualitative work to assess the reasons behind frequent changing of mobile numbers by trial participants and to identify other factors contributing to the challenges of contacting participants. Although a mixed-methods approach was employed to understand this outcome, the quantitative data produced contradictory results that did not confirm the qualitative findings as the majority of the participants had not changed their mobile phone numbers, contrary to what was observed in the qualitative data. Twenty in-depth interviews were conducted with the HeLTI cohort who were hard to reach by mobile phone. Their narrative accounts revealed that the participants predominantly changed their numbers due to mobile phone technical issues, such as poor battery life, faulty charging systems and mobile phones, and application crashes. Other challenges with contacting participants included network coverage issues, not personally owning a mobile phone, and phone (and thus sim card) theft. Participants also often left their phones at home to mitigate against theft. The significance of the daily risk of crime becomes a key data point for understanding participants' 'unreachability' and why proposed interventions may or may not work in this context.

During the implementation of HeLTI–SA, questions also arose over terminations of pregnancy among HeLTI participants, observed to occur in about 5.2 per cent of pregnancies enrolled prior to 20 weeks gestational age. This has led to a qualitative inquiry into participants' reasons for terminating their pregnancy. Using 10 in-depth interviews, the team used a socio-ecological model [26, 27] to explore how contextual and social complexities at micro- and macro-levels, including the COVID-19 pandemic, impacted participants' decision to terminate their pregnancy [28, 29]. The main reasons for termination included intra-personal factors, such as financial instability and dependency; not being emotionally prepared for pregnancy; and the impact of pregnancy on future employment and education opportunities. Reported interpersonal reasons included a lack of partner support and stability and the threat of an adverse impact on family dynamics, including abusive behaviour. In addition, participants' experiences reflected the impact of family and community beliefs around termination, accessibility, and attitudes of termination services, and the participants' sense of agency in choosing to terminate. Interestingly, the COVID-19 pandemic seemed to play a secondary and indirect role in participants' choice to terminate their pregnancy, mainly as a potential contributor to socio-economic insecurity. Exploring these factors across socio-ecological domains provides an understanding of unintended pregnancies in this setting and can help align termination services more effectively with women's needs. By extension, it also sheds light on the social and contextual elements impacting (1) the practical implementation of HeLTI in terms of pregnancy loss and (the team's understanding of) the number of participants retained in the trial through pregnancy and (2) participant experiences of (unintended) pregnancy, which can contribute to an informed interpretation of participant engagement with the intervention in its various phases. In the preconception phase, for example, a deeper understanding of participants' circumstances and priorities can help explain the degree to which intervention components resonate with young women without (current) pregnancy intent. In the pregnancy phase, insight into the experiences and challenges faced in the context of unintended pregnancy can, for instance, highlight the need for additional support among participants.

Utilising a dynamic approach means that emerging obstacles also present opportunities to address novel research questions. Attending to new questions through qualitative work with trial participants not only allows for practical adjustments to trial protocols to ensure participant retention but also illuminates social factors that might later account for or help trialists to make sense of trial outcomes. Equal investment in the gathering of biological samples and qualitative data means that integrated biosocial analyses are possible. In a nutshell then, intervention trials that adopt biosocial models are not only more likely to ensure that the trial reaches completion, but they are also more likely to offer meaningful conclusions that contextualise findings in ways that matter for learning and policy recommendation.

21.5 Discussion

The novelty of DOHaD intervention studies raises important theoretical and methodological questions that cannot be parsed without a biosocial lens. This is especially crucial for DOHaD research that employs complex public health interventions, given that these present their own unique methodological and epistemological issues [14, 30, 31]. The manner in which social context is understood and accounted for in trials has the potential to amplify or diminish attention to the social drivers of health inequities. Collaborations that encompass anthropological and science studies perspectives are more likely to account for the structural and processual factors that might offer 'real-world' explanations of trial outcomes [16]. Pragmatic and adaptive designs in DOHaD intervention trials allow for both the robust methodology and contextual relevance that are required when testing complex public health interventions [14]. Ensuring that this balance is struck is essential given that it will have a direct bearing on how recommendations are framed at the end of the trial. In sum then, a biosocial collaboration that affords 'the social' equal weight as an aspect of the trial to be studied, incorporated, and analysed means that trial outcomes are better explained and that recommendations are more suitable to local context [32].

As Béhague and colleagues described some time ago, focusing on methodological innovation without an equally rigorous approach to conceptual collaboration risks reinventing old dichotomies (deductive or inductive; specific or generalisable) that do not hold in reality, where ill-designed qualitative methods can be equally reductionist [12]. A commitment to the development of shared conceptual models that are theoretically innovative and critically informed alongside appropriate methods is thus a better hallmark of meaningful biosocial collaboration. Examples include the development of the syndemics framework (see Chapter 15 in this volume); bioethnography (Chapter 15 in this volume); and foundational work that has developed novel methods to integrate ethnography and statistics [33].

On 'doing' biosocial collaboration in practice, it is useful to borrow Anthony Stavrianakis's concept of collaboration: 'a worthwhile collaboration is one in which two kinds of participants, in their engagement, are able to name a problem or do a practice that in their position as participants (prior to engagement) they would not have been able to do ... Collaborative participation presupposes an endeavour of transformation' [34]. This is very rarely straightforward, given the necessary work required to delineate the boundaries of collaboration and to navigate pre-existing organisational and disciplinary hierarchies and the range of ethical and social demands that collaboration as a practice may introduce ([34], see also Niewöhner in this volume). However, it is critical for both the constitution of evidence in DOHaD research and the framing and communication of the DOHaD message. As outlined in the introduction, DOHaD requires an expansion of its evidence base, and in a fashion that is likely to have a policy impact. As DOHaD scientists themselves begin to take on the language of seeking evidence for 'politically palatable' solutions, it is crucial that social scientists seize the opportunity at hand – the openness of DOHaD to transdisciplinary evidence synthesis as a more productive way to find scalable solutions to the question of fostering intergenerational health. This transdisciplinary approach in HeLTI will in itself serve as a case study and will be documented so we may further learn how to better integrate these ideas in future DOHaD-inspired RCT research.

References

1. Hanson MA, Poston L, Gluckman PD. DOHaD – the challenge of translating the science to policy. J Dev Orig Health Dis 2019; 10: 263–267.

2. Penkler M, Hanson M, Biesma R, Müller R. DOHaD in science and society: emergent opportunities and novel responsibilities. J Dev Orig Health Dis 2019; 10: 268–273.

3. Müller R, Kenney M. A science of hope? Tracing emergent entanglements between the biology of early life adversity, trauma-informed care, and restorative justice. Sci Technol Hum Values 2021; 46: 1230–1260.

4. Roberts EFS, Sanz C. Bioethnography: A how-to guide for the twenty-first century. In: Maurizio Meloni, John Cromby, Des Fitzgerald, Stephanie Lloyd, editors The Palgrave Handbook of Biology and Society. London: Palgrave Macmillan, 2018, pp. 749–775.

5. Davis K, Minckas N, Bond V, Clark CJ, Colbourn T, Drabble SJ et al. Beyond interviews and focus groups: A framework for integrating innovative qualitative methods into randomised controlled trials of complex public health interventions. Trials 2019; 20: 1–16.

6. Delisle H. Programming of Chronic Disease by Impaired Fetal Nutrition: Evidence and Implications for Policy and Intervention Strategies. Geneva: WHO, 2002.

7. Dodd JM, Turnbull D, McPhee AJ, Deussen AR, Grivell RM, Yelland LN et al. Antenatal lifestyle advice for women who are overweight or obese: LIMIT randomised trial. BMJ 2014; 348: 5–7.

8. Poston L, Bell R, Croker H, Flynn AC, Godfrey KM, Goff L et al. Effect of a behavioural intervention in obese pregnant women (the UPBEAT study): A multicentre, randomised controlled trial. Lancet Diabetes Endocrinol 2015; 3: 767–777.

9. Grobler L, Visser M, Siegfried N. Healthy life trajectories initiative: Summary of the evidence base for pregnancy-related interventions to prevent overweight and obesity in children. Obes Rev 2019; 20: 18–30.

10. Stephenson J, Heslehurst N, Hall J, Schoenaker DAJM, Hutchinson J, Cade JE et al. Before the beginning: nutrition and lifestyle in the preconception period and its importance for future health. Lancet 2018; 391: 1830–1841.

11. Heslehurst N, Vieira R, Akhter Z, Bailey H, Slack E, Ngongalah L et al. The association between maternal body mass index and child obesity: A systematic review and meta-analysis. PLoS Med 2019; 16: e1002817.

12. Béhague DP, Gonçalves H, Victora CG. Anthropology and epidemiology: Learning epistemological lessons through a collaborative venture. Cien Saude Colet 2008; 13: 1701–1710.

13. Gage SH, Munafò MR, Davey Smith G. Causal inference in developmental origins of health and disease (DOHaD) research. Annu Rev Psychol 2016; 67: 567–585.

14. Winther J, Hillersdal L. Balancing methodological purity and social relevance: Monitoring participant compliance in a behavioural RCT. Biosocieties 2020; 15: 555–579.

15. Norris SL, Rehfuess EA, Smith H, Tunçalp Ö, Grimshaw JM, Ford NP et al. Complex health interventions in complex systems: Improving the process and methods for evidence-informed health decisions. BMJ Glob Heal 2019; 4: e000963.

16. Mannell J, Davis K. Evaluating complex health interventions with randomized controlled trials: How do we improve the use of qualitative methods? Qual Health Res 2019; 29: 623–631.

17. Norris SA, Draper CE, Prioreschi A, Smuts CM, Ware LJ, Dennis C et al. Building knowledge, optimising physical and mental health and setting up healthier life trajectories in South African women (Bukhali): A preconception randomised control trial part of the

Healthy Life Trajectories Initiative (HeLTI). BMJ Open 2022; 12: e059914.

18. Draper CE, Mabena G, Motlhatlhedi M, Thwala N, Lawrence W, Weller S et al. Implementation of healthy conversation skills to support behaviour change in the Bukhali trial in Soweto, South Africa: A process evaluation. SSM – Ment Heal 2022; 2: 100132.

19. Draper C, Prioreschi A, Ware L, Lye S, Norris S. Pilot implementation of Bukhali : A preconception health trial in South Africa. SAGE Open Med 2020; 8: 205031212094054.

20. Spiegel A. Introduction: Domestic fluidity in South Africa. Soc Dyn 1996; 22: 5–6.

21. Dubbeld B. How Social security becomes social insecurity: Fluid households, crisis talk and the value of grants in a KwaZulu-Natal village. Acta Juridica 2013; 13: 197–218.

22. GSMA. GSMA announces new global research that highlights significant growth opportunity for the mobile industry. GSMA Newsroom. 2012. www .gsma.com/newsroom/gsma-announces-new-global-research-that-highlights-significant-growth-opportunity-for-the-mobile-industry (accessed 7 Feb 2023).

23. Mapham W. Mobile phones: Changing health care one sms at a time: opinion. South African J HIV Med 2008; 9: 11–16.

24. Noordam AC, Kuepper BM, Stekelenburg J, Milen A. Improvement of maternal health services through the use of mobile phones. Trop Med Int Heal 2011; 16: 622–626.

25. Kaplan B, Litewka S. Ethical challenges of telemedicine and telehealth. Cambridge Q Healthc Ethics 2008; 17: 401–416.

26. Mcleroy KR, Bibeau D, Steckler A, Glanz K. An ecological perspective on health promotion programs. Heal Educ Behav 1988; 15: 351–377.

27. Bronfenbrenner U. Toward an experimental ecology of human development. Am Psychol 1977; 32: 513–531.

28. Kirkman M, Rosenthal D, Mallett S, Rowe H, Hardiman A. Reasons women give for contemplating or undergoing abortion: A qualitative investigation in Victoria, Australia. Sex Reprod Healthc 2010; 1: 149–155.

29. Rehnström Loi U, Lindgren M, Faxelid E, Oguttu M, Klingberg-Allvin M. Decision-making preceding induced abortion: A qualitative study of women's experiences in Kisumu, Kenya. Reprod Health 2018; 15: 1–12. doi:10.1186/S12978-018-0612-6.

30. Broer T, Bal R, Pickersgill M. Problematisations of complexity: On the notion and production of diverse complexities in healthcare interventions and evaluations. Sci Cult (Lond) 2017; 26: 135–160.

31. Valdez N. Weighing the Future: Race, Science, and Pregnancy Trials in the Postgenomic Era. California: University of California Press, 2021 doi:10.2307/j.ctv2j6xdzv.

32. Gibbon S, Pentecost M. Excavating and (re)creating the biosocial: Birth cohorts as ethnographic object of inquiry and site of intervention. Somatosphere 2019; November. https://somatosphere.com/2019/introduction-excavating-and-recreating-the-biosocial-birth-cohorts-as-ethnographic-object-of-inquiry-and-site-of-intervention.html/

33. Tsai AC, Mendenhall E, Trostle JA, Kawachi I. Co-occurring epidemics, syndemics, and population health. Lancet 2017; 389: 978–982.

34. Stavrianakis A. From anthropologist to actant (and back to anthropology): Position, impasse, and observation in sociotechnical collaboration. Cult Anthropol 2015; 30: 169–189.

Doing Environments in DOHaD and Epigenetics

Sophia Rossmann and Georgia Samaras

22.1 Introduction: Environment as an Elusive Concept

Every organism lives in an environment. We are able to sense, measure, experience, and even change environments. Simultaneously, environments influence and shape us. For scholars in the Developmental Origins of Health and Disease (DOHaD) field, researching environmental effects on health is a key concern: the interdisciplinary field has a long history of drawing attention to the environment and its potential influence on health trajectories by traditionally relying on observational studies in human populations [1].

As scholars from the field of science and technology studies (STS), we are especially interested in understanding what the environment 'is' that emerges in biomedical research and its interactions with our bodies. Such questions prove particularly important in the current postgenomic era, where new scientific research challenges the previous emphasis on the gene as a core explanatory concept for human development by reinvigorating the role of the environment [2].

In recent years, environmental epigenetics has emerged as a key approach towards better understanding disease aetiologies in DOHaD research, which offers scientists a molecular mechanism to trace how environments biologically inscribe themselves into bodies and change health trajectories. Epigenetic research explores how socio-material environments, such as toxicants, stress, nutrition, or poverty, induce biochemical and structural changes on the DNA that impact gene expression, without changing the genetic code itself. In contrast to permanent changes in the DNA (e.g. gene mutations), epigenetic changes are not fixed but allow us to understand bodies as dynamically shaped by the environments in which they live [3].

Although the environment is gaining renewed attention in biomedical research, it still lacks an overarching theoritisation: even in life science publications dedicated to explore the nexus between epigenetics and the environment, scientists barely offer a detailed description of how to theorise the environment that organisms live in. Broad definitions of the environment as multiple factors, for example '[c]hemical pollutants, dietary components, temperature changes and other external stresses' [4, p. 97], reveal that the environment is often conceived of as everything that surrounds cells and organisms. It is a loose definition that foremost understands the environment as distinct from anything genetic [5, 6].

In this chapter, we first discuss how DOHaD research tends to operationalise and measure environments to produce knowledge on how environmental experiences relate to health outcomes. We then show why it is important for researchers to consider how they conceive of and address the environment. We argue that what 'is' the environment is not self-evident but something that needs careful consideration. By scrutinising how environments come to matter in epigenetic DOHaD research, we aim to lay the ground for interdisciplinary critical reflections about the social and political dimensions of DOHaD.

22.2 Environments, DOHaD Research, and Environmental Epigenetics

In the twenty-first century, DOHaD has moved towards researching the health effects of a variety of environmental factors. Looking at how complex socio-material environments enter DOHaD research reveals how environments as research objects are not just 'out there'; instead, researchers have to actively *do* environments in the laboratory. For example, in population-based research, DOHaD scientists use measurements such as body mass index or birthweight as indicators for the food environment of cohort participants [7], while in experimental rodent models, food becomes operationalised as a nutrient component [8]. We therefore suggest that how DOHaD researchers are *doing* environments needs careful consideration to understand the consequences that these *doings* might have and for whom.

Social sciences' and humanities' conceptualisations of the notion of environment offer theoretical avenues for how to conceive of the relationship between organisms and the environment in which they live [9]. Understanding this relationship as dynamic and mutually influencing renders stressors not as stressors per se but as phenomena that become stressors *in relation* to an organism. In theory, DOHaD has the potential to provide evidence on how diverse biological and socio-material environments spanning across different scales (intrauterine environment to neighbourhoods to social and economic structures) interact with organisms in a non-linear fashion and impact developing organisms and populations across different temporal horizons (preconception, prenatal periods, infancy, childhood, adolescence, adulthood, and generations). However, operationalising and measuring these dynamic, perhaps 'unfinalizable relations' [10, p. 708] between environments, bodies, spaces, and times is proving to be a challenging task for DOHaD researchers [11].

Social scientists appreciate the potential of epigenetic research to unpack what counts as environments and to reconsider questions of individual and collective responsibility towards these environments, potentially furthering political quests for health equity and social and environmental justice [12, 13]. At the same time, they frequently criticise that concepts of environments in the life sciences tend to be too simplistic [14] or lack consensus over what is meant by 'environment' [15]. There are three central social science critiques on how epigenetic DOHaD research operationalises the environment.

First, social science scholars have pointed out that epigenetic research tends to reduce complex environments to how environmental factors have an effect on the molecular level. For example, Landecker [16] demonstrates how research in nutritional epigenetics reconfigures the complexity of food to a molecular exposure capable of changing epigenetic mechanisms and the metabolism: what we eat has come to be framed as an epigenetic environment, that is an external exposure that conditions the (prenatal) body for later-life health outcomes such as diabetes or heart diseases.

This 'molecularization of biography and milieu' [3] that is rendering complex environments, relationships, and histories in terms of their molecular effects on bodies has been cautioned against also by DOHaD researchers in interdisciplinary collaboration.

Social and life scientists together have argued how such an understanding might obscure how these exposures are socially patterned and unequally distributed across the social worlds we live in [17, 18].

Second, social science scholarship has discussed the potential of DOHaD research to individualise environments. As Chiapperino et al. extensively discuss in this handbook, epigenetic DOHaD research tends to focus on individual behaviours and traits as primary sites to make environmental exposure visible. This focus can be problematic as neglecting how structural factors impact health beyond individual decisions can lead to rendering exposure situations as products of lifestyle decisions, thereby favouring behavioural over structural health interventions. Thus, individuals might be responsibilised for managing their health risks and diseases [17].

Interestingly, as Warin et al. [19] outline, DOHaD research originally had a focus on how gendered socio-economic effects of maternal undernutrition impact the disease susceptibilities encountered in adulthood. However, with an increasing focus on overnutrition, maternal obesity, and diabetes, DOHaD's notions of the environment have become narrower over time, 'telescoping' on the uterus as '"the environment" of scrutiny; ... the social environment [became] an independent and secondary context'. [19, p. 456]. Such tendencies to become more concerned with individual-level factors and choices also speak to a gendered stereotype of female caregiving that is especially prevalent in the Global North and perpetuates culturally situated concepts of the environment as singular and bounded [12].

Lastly, social scientists have argued how specific experimental set-ups in epigenetic DOHaD research give more attention to some environments than others [20]. Studying clinical trials in the UK and USA, Valdez [14] demonstrates how with selecting some experimental set-ups (e.g. animal models and randomised clinical trials), researchers choose certain environmental factors as significant over others, ultimately influencing what public health professionals regard as central for designing and implementing interventions. These choices often stem from the epistemological traditions of scientific fields. For example, in social epidemiology, diet might be access to different types of food shaped by socio-economic structures [20]. In comparison, nutritional epigenetics operationalises diet as environmental exposures in the form of nutrients [16], whereas in the mundane experiences of family meals diet, even if considered unhealthy, might be interpreted as expressing love to one's family members [21].

22.3 Caring for More Complex Environments in DOHaD Research

With environments playing a central role in DOHaD research, we believe it is important to consider *how* scientists measure and operationalise environments. As findings are increasingly taken up in healthcare and global policy guidelines [22], they have social and political consequences for wider society. They shape how society understands diseases, (re-)assigns responsibilities towards tackling them, and what health strategies and interventions are imagined possible. If framings of the environment are mostly done on the individual level and as simplistic factors, they steer interventions in the direction of educational public health messaging and lifestyle changes rather than examining the structures that undergird certain choices (cf. Chapter 16).

However, this does not mean that DOHaD researchers do not engage in reflections on the complexity of human lives. Penkler [11] shows how the simplistic environments emerging in DOHaD study designs are sometimes 'at odds with the researchers' own normative commitments and aspirations' and their aim to position themselves against the 'reductionist science' (p. 2) of gene centrism in the 1990s and 2000s.

Looking at very recent developments in DOHaD fields provides interesting cases of researchers' attempts to conceptualise environments in more complex ways and to shift attention to environments that might have a positive effect on health trajectories. Informed by our own ethnographic fieldwork in environmental epidemiology (Rossmann) and neurobiology (Samaras), we briefly discuss two examples: green spaces and stress as a complex experience. Both examples exhibit a fundamental question that receives renewed attention with environmental epigenetics: how can DOHaD research account for the entangled relationship between organisms and environments?

22.3.1 Green Spaces

Green spaces (e.g. parks) have been associated with a plethora of beneficial health outcomes such as improved physical and mental health and a lowered risk of cardiovascular and respiratory diseases. Treated as an exposure variable, green spaces tend to be operationalised using established variables available and harmonised across different cohort studies. These variables currently include (1) surrounding greenness using satellite-derived indices to quantify the intensity of greenness; (2) access to a green space within 300 metres of residence; (3) straight line distance to the nearest green space; and (4) area of the closest green space.

Yet, what green spaces 'are' at the specific institute for epidemiology and public health at which Rossmann conducted her fieldwork is not fixed from the start but instead the outcome of a series of negotiations among the researchers. Rossmann could observe how green spaces are done in practice: in scientific articles, international guidelines, through infrastructures and their available data sets, and in scientific meetings. Researchers actively assemble the variable 'green spaces' using different types of aggregated data, including satellite images, topographical maps, questionnaires, measurements, and experiences through particular modes of calculation. They reflect upon its *temporal* dimension measured as the greenest moment of the year and time spent in green spaces; *spatial* dimension measured quantitatively as distance, access, and size and qualitatively emphasising the importance of local environments; and *social* dimension considering how people might experience and use these spaces differently, where green spaces can create both restorative effects and stressful experiences when perceived as dangerous.

At the end of these negotiation processes, the group Rossmann followed will have decided to focus on two variables to analyse for one of their first publications on epigenetic changes in relation to exposure to green spaces: greenness and access. These two variables will appear as clear-cut definitions of green spaces in their publication, momentarily stabilising a specific version of green spaces reintegrated into the classical terminology of exposure variables while excluding the process that went into deciding upon them.

22.3.2 Stress as a Complex Experience

The experience of stress has long been a subject in neurobiological research. This branch of research describes stress as having a potential pathogenic effect, leading to depression or anxiety, especially when considered severe or occurring over a long period of time.

Rendered as an environmental exposure, neurobiologists tend to operationalise stress by eliciting a systemic response, for example by placing mice into a narrow tube to measure the traces stress leaves behind as changes in DNA methylation or histone modifications. In these re-enactments, stress is reduced to (a series of) singular measurable events that challenge organisms, obscuring how stress is omnipresent in a lab rat's life, for example through differences in their handling or housing.

The work of the research group with which Samaras conducted her ethnographic fieldwork contrasts with this reductionist approach. The group attempts to invite a more complex notion of environment into the mouse model by including what they term 'social' factors: they create a completely new experimental arena for the mice to live in to construct a 'semi-natural' or 'enriched' environment that allows the researchers to test the mice in groups. This highly sophisticated experimental arena, termed 'complex behaviour', consists of various interconnected cages in which the mice are offered toys, food, and water at all times. By extending the experiment over several days during which the mice experience exposure to stress, undisturbed phases, and even positive environments (toys), researchers attempt to emphasise the temporal dimension of the environment and to account for the dynamics of experiencing stress. Stress emerges as a processual experience that spans across life instead of singular events that are disconnected from most parts of an organism's life. The 'complex behaviour' set-up therefore allows researchers to understand stress as an environmental phenomenon proceeding in action, where the mouse is triggered and then equilibrated, triggered again, and so forth.

Both examples demonstrate that it matters to care for constructing more complex exposure variables and research arrangements. First, these examples illustrate current developments in DOHaD to move away from a historically strong emphasis on 'damaged-centred' [23] research towards environments with buffering and restorative effects. Green spaces, for example, are assembled as elements of the urban environment that can have buffering effects, counterbalancing adverse health trajectories. Similarly, the 'complex behaviour' experiment offering 'enriched environments' encourages conversations on how positive social interventions, especially early in life, might have therapeutic effects [cf. 24]. Taking seriously the dynamic and processual character of environments across time increasingly means for DOHaD researchers to also consider 'positive' environments.

Second, these more complex renderings of environments shift attention away from dominant interventions on the individual level towards understanding organisms embedded in the ecologies in which they live. Evidence on green spaces is directed at policymakers to raise questions on how to design the cities where we want to live. 'Complex behaviour' experiments shift attention to how certain variables of interacting life circumstances shape health outcomes.

22.4 Obstacles to Put Complex Environments into Practice

As outlined in the previous section, DOHaD researchers discursively care about acknowledging the dynamicting character of environments, with some moving towards incorporating more complexity into the study designs. Simultaneously, most DOHaD researchers grapple with this complexity: being embedded in institutional contexts and established infrastructures hampers scientists to put their complex understanding of environments into practice [11]. We see three obstacles arising from the current disciplinary and research policy structures from putting main drivers of this challenge.

First, while constructing environments as phenomena taking place over time carries more ecological validity, this poses new challenges as to how to turn these considerations into research set-ups that capture the dynamic relations. Ackerman et al. [25] identify a 'moral economy of quantification', which arises from the dominant and collectively negotiated virtues in science that 'shape ... how knowledge about complex causality can be produced.' (p. 213). This moral economy favours operationalisations of environments that can be turned into 'precise measurements' and data to be harmonised and traded across laboratories. Such aspirations to produce universal data incentivise researchers to focus on environments that are easier to manage in the laboratory, making it unrewarding to operationalise environments as experiences arising from structural circumstances.

Second, these epistemological reasons are intertwined with the power of current research infrastructures and framework conditions in the life sciences [26]. As Pinel [27] points out, the biological environment to trace how exposures and experiences produce epigenetic changes is embedded within a social environment of the entrepreneurial university where research is conducted. This environment is structured and influenced by multiple overlapping scales of funding bodies, audit cultures, peer-reviewed journals, and scientific communities and their established practices. Thus, decisions on how to operationalise environments are not only guided by the research questions but also depend on institutional settings, economic aspects (e.g. time and material resources), and technical infrastructures (e.g. computing power available for statistical analyses) [27].

Third and relatedly, the current and rather rigid logic of publishing may not allow to include how researchers negotiate which environments to re-enact and how. Life science publication culture is mostly geared towards representing research as linear and producing unambiguous results. We know from STS that research practices are tedious processes in which scientists have to negotiate what materials and methods they in-/exclude, how, and why [28]. To account for these local and situated experimental conditions that bring about the final research results, as discussed above with green spaces and stress, would require a new publication ethos that allows research to be portrayed as a dynamic and social process, for instance, in the form of an extended Materials & Methods section [29].

22.5 Conclusions: Avenues for Interdisciplinary Conversations

The environment represents an elusive concept to capture for biomedical research. With findings from DOHaD research becoming increasingly relevant for policy and healthcare [22], it matters how scientists conceive of and address the environment. In order to conceptualise environments that allow for more complexity in research designs, we discuss the merits of interdisciplinary collaboration in which social and life scientists *together* engage in critical reflections about the social and political dimensions of DOHaD.

On the epistemological level, including certain environments in research designs is necessarily selective to become workable: most research has to be reductionist to a certain degree to be feasible. Engaging in these kinds of 'pragmatic reductionisms' [30] demands reflections on the strategic choices and trade-offs made and their potential political consequences outside the scientific arena. To take this task seriously, we consider it important for both, DOHaD researchers and social scientists, to critically and responsibly question their own practices: being aware of which reductionisms they want to engage in, that is which reductionisms they potentially reproduce with their research and still comply with.

On the practical level, interdisciplinary collaborations could help provide more complex accounts of the biosocial environments that shape health trajectories across the lifespan and generations. Examples of the forms that these collaborations can take can be found in this handbook (Chapters 15 and 29). Roberts et al., for example, propose the method of *bioethnography*, which combines ethnographic observation and biochemical sampling and encourages both social and life scientists to engage in an open-ended and iterative process of doing research.

Niewöhner advances the term 'co-laboration' to think about interdisciplinary collaborations, as he argues elsewhere, in terms of 'temporary, non-teleological, joint epistemic work aimed at producing disciplinary reflexivities not interdisciplinary shared outcomes' [31, p. 2]. In other words, interdisciplinary work is not about giving up on one's own disciplinary positioning but encouraging spaces to think differently about one's own knowledge practices. Such spaces to engage in processes of mutual learning emerge from encounters in 'reading groups, joint empirical work, visiting conferences together, writing together, designing and conducting experiments together' [31, p. 18].

We propose that such interdisciplinary collaborations, even when situated in divergent research ecologies, prove fruitful to further discussions on *doing environments*. We suggest five (non-exhaustive) reflections for these discussions to account for the different epistemological and socio-political dimensions environments are made up of in DOHaD research:

1. to discuss *doing* environments as an active achievement, that is as a product of the decisions made and methods used to know and measure environments (performative dimension);
2. to take seriously the temporal dimensions of environments beyond their re-enactments as singular damage in the laboratory (processual dimension);
3. to carefully consider how environments as research objects are embedded in the (research) contexts in which they occur, that is to acknowledge accounts of environments as historically, socio-politically, and economically influenced (situational dimension);
4. to understand *doing* environments as political, bearing potential consequences for which environments become relevant outside the scientific arena (political dimension);
5. and to allow for interdisciplinary reflexivity to identify blind spots in defining environments across disciplines (reciprocal dimension).

We hope that these reflections further encourage interdisciplinary conversations about the importance of carefully attending to how environments are done in DOHaD research. We consider it necessary to acknowledge *doing environments* as a concrete research practice and as a repertoire in scientific discourse, instead of leaving this central scientific task undiscussed. In doing so, DOHaD researchers could, for example, take into account environments beneficial to organisms and invest in studying the effects of 'enriched' environments [24]. This could open up discussions about the restorative effects of social interventions and help address structural problems in public health policy [cf. 13]. Here, we see a great opportunity to go beyond individualised and damage-centred narratives in DOHaD research in order to tell scientific stories that account for the complexity of biosocial worlds.

References

1. Gluckman PD, Buklijas T, Hanson M. The Developmental Origins of Health and Disease (DOHaD) concept: Past, present, and future. In: Rosenfeld CS, ed. The Epigenome and Developmental Origins of Health and Disease. Boston, MA, Academic Press. 2016; 1–15.

2. Richardson SS, Stevens H, eds. Postgenomics: Perspectives on Biology after the Genome. Durham, NC, Duke University Press, 2015.

3. Niewöhner J. Epigenetics: Embedded bodies and the molecularisation of biography and Milieu. BioSocieties 2011; 6(3): 279–98.

4. Feil R, Fraga MF. Epigenetics and the environment: Emerging patterns and implications. Nature Reviews Genetics 2012; 13(2): 97–109.

5. Pinel C, et al. Markers as mediators: A review and synthesis of epigenetics literature. BioSocieties 2018; 13(1): 276–303.

6. Darling KW, Ackerman SL, Hiatt H, Lee SS-J, Shim JK. Enacting the molecular imperative: How gene-environment interaction research links bodies and environments in the post-genomic age. Social Science & Medicine 2016; 155: 51–60.

7. Uchinuma H et al. Gestational body weight gain and risk of low birth weight or macrosomia in women of Japan: A nationwide cohort study. International Journal of Obesity 2021; 45(12): 2666–74.

8. Jirtle RL, Skinner MK. Environmental epigenomics and disease susceptibility. Nature Reviews Genetics 2007; 8(4): 253–62.

9. Ingold T. The Perception of the Environment: Essays on Livelihood, Dwelling and Skill. London, Routledge, 2000.

10. Warin M, Martin A. Emergent postgenomic bodies and their (non) scalable environments. In: Meloni M, Cromby J, Fitzgerald D, Lloyd S, eds. The Palgrave Handbook of Biology and Society. London, Palgrave Macmillan. 2018; 703–25.

11. Penkler M. Caring for biosocial complexity. Articulations of the environment in research on the Developmental Origins of Health and Disease. Studies in History and Philosophy of Science 2022; 93: 1–10.

12. Warin M, Kowal E, Meloni M. Indigenous knowledge in a postgenomic landscape: The politics of epigenetic hope and reparation in Australia. Science, Technology, & Human Values 2020; 45(1): 87–111.

13. Müller R, Kenney M. A science of hope? Tracing emergent entanglements between the biology of early life adversity, trauma-informed care, and restorative justice. Science, Technology, & Human Values 2021; 46(6): 1230–60.

14. Valdez N. The redistribution of reproductive responsibility: On the epigenetics of 'environment' in prenatal interventions. Medical Anthropology Quarterly 2018; 32(3): 425–42.

15. Shostak S, Moinester M. The missing piece of the puzzle? Measuring the environment in the postgenomic moment. In: Richardson SS, Stevens H, eds. Postgenomics: Perspectives on Biology after the Genome. Durham, NC, Duke University Press. 2015; 192–209.

16. Landecker H. Food as exposure: Nutritional epigenetics and the new metabolism. BioSocieties 2011; 6(2): 167–94.

17. Penkler M, et al. DOHaD in science and society: Emergent opportunities and novel responsibilities. Journal of

Developmental Origins of Health and Disease 2019; **10**(3): 268–73.

18. Müller R, et al. The biosocial genome? Interdisciplinary perspectives on environmental epigenetics, health and society. EMBO Reports 2017; **18**(10): 1677–82.

19. Warin M, Moore V, Zivkovic T, Davies M. Telescoping the origins of obesity to women's bodies: How gender inequalities are being squeezed out of Barker's hypothesis. Annals of Human Biology 2011; **38**(4): 453–60.

20. Shostak S, Moinester M. Beyond geneticization: Regimes of perceptibility and the social determinants of health. In: Bell SE, Figert AE, eds. Reimagining Biomedicalization, Pharmaceuticals, and Genetics: Old Critiques and New Engagements. New York, Routledge. 2015; 216–38.

21. Roberts E. Food is love: And so, what then? BioSocieties 2015; **10**: 247–52.

22. Pentecost M, Ross F. The first thousand days: Motherhood, scientific knowledge, and local histories. Medical Anthropology 2019; **38**(8): 747–61.

23. Tuck E. Suspending damage: A letter to communities. Harvard Educational Review 2009; **79**(3): 409–27.

24. Chiapperino L. Environmental enrichment: An experiment in biosocial intervention. BioSocieties 2019; **16**(1): 41–69.

25. Ackerman SL, Darling KW, Lee SS-J, Hiatt RA, Shim JK. Accounting for complexity: Gene–environment interaction research and the moral economy of quantification. Science, Technology & Human Values 2016; **41** (2): 194–218.

26. Müller R, de Rijcke S. Thinking with indicators. Exploring the epistemic impacts of academic performance indicators in the life sciences. Research Evaluation 2017; **26**(3): 157–68.

27. Pinel C. What counts as the environment in epigenetics? Knowledge and ignorance in the entrepreneurial university. Science as Culture 2022; 1–23: 311–33.

28. Knorr-Cetina KD. The Manufacture of Knowledge: An Essay on the Constructivist and Contextual Nature of Science. Oxford: Pergamon, 2013.

29. Samaras G. Re-Enacting Stress in the Lab. On Environmental Epigenetics, Social Adversity and the Molecularisation of Mental Health. Unpublished PhD thesis, Technical University of Munich, 2020.

30. Beck S, Niewöhner J. Somatographic investigations across levels of complexity. BioSocieties 2006; **1**(2): 219–27.

31. Niewöhner J. Co-laborative anthropology: Crafting reflexivities experimentally. In: Jouhki J, Steel T, eds. Ethnologinen Tulkinta ja Analyysi. Kohti Avoimempaa Tutkimusprosessia. Helsinki, Ethnos. 2016; 81–125.

Narrative Choreographies
DOHaD, Social Justice, and Health Equity

Martha Kenney and Ruth Müller

Communicating research findings is a storytelling practice. The stories we tell as researchers are important to how publics understand research findings and how research circulates in society. This is especially true for fields that have important social, political, or policy implications, such as the Developmental Origins of Health and Disease (DOHaD). In its emphasis on gestation and early childhood, DOHaD research often focuses on the behaviours of parents (especially mothers) as crucial to the development and health of their children. Depending on how the story is told, this can lead to blaming mothers for future diseases [1]; however, this is not the only possibility. If we zoom out and focus the narrative not on the individual, but on the larger social, economic, and political environment, it is also possible to use DOHaD research to problematise the structural conditions that shape health across generations [2, 3]. In this case, the upstream social determinants of health such as wealth inequality, economic exploitation, sexism, and systemic racism become targets for public health intervention. The stories we tell about the research matter to how research questions are framed, how studies are conducted, how findings are interpreted, and what kinds of interventions are proposed. Thus, it is important to understand storytelling as crucial to the practice of doing responsible research at the science–society interface.

We use the term 'narrative choreographies' [4] to capture the way researchers, clinicians, science journalists, and other actors conceptualize and embed DOHaD knowledge claims as part of larger scientific, social, and political narratives. Sometimes narrative choreographies are strategic, where we deliberately choose language to encourage certain interpretations of research findings and discourage others; however, more often than not we employ narrative choreographies unconsciously, using scientific and cultural narratives that are available to us in our wider social environment – which can have unintended consequences. For example, DOHaD narratives are often focused on the effects of maternal obesity[1] and gestational diabetes on fetal development. Feminist science studies scholar Sarah Richardson argues that this narrative focus can lead to self-rapprochement in mothers who have a BMI classified as 'obese' and a lower standard of

---

Ruth Müller's work on epigenetics and DOHaD has been supported by the German Research Foundation DFG through the project grant "Situating Environmental Epigenetics" (403161875; PI: Ruth Müller). Ruth Müller's and Martha's Kenney's work on this chapter has further been supported by a collaborative research residence fellowship at the Brocher Foundation in Hermance, Switzerland, in 2022. Please see their website for information on their mission and programs: https://www.brocher.ch/en/?

[1] We use the terms obese and obesity in this article because they reflect scientific discourse. We would like to note though that these terms have been criticized and rejected by many fat rights activists and fat studies scholars because they are understood as pathologizing fat bodies (e.g., [5]).

care in clinical encounters. Furthermore, framing obesity in children as a negative outcome of maternal obesity runs the risk of 'replicating harmful stereotypes and misconceptions that contribute to stigma about fat children, which in itself can harm their mental and physical health and imperil their safety' [6, p. 215]. These narratives could be productively rescripted to focus on access to tasty, culturally appropriate, nutritious, and affordable food for parents and children rather than pathologising the size of their bodies. When we rely on narrative conventions we inherit from our field, we can miss the opportunity to ask critical questions about how to tell responsible stories about our research. While we don't always have control over how our research is interpreted in other arenas, carefully constructing narrative choreographies increases the likelihood that our research will have the social impact we desire.

Our years of working with DOHaD researchers have taught us that many researchers in this field do research explicitly with the intention of affecting positive changes in the world: they want to increase the health and well-being of people, especially those who have historically been disadvantaged, marginalised, and underserved. However, current narratives emerging from DOHaD often unintentionally serve to further stigmatise these groups rather than support their health and well-being [7, Chiapperino et al. in this volume].

In this chapter, we advocate for deliberately choreographing DOHaD narratives to address structural inequality and support struggles for social justice and health equity. In order to do this, we suggest moving away from focusing on individual responsibility, and instead, emphasising the social determinants of health. A narrow focus on individual responsibility can unduly blame people for their health status and the health status of their children, without addressing the causes of inequality, which are structural and socially determined. We further recommend crafting narrative choreographies that avoid pathologising people who have experienced early life adversity, and instead focus on possibilities for healing, growth, and health throughout the lifecourse.

In your own research area, you will likely have a sense of some of the harmful narratives that circulate among researchers, in policy, and in the wider media; these may be different than those we present here. We encourage you to reflect on how to choreograph your DOHaD narratives to avoid harmful social and political implications and to suggest policy interventions that better support parents, children, and communities. We offer three examples from our own research to demonstrate how to recognise narrative choreographies at work in DOHaD and neighbouring fields with an eye towards avoiding potential pitfalls and connecting research with the real-life challenges that communities face due to inequality and discrimination. We conclude by offering recommendations for DOHaD researchers who are interested in workshopping their own narrative choreographies.

23.1 Example #1: Epigenetics of Maternal Care

Our first example comes from a research area that has emerged from a series of experiments on the epigenetic effects of maternal care in rats conducted at McGill University. These experiments have not only been influential within the field of environmental epigenetics but also in fields like DOHaD that have significant policy implications. The McGill group found that when a mother rat licks and grooms her pups regularly, it leads to the stronger expression of a glucocorticoid receptor gene in the pups' brains, which makes them calmer and easier to handle as adults [8]. When there is less licking and grooming behaviour, they found that the rat pups become more anxious and aggressive, a change in behaviour that is considered to be epigenetic in origin and is thought to last throughout the lifecourse. When this research is translated into claims about human behaviour and health, it is often embedded in narrative choreographies that blame mothers for undesirable epigenetic changes that affect the health and well-being of their offspring [1, 9, 10]. Despite the fact that rats do not practise bi-parental care, the model organism findings are used to argue that human mothers are responsible for the future health and disease of their children, without paying attention to the role of fathers, extended family, paid caregivers, and the environment beyond the home [11]. This too-quick translation between model organisms and humans leads to narratives that focus on mothers' parenting behaviours without considering the larger social and economic environment in which parenting occurs [10].

For example, in the article, 'Maternal warmth buffers the effects of low early-life socioeconomic status on pro-inflammatory signaling in adulthood' [12], Chen et al. use the McGill experiments to frame their research on 'maternal warmth' in humans.[2] They find that in low socio-economic status (SES) households, high levels of maternal warmth protect children against the negative health effects of poverty, which they measure via biomarkers of immune activation and systemic inflammation. At the end of the article, they discuss the policy implications of this research:

> Working to alleviate poverty, as lofty and important a goal as this is, has remained an intractable problem in our society. Complementing this effort, encouraging and teaching parenting behaviors that facilitate warm emotional climates, even in the face of adversity, might prove to be a supporting, effective target of intervention (as suggested by cross-fostering and environmental manipulation studies in previous animal research).
>
> [12, p. 735]

By framing poverty as 'intractable', these researchers advocate instead for interventions on the individual level, such as parenting classes for low-SES women. This narrative choreography precludes interventions that target the upstream social determinants of health, and instead places the burden of social transformation on low-SES mothers to protect their children from a world that is stacked against them from the start. Furthermore, they do not discuss the structural reasons for low-SES status such as racism, discrimination against people with disabilities, and xenophobia.

Individual interventions are popular in a neoliberal policy climate that seeks the most cost-effective solutions to public health problems. However, these interventions do not target the root cause of health inequity and put the burden for change on the most vulnerable. In the US context, where systemic racism limits life chances for Black Americans, prominent political activist and scholar Angela Davis and her sister, Fania Davis – a leader in the restorative justice movement – write:

> While the difficulties besetting the family should by no means be dismissed, any strategies intended to alleviate the prevailing problems among poor Black people that methodologically target the family for change and leave the socioeconomic conditions perpetuating Black unemployment and poverty intact are doomed to failure at the outset.
>
> [13, p. 81].

---

[2] See Kenney 2022 [11] for a longer discussion of this article and the problem of interventions that target individuals.

Following Davis and Davis, public health interventions that focus on poor and racialised mothers[3] fail to support efforts for anti-racism and economic equality [see Valdez and Lappé in this volume]. Rather than parenting classes and other forms of public health surveillance, Chen et al. could advocate for more parenting *resources*, such as paid parental leave, free daycare, and affordable food and housing. Local activists and organisations as well as researchers in sociology and social work who support low-SES parents might be able to offer specific policy recommendations that would be relevant to their goals. Seeking out the necessary experts and expertise for crafting responsible narratives and policy recommendations is essential for DOHaD research to have a positive impact on the life worlds of the people they study. We include specific recommendations for interdisciplinary inquiry and collaboration at the end of our chapter.

23.2 Example #2: NEAR Science Trainings

In our work on the McGill experiments on the epigenetics of maternal care in rats [10], we became concerned by narrative choreographies that focused almost exclusively on the *damage* caused by early-life adversity. We felt that a focus on damage without a concomitant discussion of healing and reversibility could run the risk of pathologising those who have experienced childhood adversity and increase stigmatisation and discrimination [14; see also Meloni et al. in this volume]. However, in our later fieldwork in the US Pacific Northwest, we were surprised to find that this research had been taken up by actors outside of DOHaD and public health and placed into a different narrative choreography that emphasised how widespread early-life adversity is and that focused on possibilities for healing, health, and well-being throughout the lifecourse.[4]

At our field site, actors reported a crisis in schools, which was characterised differently depending on who we spoke to. This is how the crisis was framed by a community leader at a local nonprofit:

> We have a very high teen suicide rate here. The school district, the reason that they became motivated for trauma-informed practices [was that] they had two high school students the same year [die by] suicide. It's a small school, right? The then-superintendent was just devastated. And she goes to her school board and says, 'We had two kids kill themselves. We've got to do things differently.' They didn't know what to do differently, but she and her district became kind of like this learning community.
>
> (NEAR-org 2)

One of the novel approaches they adopted to address this crisis was NEAR Science trainings. These trainings are based on the findings of the CDC-Kaiser Adverse Childhood Experience (ACE) Study, which shows that the more ACEs a person has experienced out of an ACE score of 10,[5] the more likely a person is to develop negative

---

[3] It is also important to note that policy interventions that focus on the poor mothers are often covertly targeting racialised mothers in the United States and other national contexts. This can inflect how the problems and the solutions are framed, even if race is not explicitly mentioned in the article.

[4] For more information on our findings, see Müller and Kenney 2020 [4].

[5] The ten Adverse Childhood Experiences (ACEs) that make up the ACE score are as follows: emotional abuse, physical abuse, sexual abuse, mother treated violently, household substance abuse, mental illness in household, parental separation or divorce, criminal household member, emotional neglect, and physical neglect.

physical and mental health outcomes across the lifecourse. In the trainings, trainers combine the ACE Study with more recent research findings in epigenetics and neuroscience to explain how ACEs can lead to negative health and behavioural outcomes. The NEAR acronym brings these different research strands together; it stands for Neuroscience, Epigenetics, ACEs, and Resilience.

Although the findings of the CDC-Kaiser ACE Study can be discouraging for those with ACEs, the trainers frame the NEAR Sciences as 'sciences of hope'. They employ narrative choreographies that deliberately avoid biological determinism (i.e. ACEs always lead to negative health outcomes) and pathologisation (i.e. stigmatising people with ACEs). For example, after saying that toxic stress can rewire the brain to expect danger everywhere, the trainers make clear that this is not necessarily negative or a disease state; they explain that people with ACEs have 'protector brains' and are well suited for high-stress careers such as 'first responder'. Trainers emphasise that ACEs are common and that having ACEs does not necessarily mean future ill health. They tell the story of a doctor who was highly successful and respected in her community. When she attended a NEAR Science training, she raised her hand during the discussion and said, 'I have all ten ACEs; why did I turn out so well?'; she went on to talk about the support she received in her life that led to her success. This story is used to illustrate how resilience – which is often defined as interpersonal – can protect people against the potential negative health effects of ACEs. One adage that trainers repeat frequently is that a positive relationship with 'one caring adult' can support resilience. Although this at first may appear similar to the notion that maternal warmth can 'buffer' against early childhood adversity, the NEAR Science trainings move the locus of responsibility out of the home and into the community and the institutions that support children (e.g. schools). They emphasise that this "one caring adult" does not have to be a mother or parent to be effective. Thus, in the NEAR Science trainings, the biology of early life adversity is framed as actionable with community support, rather than dooming people to a life of poor mental and physical health.

When ACEs are framed as deterministic, prevention becomes the only solution to the problem of ACEs. And while prevention is important, it does not help those who have already experienced early-life adversity live healthy and fulfilling lives. The narrative choreographies of the NEAR Science trainings emphasise that ACEs are common and assert that it is possible to intentionally build resilience in individuals and communities. For example, inspired by the NEAR Science trainings, schools are making changes to how they address difficult behaviours. In the NEAR Science framing, these behaviours are understood to be as a result of ACEs rather than wilful disobedience. Therefore, schools are intentionally reducing punitive disciplinary measures, such as suspension and expulsion, and introducing practices from restorative justice and trauma-informed care [4].[6] Restorative justice is an established alternative to punitive justice that focuses on building and maintaining relationships and repairing harm. This approach allows children to engage in social-emotional learning and mend relationships rather than be excluded from the community when they harm others. This rejection of received forms

---

[6] This is especially important in the US context as suspensions and expulsions are strongly correlated with adult incarceration. The disproportionate punishment of Black children in schools contributes to the disproportionate incarceration of Black adults – a phenomenon known as the school-to-prison pipeline [25].

of punitive discipline and this new focus on maintaining strong interpersonal relationships creates novel possibilities for children with ACEs – and indeed all children – to flourish in the school environment. The narrative choreography of the NEAR Science trainings, with its emphasis on growth, learning, and healing throughout the lifecourse, makes these kinds of novel interventions possible.

23.3 Example #3: An Obesity Epidemic in the Global South?

The last example we will discuss concerns the effects of maternal nutrition on children's health. While maternal nutrition is a broad topic of concern within DOHaD [15], here we specifically focus on discourses within DOHaD that engage with the rise in average BMI in the Global South [16]. Researchers in DOHaD have been warning that obesity is on the rise in nations such as India where eating habits are changing, and more people are adopting a so-called 'Western diet'. This shift is thought to increase the risk of non-communicable diseases (NCDs) in the population. In the popular science book, *Mismatch: Why Our World No Longer Fits Our Bodies*, Gluckman and Hanson have argued that this dietary transition constitutes a ticking 'lifestyle disease timebomb' [17], while others have called India the new 'diabetes capital' of the world [18]. The DOHaD explanation for India's rise in average BMI and NCDs is that there is a mismatch between the current nutritional environment and the nutritional environment of the previous generation. In utero, the current generation was exposed to their mothers' diet, which is assumed to be variously 'less processed', 'traditional', or contributing to 'undernourishment'. Experiencing their mother's diet as a fetus would have programmed the bodies of the current generation to anticipate low-caloric foods through their lifecourses. Thus, their bodies would exhibit a 'thrifty' metabolic phenotype that gains body weight easily when transitioning to a calorically dense 'Western diet', putting them at an elevated risk of NCDs.

Narratives in the DOHaD literature about why eating patterns change in postcolonial contexts such as India are often focused on individual choices: adopting a Western diet is thought to be a sign of wealth and cosmopolitanism, particularly in the growing Indian middle class (see, e.g. [19]). Indians in this context are often framed as eager to catch up with the West and unaware of the possible health consequences of their new diet. At the same time, phrases like 'lifestyle disease timebomb' construct Indian bodies as a threat to themselves as well as to global health. By adopting these paternalistic and alarmist narrative choreographies to discuss emerging health challenges in India, DOHaD inadvertently perpetuates colonial tropes that serve to obfuscate histories of colonial violence and persistent post-colonial power differentials. It also upholds the notion that it is the role of Western science to educate and manage non-white bodies in the Global South – an ongoing legacy of colonial science.

There are different narrative possibilities, however. When discussing a rise in median BMI in India, DOHaD researchers could draw attention to how Western food corporations have come to colonise food markets in the Global South and increasingly control the foods that are available to the local population, as well as large-scale industrial agriculture that encourages monoculture. They could also discuss the shift in priority setting in local agriculture towards crops for export rather than traditional foods for local consumption. In this context, researchers could partner with local social movements and activists who work to achieve food sovereignty and access to healthy, affordable foods and follow their lead in how to define problems, solutions, and interventions.

23.4 Recommendations for Narrative Choreographies

Drawing on the three examples listed above, we have compiled two sets of recommendations for DOHaD researchers who are interested in connecting their research to social justice and health equity goals. The first is a set of suggestions for developing an active practice of choreographing DOHaD narratives. The second is a list of pitfalls we have observed in commonly circulating DOHaD narratives. These lists are not exhaustive, and we fully expect pitfalls to change over time as the research field grows and narratives change. The important part is to recognise that storytelling is a consequential scientific practice and to reflect on the social and political effects of the stories we tell about our research.

23.5 How to Make and Revise Your Narrative Choreography

- Reflect on the narratives you are currently using when communicating your research. Consider why you are using these narratives and how they could be reimagined to better support positive change. Ask yourself: who is included in the narrative, and who is excluded? Who is held responsible for healthy/unhealthy development, and do they have the resources and support needed to effect change? Does this narrative reinforce or challenge existing inequalities? Are there any implicit stereotypes about gender, race, sexuality, disability, fatness, or other categories of difference that should be addressed? Which policy positions does this narrative support or undermine? Does this narrative explicitly advocate for social justice and health equity goals?
- Partner with stakeholders, communities, and organisations that represent and support vulnerable people. Learn about the real-life problems that parents, children, and communities face and what kinds of interventions and resources would most benefit them. If possible, connect your research findings with these goals.
- Reach out to colleagues in other fields such as science and technology studies, education, social work, history, women and gender studies, and ethnic and area studies as potential research partners to benefit from their expertise and to learn viable alternatives to dominant narratives.
- Deliberately plan your narrative choreographies. Decide which framings and interventions you want to promote and which might be harmful and should be avoided. Consider whether the language you are using supports this plan or surreptitiously works against your goals. Practise your narrative in front of different audiences to learn how it is received and make changes accordingly.
- Revise your narratives. Storytelling is situated. What might work well in one context may not work in another [20]. Re-choreograph narratives for different audiences and as political language and awareness changes. For example: what does it look like to talk about racism and health in the wake of the Black Lives Matter movement? Or childhood sexual abuse after the #MeToo movement?

23.6 Pitfalls to Avoid

- Avoid policy recommendations that identify marginalised individuals and families as the singular target of intervention. Employ narrative choreographies that emphasise structural issues such as racism, wealth inequity, and the upstream social determinants of health. Connect DOHaD findings to key issues in social justice and health equity. Advocate for resources that support parents and children's healthy development.

- Avoid narratives that pathologise those with ACEs or perinatal exposures. Instead, use non-deterministic frameworks that acknowledge opportunities for health and resilience across the lifecourse. Recognize that early-life adversity is common; when early-life adversity is framed as rare and pathogenic, it can alienate and shame people with these experiences. Partner with educators and others who work with children to create institutions and programmes that support social-emotional growth.

- When doing research that involves a different national or social context, pay attention to power differentials and to how global histories shape the available narratives. No matter what our social position and national context, it is important to avoid imposing our own problem/solution framework on the lives of others. Often people themselves are the best experts on their own lives and can readily identify which problems are important/unimportant and which interventions are helpful/harmful [21]. Avoid using alarmist language and terms like 'obesity epidemic' or 'disease timebomb' to speak about entire populations, and thereby, implicitly framing them as a danger to themselves and to global health writ large.

- Avoid pathologising obesity in pregnant women/people and in children in both research and clinical encounters. Making people feel shame about their bodies is an 'affective determinant of health' [22] that can negatively impact pregnancy and health outcomes [23]. DOHaD narratives should support people's health goals regardless of their body weight, disabilities, mental health status, etc. Health can act as a moral category [24] that is used to shame people who 'deviate from an imagined ideal norm of health, youth, fitness and . . . attractiveness' [22]. It is important to avoid shaming and blaming those who fall outside of a perceived norm. Question your own assumptions about health and listen to those who have had negative experiences with the healthcare system.

- Reflect on your own research area and add any additional pitfalls you haven't seen to this list.

We believe that many researchers in DOHaD are committed to strengthening social justice and health equity worldwide. We offer these recommendations in a spirit of collaboration and hope that they open more opportunities for partnership across disciplines and sectors as we attempt to address the significant public health implications of DOHaD. Deliberate narrative choreographies, narrative choreographies that link NCDs back to structural violence and avoid individual blame, constitute one important practice in the co-creation of responsible biomedical research and clinical practice.

References

1. Richardson SS, Daniels CR, Gillman MW, et al. Society: Don't blame the mothers. Nature 2014; 512(7513): 131–32.

2. Müller R, Hanson C, Hanson M, Penkler M, et al. The biosocial genome? Interdisciplinary perspectives on environmental epigenetics, health and society. EMBO Reports 2017; 18: 1677–82.

3. Penkler M, Müller R, Kenney M, Hanson M. Back to normal? Building community resilience after COVID-19. The Lancet Diabetes and Endocrinology 2020; 8(8): 664–65.

4. Müller R, Kenney M. A science of hope? Tracing emergent entanglements between the biology of early life adversity, trauma-informed care, and restorative justice.

Science, Technology, & Human Values 2021; **46**(6): 1230–60.

5. Gordon A. "You Just Need to Lose Weight": And 19 Other Myths About Fat People. Beacon Press, 2023.

6. Richardson SS. The Maternal Imprint: The Contested Science of Maternal-Fetal Effects. Chicago, University of Chicago Press, 2021.

7. Penkler M, Hanson M, Biesma R. DOHaD in science and society: Emergent opportunities and novel responsibilities. Journal of Developmental Origins of Health and Disease 2019; **10**(3): 268–73.

8. Weaver ICG, Cervoni N, Champagne FA et al. Epigenetic programming by maternal behavior. Nature Neuroscience 2004; **7**: 847–54.

9. Richardson SS. Maternal bodies in the postgenomic order: Gender and the explanatory landscape of epigenetics. In: Richardson SS, Stevens H, eds. Postgenomics: Perspectives on Biology after the Genome. Durham, NC, Duke University Press. 2015; 210–31.

10. Kenney M, Müller R. Of Rats and Women: Narratives of motherhood in environmental epigenetics. BioSocieties. 2017. **12**; 23–46.

11. Kenney M. Daphnia and Apollo: An epigenetic fable. Catalyst: Feminism, Theory, Technoscience. 2022; **8**(2); 1–24. https://catalystjournal.org/index.php/catalyst/article/view/36728/version/25426.

12. Chen E, Miller GE, Kobor MS et al. Maternal warmth buffers the effects of low early-life socioeconomic status on pro-inflammatory signaling in adulthood. Molecular Psychiatry 2011; **16**: 729–37.

13. Davis A, Davis F. Slaying the dream: The Black Family and the crisis of capitalism. In: Davis A, ed. Women, Culture and Politics. New York, Vintage Books. 1984: 73–90.

14. Tuck E. Suspending damage: A letter to communities. Harvard Educational Review 2009; **79**(3): 409–27.

15. Valdez N. Weighing the Future: Race, Science, and Pregnancy Trials in the Postgenomic Era. Oakland, University of California Press, 2021.

16. Pentecost M. The first thousand days: Epigenetics in the age of global health. In: Meloni M, Cromby J, Fitzgerald D, Lloyd S, eds. The Palgrave Handbook of Biology and Society. London, Palgrave Springer. 2018; 269–94.

17. Gluckman P, Hanson M. Mismatch: Why Our World No Longer Fits Our Bodies. Oxford, Oxford University Press, 2006.

18. Solomon H. Metabolic Living: Food, Fat, and the Absorption of Illness in India. Durham, NC, Duke University Press, 2016.

19. McMurry HS, Shivashankar R, Mendenhall E, Prabhakaran D. Insights on overweight and obesity. Economic & Political Weekly. 2017; **LII**(49): 84–88.

20. Kenney M, Müller R. Biology for racial justice? Building biosocial responses to trauma and inequality. Forthcoming.

21. Johnson MA, Niemeyer ED. Ambivalent landscapes: Environmental justice in the US–Mexico borderlands. Human Ecology 2008; **36**: 371–82.

22. Dolezal L, Lyons B. Health-related shame: an affective determinant of health? Medical Humanities 2017; **43**(4): 257–63.

23. Moore V, Warin M. The reproduction of shame: Pregnancy, nutrition and body weight in the translation of developmental origins of adult disease. Science, Technology, & Human Values 2022; online first: https://journals.sagepub.com/doi/abs/10.1177/01622439221108239.

24. Metzl JM, Kirkland A. Against Health: How Health Became the New Morality. New York, New York University Press, 2010.

25. Gonzalez, T. Keeping Kids in Schools: Restorative justice, punitive discipline, and the School to Prison Pipeline. Journal of Law & Education 2012; **41**(2): 281–335.

Chapter

24

Interdependence
Reworking Ontogeny through
Tendrel Fishbones and Dirty Chickens

Shivani Kaul and Emily Yates-Doerr

24.1 Introduction

In 2008 and 2013, *The Lancet* published a series on maternal and child undernutrition that laid the groundwork for public health policymakers to approach nutrition as a foundational component of global development. In the series introduction, Robert Black and his co-authors emphasise a hierarchy of medical and monetary factors that cause malnutrition and serve as sites for intervention. Using a framework developed by UNICEF, they list eight color-coded risk factors, all stacked vertically [1]. 'Basic' causes of malnutrition like 'social and economic conditions' and 'lack of capital' sit at the bottom of the stack (see Figure 24.1). Then come monetised 'underlying' conditions like 'income poverty', which is listed prior to and distinct from conditions like 'unhealthy household environment'. At the top of the stack, closest to undernutrition, are 'immediate' causes such as 'inadequate dietary intake' and 'disease'. In the first article of the series, Geneva and US-based authors emphasised the period from conception to the second birthday – a period of roughly 1000 days – as a 'crucial window of opportunity' to address undernutrition [2, p. 510]. The series' second article emphasises the health and 'human capital' consequences of malnutrition. Here, the multidisciplinary authors draw on the Developmental Origins of Health and Disease (DOHaD) hypothesis to argue that poor fetal nutrition in early life leads to 'irreversible damage' to future adult health, school achievement, and adult income for up to three generations [3, p. 340].

The dominant logic woven through this publication series is that a narrow window of physiological development has profound implications for future health and economic productivity, which neoclassical economists value for its contribution to gross domestic product (GDP). Though the potential nutrition interventions discussed in these papers range from land reform to rest during pregnancy, most 'proven' nutrition interventions the authors recommend focus on what they call immediate causes. The third article illustrates the overarching message of the series: that policy actions on maternal and child undernutrition can include a wide range of interdependent interventions while excluding 'important interventions that might have broad and long-term benefits'

The writing and research for this chapter were supported by European Starting Council Grant #759414 for research on Global Future Health. We thank Stephanie Lloyd, Pierre-Eric Lutz, and Andie Thompson for thorough and incisive feedback on an early version of this chapter; Noel W. Solomons and Michi Penkler for their close readings; and all of the editors for their care through the process of review. Noel Solomons died on March 23rd, 2024, as we were reading the page proofs for this chapter. We dedicate it to his commitment to rethinking the fields of biology and nutrition through insights from science in the Global South.

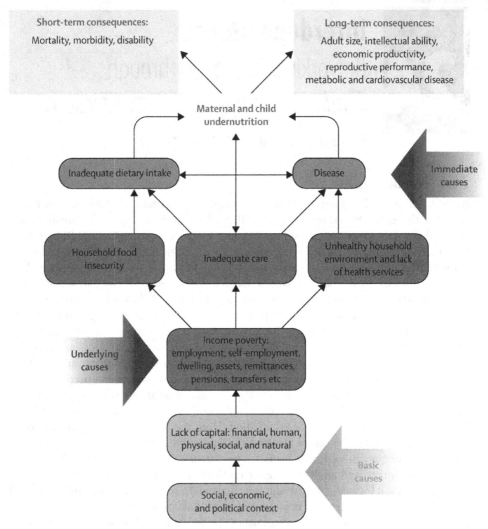

Figure 24.1 The *Lancet* model of causal interdependence
[1, p. 244]

because they are 'outside the scope' of review, or because they lack an appropriate evidence base appropriate evidence like randomised control trials [4, p. 418]. 'We must be targeted in our approach', one US-based politician has said about the need to address malnutrition during the early developmental stages (see also Jacob et al. in this volume).

In our chapter, we draw upon research on child development that inspires a reworking of *The Lancet*'s causal models and the policies that result. The DOHaD scientists in Bhutan and Guatemala whose work we describe are in conversation with *The Lancet*'s series on child development. But whereas *The Lancet*'s authors place 'social, economic, and political' factors at the edge of the conversation about child development, these scientists place cultures, economics, politics, and ecologies squarely at the heart of development, advancing a theory of ontogeny that insists on a complex and interdependent web of causation.

Ontogeny (from the Greek words onto/being and genesis/birth) is a term biologists use to describe physiological growth and development. It emphasises how an organism's form emerges through a process of temporal maturation, with early-life inputs coming to shape later-life physiological structures. This chapter illustrates how different scientific models for ontogenic (biological) development shape the terrain of possibility for global (economic) development, which warrants attention since scientists' vision of development impacts the interventions they design. In Bhutan, we highlight the example of 'fishbone' modelling that unfolds child development factors along multiple, horizontal, spatial, and temporal themes. That child development is the effect of collective well-being amplifies Buddhist relational logics of *tendrel*, or interdependent origination. In Guatemala, we highlight the example of the 'dirty chicken hypothesis', which directs attention to ecological relations. In the Guatemalan case, the normative question of how the organism should develop is one that requires also asking whether the environments that shape and surround this development are well supported.

While *The Lancet*'s models and the Bhutanese and Guatemalan models for malnutrition all emphasise interdependence between humans and their surroundings, they differ in how they organise this interdependence, and, as a result, where the work of intervention must fall. Whereas *The Lancet*'s models are linear and hierarchical, resulting in a policy focus on what and how mothers eat, the theories of interdependent ontogeny that we describe in Bhutan and Guatemala insist upon the value of an ecological approach to health policy, where any given intervention must be reformulated away from targeting individuals to instead amplify caring coalitions. 'Target', we learn from this theory of ontogenesis-as-interdependence, is frequently the wrong metaphor: human communities and landscapes must be cared for together.

24.2 Bhutan: The Fishbone Model

24.2.1 The Golden 1000 Days

Since 2008, the Geneva-based organisation Scaling Up Nutrition (SUN) has been rallying governments, multinational corporations, and non-profit organisations to fund 13 'high impact' interventions selected from *The Lancet* series. The organisation has become 'the most important symbol for the increased interest in nutrition' in global development today [5, p. 552]. Leaders in food policy from 65 countries have joined SUN so far. But some governments have not been so quick to sign up for this targeted approach to intervention and financing. In 2016, the Royal Government of Bhutan sent three representatives to Bangkok to attend the SUN workshop on public finance for nutrition in Asia. Bhutanese representatives did not join SUN, instead citing the need to complete more research on broader actions that follow different pathways of maternal health.

Scientists and policymakers in Thimphu, the capital of Bhutan, have been mobilising over the last decade around a range of interventions related to the first 1000 days agenda, known locally as the 'Golden 1000 Days'. This agenda has generated passionate public discourse within Bhutan – a country never directly colonised, in which an alternative philosophy of economic development circulates named Gross National Happiness (GNH). The agenda's proposed interventions include standard actions like micronutrient powders, breastfeeding and nutritional counselling, and conditional cash transfers, but also broader socio-economic interventions such as six months of paid maternity leave for all civil servants. Additionally, the Golden 1000 Days builds on existing development policies to ensure GNH or collective well-being, including the constitutional protection of 60 per cent

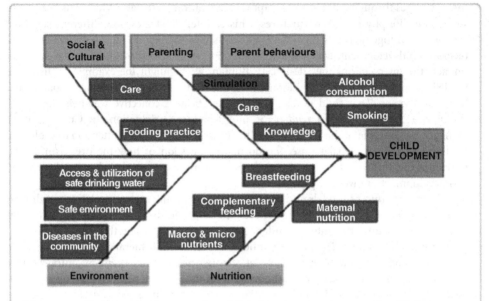

Figure 1: Fish bone diagram for child development causality. Fish bone diagram presenting the factors affecting child development.

Figure 24.2 The 'fishbone' model of causal interdependence
[6, p. 2]

of the country's forest coverage, free education, and fully state-funded biomedical and Sowa Rigpa (Tibetan) healthcare, with an emphasis on primary care [6].

24.2.2 Developing Differently

While *The Lancet* authors model the causes of malnutrition through hierarchical, monetary, and medicalised factors, Bhutanese scientists emphasise interdependence across causal domains – adopting a more horizontal and multidisciplinary approach to addressing undernutrition. Take, for example, the work of Deki Pem, Deputy Dean of Nursing & Midwifery at Khesar Gyalpo University of Medical Sciences in Bhutan. When conceptualising The Golden 1000 Days agenda in Bhutan in 2015, Deki published a 'fishbone' diagram for child development designed to model cause and effect [7]. The 'fishbone' is a conceptual tool that identifies multiple factors that could be contributing to unanticipated outcome variation developed by Japanese organisational theorist Kaoru Ishikawa in the 1970s. Deki used this modelling technique to fan out the potential risk factors for undernutrition to 14 factors (see Figure 24.2). She organised these factors horizontally, not vertically. Instead of separating and then ordering undernutrition's causes into basic, underlying, and immediate causal classes, the 'fishbone' model brings concerns for the environment, society, and culture, parental care, and eating into the conversation of ontogeny. Collective norms of care appear along the sociocultural rib, and safe drinking water features in the environmental rib. What women themselves eat or feed their children becomes a small part of this causal map.

Multiplying the causal origins of child development opens up alternative strategies for nutrition intervention and research. Approaching the Golden 1000 Days through the 'fishbone' model, it becomes difficult to imagine designing effective interventions targeting what women eat – though economists and nutritionists working for the Ministry of Health and international organisations like the World Bank do promote micronutrient sachets and behaviour change interventions in Bhutan [8, 9]. As a nursing practitioner and medical university instructor, Deki has been concerned about customary alcohol use during pregnancy and first food practices that might disrupt exclusive breastfeeding, but her horizons were open. A wide range of remaining known unknowns compel her work – from intergenerational changes in the relationship to food and childcare due to rural-urban migration to the capital Thimphu, to potential sources of environmental lead exposures.

Over a shared plate of *omurice*, Deki explained to Shivani her recent collaborative research on elevated blood levels among children in Thimphu and Phuntsholing. The specific concern in this study on undernutrition was anaemia, 'a critical public health problem in Bhutan', with indicators that had not improved in over 18 years [7, p. 2]. The multiplication of causal factors involved in ontogenetic development also invites multidisciplinary collaboration. With a coalition including physicians, medical statisticians, nursing faculty and anthropologists, Deki has pivoted from studying feeding practices to studying environmental exposures.

Their recent research showed that about 44 per cent of a sample of children between two months and five years of age from the capital city Thimphu and the industrial border town of Phuntsholing had elevated blood lead levels [10]. Deki and her co-authors were surprised to find a significantly higher prevalence of elevated blood lead levels among the children living in otherwise 'clean' Thimphu, in spring, and those who regularly eat with their hands. Their findings indicate the need for more research on the role of 'demolition and construction, weather differences, and possible water contamination', in childhood malnutrition [10, p. 12]. Environmental exposures potentially have knock-on effects on iron deficiency, anaemia, and undernutrition, confirming the need to multiply the sites of research and to rethink the strategy for nutrition interventions during the Golden 1000 Days.

24.2.3 *Tendrel* Interventions

The Lancet's diagram for ontogeny dismissed 'social, economic, and political context' factors for development as too difficult to operationalise in health interventions. Meanwhile, Deki Pem and other malnutrition researchers in Bhutan have highlighted the need to care about what and how different generations of people eat, what social supports they encounter, and the unevenly contaminated environments in which they live. Rather than causally write off ecology and history as 'distant', the scientific practice of Deki Pem and her colleagues enacts a vision for development where socioeconomics, culture, history, diet, safe living environments, water quality, and so on could all be understood as 'immediate' contributors to conditions of inequitable nutrition outcomes. One factor does not precede another in importance; likewise, quick or targeted interventions are not necessarily more effective than those with a slower temporal horizon.

The 'fishbone' diagram of child development amplifies the causal logic of *tendrel* or interdependent origination, which informs health practice in Bhutan. Physician historians Tandi Dorji and Bjorn Melgaard articulate how Buddhist theories of causality facilitate health interventions that open a multiplicity of interdependent factors:

The concept of interdependence of all phenomena, that nothing exists as a separate entity but as a part of the whole, is one of the fundamental beliefs in Buddhism. When considering health and disease, this concept implies that the person with the illness must be viewed in relation to the whole, i.e. all internal and external factors that the person is dependent upon, such as physical, mental, social, moral, environmental, familial, work, diet, etc. [11, p. 25].

While this may sound romantic, *tendrel*, in its evocation of being dissimilar but related, emphasises the need to cooperate across difference – across scales and sites. *Tendrel* emphasises the co-arising of beings as an impermanent and indeterminate process of relationship, according to the cultural historian Karma Phuntsho [12]. From this causal logic of interdependence, it is important to discern which relations are generative and which relations are harmful. As much as connecting or adding relations, identifying and refusing toxic attachments becomes key for development and collective well-being. Human interdependence with landscapes is a distinguishing causal feature of Sowa Rigpa and healing practices in Bhutan [13] and has also influenced how complex global health problems like pandemics have been addressed through coalitions and careful refusal of global market relations [14].

Incorporating *tendrel* into child development policy shifts how DOHaD-informed nutrition interventions might be designed. In contrast to short-term interventions to address immediate causes, policymakers must identify and act upon the multiple conditions that contribute to a given goal. From the interdependent causal logic of *tendrel*, effectively intervening in the ontogenesis of undernourished bodies requires working in multidisciplinary coalitions to address a wide range of cultural, political, and ecological conditions. This attention to the 'gradual unfolding' of child development is what Deki Pem's fishbone diagram and scientific practice opens up [7, p. 1], reminding policymakers why the Golden 1000 Days in Bhutan would not be possible without development actions as expansive as tending to natural resources like forests, providing free biomedical and Tibetan healthcare, and free public education.

24.3 Guatemala: The Dirty Chicken Hypothesis

24.3.1 Nutrition as an Interdisciplinary Science

In the mid-1970s, Dr Nevin Scrimshaw, the founding director of the United Nations' *Institute of Nutrition of Central America and Panama* (INCAP), recommended one of his former students, Noel Solomons, for a research position at the institute's headquarters in Guatemala City. In operation since 1949, INCAP has become a key international centre for science and policy on child development. Guatemala, a country that was roughly half-Maya with a long history of resistance to colonial conquest, is also reported to have high rates of hunger and malnutrition. Americas. INCAP was founded with the goals of learning about the biology of nutrition and carrying out policy interventions to act upon this knowledge.

Both Solomons and Scrimshaw held medical degrees, with specialisation in clinical nutrition, but they were also both interdisciplinary and expansive thinkers. Scrimshaw was widely known for his knowledge of biochemistry, but after a decade at INCAP he took a sabbatical break at Harvard to complete a master's degree in Public Health. His 1959 thesis examined the 'Interactions of Nutrition and Infection' to make the argument that malnutrition enhanced the susceptibility to infection, while the burden of infection impaired the acquisition and retention of nutrients. Solomons would later call this Scrimshaw's 'most transcendental conceptual synthesis', [15] celebrating Scrimshaw's talent for making crucial connections across vastly different domains of expertise.

Solomons, a Black man from Boston whose paternal grandparents were raised on the Dutch island colony of Aruba and who self-identifies in policy spaces as a feminist, was also accustomed to linking diet to broader social contexts, including those of imperialism, colonialism, and social oppression. In addition to holding a medical degree from Harvard, he was trained in internal medicine and infectious disease at the University of Pennsylvania and in gastroenterology and clinical medicine at the University of Chicago. His inclination towards systems thinking afforded him insight into the shortcomings of studying nutrients in isolation. He is fond of pointing out that an understanding of the human body requires a deep understanding of the surrounding environment. To the adage that people eat food, not nutrients, Solomons has added his insight that people don't just eat food, but they ingest adverse influences from certain social and ecological environments.

24.3.2 Contaminated Ecologies

In 1985, Solomons split with INCAP to found his own nutrition research centre in Guatemala City, named the *Center for Studies of Sensory Impairment, Aging, and Metabolism* out of the recognition that nutrition was linked to the development of metabolic and sensory integration processes. Among the hundreds of scientific articles and briefs Solomons has published over the last half-century, he is especially fond of a 1993 paper titled 'The Underprivileged, Developing Country Child: Environmental Contamination and Growth Failure Revisited', which advances what he calls 'the dirty chicken hypothesis'. This is an allusion to the phenomenon well known by poultry scientists that chickens would not grow or put on meat when reared in unsanitary surroundings despite an abundance of feed. A background concern animating the publication is that the public health nutrition community is overly focused on diet. In contrast, Solomons et al. write that 'poor growth appears to be strongly influenced by environmental factors as well as nutrition' [16, p. 327].

With an eye to veterinary science, Solomons observed that veterinarians had long known that animals raised in cleaner conditions – or, alternatively, animals who were fed a low-dose supply of antibiotics to ward off repeated inflections – grew bigger than those raised in contaminated growing conditions. Growth failure in humans, he and his co-authors argued in this 1993 paper, might similarly be more influenced by 'recurrent, overt infections of the respiratory and gastrointestinal tracts', than by whatever foods people are, or are not, eating. He explained that frequent microbial infections brought about by poor sanitation will 'result in continual activation of the immune system and specific metabolic changes' [16, p. 329]. These infections were often 'inapparent' – that is they were not visible to the naked eye or perceived by the person living in these conditions – but they nonetheless led to the condition of 'immunologic stress' and hampered growth. The paper proposed that monokines such as interleukin, tumour necrosis factor-α, or interleukin-6 become caught up in an immune response that alters metabolism. They write,

> The metabolic changes represent a homeorrhetic response that alters the partitioning of dietary nutrients away from growth and skeletal muscle accretion in favour of metabolic processes that support the immune response and disease resistance. These changes form the basis for impaired growth and feed utilization, and for altered nutritional requirements in chicks [16, p. 329].

A human child is, of course, not a baby chicken, but the scientists saw that their observation about chicks might influence the science and policy of human development.

In the background of the dirty chicken article is Solomons' critique of the field of public health nutrition for taking a 'monolithic' approach to malnutrition, overly focused on dietary supplementation. One of Solomons' scientific domains of expertise is the metabolism of anaemia, and he frequently points to the short-sighted impulse to treat anaemia with iron supplementation. This is not only a largely ineffective route to improving the amount and circulation of iron in the blood, he argues, but can affect the production and circulation of haemoglobin that can, in regions where malaria is common, exacerbate this blood-borne illness. Targeting deficient nutrients and not environmental toxicity will throw interdependencies between human biologies and ecological systems out of balance. The challenge, he writes, is to reduce recurrent harmful stimulation to the immune system by addressing environmental damages associated with living in communities that have been forcibly held in toxic poverty. In other words, the 'developmental origins' of malnutrition may be more tightly linked to growing up in toxic environments than to conventional approaches to food security focused on insufficient access to food.

Although Solomons does not write explicitly about racism and sexism in his paper, his conclusion poses challenges for these systems of oppression. When the origins of malnutrition lie in prenatal nutrition, it becomes women – and, especially, Indigenous women who experience Guatemala's highest rates of chronic malnutrition – who are marked as deficient and targeted for supplementation. Similarly, when the problem of malnutrition lies in what people are eating, it is women's expertise that is undermined, given that they primarily run their families' kitchens. In contrast, when malnutrition becomes understood as originating in toxic water and sanitation systems, the burden of treatment might shift to governments, who have the responsibility to provide healthy infrastructures.

24.3.3 Care for the Context

In the years since the publication of the dirty chicken hypothesis, Solomons' critique of nutrient-based development interventions has grown more pronounced [17, 18]. He wants his colleagues in nutrition and public health to see human growth as an adaptive and ecologically interdependent process of development. Human growth on its own is not an obvious or intrinsic good, he argues; environments must also be conducive to this growth. As he explains, in an article titled 'Environmental Contamination and Chronic Inflammation Influence Human Growth Potential',

> [P]ushing dietary interventions to achieve faster growth in the absence of other measures to improve living conditions could prove to be futile (and expensive), counterproductive (and dangerous) or both, depending upon the specifics of ethnicity, climate, cultural practices and human ecology in a given underprivileged setting [18].

The resultant argument is that along with care for diet, the public health community must care about environmental antigens, including toxicities and contamination that impede growth, and cultural and political systems that shape urban planning and family planning alike.

Solomons critiqued a narrow understanding of development that pushed mothers and babies to grow larger while ignoring the environments in which they lived, including not only questions of hygiene but also questions of whether women birthed with midwives or in hospital settings, and whether there were resources to support obstructed labour. He was particularly concerned that the field of public health nutrition's goal of producing large babies, and its reliance on prenatal supplemental nutrition as a means of achieving this goal, would set up conditions of obstetric violence, increasing rates of maternal and child mortality. The implication, building upon Scrimshaw's long-standing interest in the interdependence of bioecological systems, was that the public health and development communities should direct more attention 'to the material environment than to the infant/toddler diet' [15]. As Solomons had earlier written, 'Such a comprehensive public health approach should permit children to be bigger under environmental circumstances in which becoming bigger is truly better' [18].

24.4 Conclusion

In this chapter, we have asked how the field of global development might change by adopting models for DOHaD that emphasise how human ontogeny is interdependent on social and ecological conditions. In our two cases, scientists in Bhutan and Guatemala concern themselves with how relational and systemic interactions shape child development. In the Bhutanese case, Deki Pem observes that maternal and child nutrition, substance abuse, intergenerational eldercare, and environmental toxicities might also be interdependently addressed in DOHaD interventions. Caring for one input of the 'fishbone' while neglecting others makes little sense, since they all contribute to the child's development. In the Guatemala case, interdisciplinary interest in the immunological impact on metabolic processes leads scientists to advocate for the importance of addressing environmental contamination. While the cases differ in their historical and cultural specificities, the scientists in Bhutan and Guatemala both argue that equating nutrition primarily with nutrients misses out on the dynamic, systemic interdependencies that give shape to development.

To be sure, biological models of interdependent ontogeny pose their own challenges. Solomons found the science of ontogeny inspiring because it shifted attention away from how mothers cooked and what they ate and towards environmental contaminants, ranging from microbes to chemical pollutants. In practice, however, a focus on ontogeny can risk cementing the notion that mothers are responsible for the future development of their children [19, 20]. Natali Valdez illustrates how theories of the interdependency of development that might inspire policymakers to act capaciously become foreclosed by reductionist – and frequently racist and sexist – policy imperatives [21]. For example, in The Lancet's hierarchical modelling, development may depend on a great many factors, but it's the mother's behaviours (what and how she eats) that matter most. This model risks reinstating the oppressive mother-focused interventions that some DOHaD scientists wielding models of interdependent growth endeavoured to overcome.

Although interdependence is not a virtue in its own right, we have shown how scientific analyses of interdependent ontogeny from Guatemala and Bhutan can offer a pathway for reworking development interventions. Amber Benezra, in her research on nutrition science, points to the need for policymakers to recognise how they are engaging with interdependent, intergenerational, interdisciplinary, interactive, and intersectional processes [22]. We have likewise described a pathway for conceptualising development through selectively unfolding relations. Rather than understand development as hierarchical, teleological, or following a pre-programmed trajectory, we might rather see the development of the child as part of an adaptive ecological system that coalitions of actors can work to shape. Politics, culture, and environments must all be cared for together.

Expanding the conceptual vocabulary surrounding development to think of ontogeny as an interdependent process helps to cultivate new possibilities for health intervention, inspiring what Hannah Landecker has described as 'different biologies than otherwise would have existed' [23, p. 149]. *The Lancet*'s hierarchical and linear models of development encourage health policymakers to focus primarily on malnutrition's most proximate causes. Taking a page from the sciences of ontogeny in Bhutan and Guatemala, however, may help inspire policymakers to consider that which appears neither immediate nor urgent, but which nonetheless has a structuring influence on global development and human health alike. They might prioritise, for example, the virtue of a clean water system (see also Roberts in this volume). When water is clear, affordable, and contaminant-free, its flow can allow an entire community to flourish. When it comes to implementing health interventions, policymakers might ask if these interventions attenuate stress and build strong communities. Is the land people live in on safe, and do they have sovereignty over this land? Are people encouraged to engage in political and social advocacy and taught how to organise themselves to refuse sources of hunger and exploitation? A lesson from the tendrel fishbone model and the dirty chicken hypothesis is that DOHaD-informed child development policies must look far beyond the child, caring not just for the nutrients this child eats but for its relations. The questions are at once scientific and political: how do we strengthen those relations that are nourishing and detach from those that further toxicity?

References

1. Black RE, Allen LH, Bhutta ZA, et al. Maternal and child undernutrition: Global and regional exposures and health consequences. The Lancet 2008; **371** (9608):243–260.

2. Bryce J, Coitinho D, Darnton-Hill I, et al. Maternal and child undernutrition: Effective action at national level. The Lancet 2008; 371(9611):510–526.

3. Victora CG, Adair L, Fall C, et al. Maternal and child undernutrition: Consequences for adult health and human capital. The Lancet 2008; 371(9609):340–357.

4. Bhutta ZA, Ahmed T, Black RE, et al. What works? Interventions for maternal and child undernutrition and survival. The Lancet 2008; 371(9610):417–440.

5. Gillespie S, Haddad L, Mannar V, et al. The politics of reducing malnutrition: Building commitment and accelerating progress. The Lancet 2013; **382** (9891):552–569.

6. Wangmo D. The evolution of primary healthcare in Bhutan. DrukRig Colloquium. Thimphu, Bhutan. Paper presentation. 20 January 2021.

7. Pem D. Factors affecting early childhood growth and development: Golden 1000 days. Advanced Practice Nursing 2015;**1** (101):2573–3347.

8. Dzed L, Joshi V, Zangpo L, et al. Creating an enabling environment for delivering maternal nutrition interventions in Bhutan. Nutrition Exchange Asia 2019; **1**:12.

9. Leao I, Lhaden, T. Promoting better nutrition in Bhutan. World Bank. 14 May, 2018. https://blogs .worldbank.org/endpovertyinsouthasia/ promoting-better-nutrition-bhutan (Accessed 14 December 2022).

10. Erbele P, Pem D, Tobgay P, et al. Blood lead levels in children 2 through 59 months old in Bhutan. Bhutan Health Journal 2019; 5(2):7–14.

11. Dorji T, Melgaard B. Medical history of Bhutan: Chronicle of health and disease from Bon times to today. Thimphu: Centre for Research Initiatives, 2018.

12. Phuntsho K. Tendrel: Interdependent Causation. Bhutan Cultural Library. 2017.

https://texts.mandala.library.virginia.edu/text/tendrel-interdependent-causation (Accessed 14 December 2022).

13. Choden K. Chilli and Cheese: Food and Society in Bhutan. Delhi: White Lotus; 2008.

14. Kaul S, Pelden S, Tobgay Y, et al. Post-growth pandemic policy from the Himalayas? De-growth or Reinventing Life: Prospects and Projects Conference. Delhi, India. Paper presentation. 4–6 October 2021.

15. Solomons NW. Obituary Nevin Stewart Scrimshaw, PhD, MD, MPH, 1918-2013. Annals of Nutrition Metabolism 2013; 62:277-278.

16. Solomons NW, Mazariegos M, Brown KH, et al. The underprivileged, developing country child: Environmental contamination and growth failure revisited. Nutritional Review 1993; 51 (11):327–332.

17. Solomons NW. Developmental origins of health and disease: Concepts, caveats, and consequences for Public Health Nutrition. Nutritional Review 2009; 67 (Suppl 1): S12–S16.

18. Solomons NW. Environmental contamination and chronic inflammation influence human growth potential. The Journal of Nutrition 2003; 133(5):1237.

19. Colom A. Forced motherhood in Guatemala: An analysis of the 1000 days initiative. In Chary A, Rohloff P, eds. Shifting Healthcare Landscapes in Maya Guatemala. London: Lexington Books, 2015.

20. Pentecost M, Ross F. The first thousand days: Motherhood, scientific knowledge, and local histories. Medical Anthropology 2019; 38(8):747–761.

21. Valdez N. Weighing the Future: Race, Science, and Pregnancy Trials in the Postgenomic Era. Oakland: University of California Press, 2022.

22. Benezra, A. 2023. Gut Anthro: An Experiment in Thinking with Microbes. Minneapolis: University of Minnesota Press.

23. Landecker H. It is what it eats: Chemically defined media and the history of surrounds. Studies in History and Philosophy of Biological and Biomedical Science. 2016; 57:148–160.

Chapter

25

Modelling in DOHaD
Challenges and Opportunities in the Era of Big Data

Julie Nihouarn Sigurdardottir and Salma Ayis

25.1 Introduction

Public health data available for research are booming with the expansion of Big Data sources, shifting the landscape of DOHaD research. These new forms of data offer ample opportunities to advance epidemiological modelling within the DOHaD framework. Big Data is often described by the '3 Vs': high volume, high velocity, and wide variety and refers, for example, to the large volumes of Electronic Health Records (EHRs) now stored as many nations move towards the routine electronic recording and centralising of health data. The term Big Data also applies to data derived from wearable devices and phone applications, increasingly affordable technologies that allow for the collection of new kinds of data, in larger volumes, and almost in real time. Such technologies, along with improved data processing speed and advanced computing capacity, grant access to the lifestyle and health information of millions of individuals who can be followed through the lifespan.

However, within heterogeneous and dynamic socio-demographic contexts and a fast-moving technological landscape, these new forms of data raise a plethora of methodological challenges related to accurately characterising population health trajectories and biological mechanisms. In addition, while the current inferential potential of DOHaD research depends on which variables are collected, at what frequency, and at what time points, it is also closely shaped by the theoretical model(s) chosen for a given study: a framework implicating critical and sensitive windows in development shaped the early DOHaD literature, but other models were added such as the *accumulation of risk model*, the *chain of risk model*, and a hybrid of those [1]. These frameworks shape study designs, data collection practices, and the interpretation of results and set the scene for how Big Data is likely to be taken up in the field.

In this chapter, we provide an overview of DOHaD modelling methods and consider the emerging place of Big Data in investigating multidimensional research questions in the field. To do so, we discuss various methodological aspects of modelling, such as operationalisation, sampling, population representation, ethics, and the accuracy of tools used to acquire and analyse data. We also discuss the current landscape of artificial intelligence-derived methods, judging their utility against the validity of findings, and their potential when compared to 'traditional' empirical data sources and analytical approaches.

25.2 Current DOHaD Modelling and Methodological Challenges

A myriad of methodological challenges are present in DOHaD research even prior to Big Data, in particular, the issues of validity across time and space, characterising causal links, and identifying sources of bias. Physiological processes are difficult to model because they are integrated into non-static systems. These refer to the less quantifiable and less predictable behavioural, lifestyle, environmental, and socio-economic systems interacting with biology. The moderating or mediating effects of culture, health inequalities, medical systems, and health policy on health outcomes must be clarified to assess the generalisability of any given model. Even in gold-standard birth cohort research designs, epidemiological models need to account for the fact that, for example, through societal restructuring and climate change, the properties of exposures can change over time and across generations [2]. As a result, it is difficult to produce predictive DOHaD models and interventions that remain valid and useful across time for a given population. Alternative designs such as the observational study design in humans cannot, however, capture the complexity of all important causal links.

A further challenge for aetiological and epidemiological models of DOHaD is how to define the sources of individual differences in health outcomes with a robust degree of certainty. Some examples include disentangling antenatal and postnatal exposure and their interactions [3]; accounting for sex and gender-based differences in biology and behaviour; inter-organ variation in adaptability to maternal ill health (e.g. the placenta response to stress) [4, 5]; and evaluating disparities in outcomes across diverse groups given that the bulk of data is from a small number of middle- to high-income and white-dominated contexts [6, 7].

Prediction models are also prone to confounding and collider bias [8] (a variable in a causal pathway that is a shared effect of more than one cause). For DOHaD research, the primary exposures studied in the developmental pathway are nutrition, parental physiological and psychological health, the environment and toxicants, and social and demographic determinants [7]. Intuitively it is easy to assume that many of these exposures can co-occur and may moderate one another. While confounding can often be resolved by taking these variables into account, residual confounding remains a risk when those influencing factors are unknown or unmeasurable. In the case of collider bias, this can also lead to counter-intuitive conclusions. Such counter-intuitive conclusions are exemplified by the 'birthweight paradox', where babies born with low birthweight (LBW) to smoking mothers (exposure) appear to have a lower risk of neonatal mortality (outcome) compared to those born with LBW to non-smoking mothers [9].

Here, tools such as directed acyclic graphs (DAGs) that portray causal relationships graphically can help a researcher explore a model's functional assumptions and conceptualise any mechanisms of causality. DAGs help recognise mediators, moderators, confounders, and colliders [10] and have helped to illustrate the collider role of LBW in the above paradox [9]; that is, when maternal smoking is absent, other unobserved causes (malnutrition and congenital defects) can lead to LBW and more severe health problems and thus higher infant mortality. Therefore, while the above research question appeared 'simple' initially and involves few measurable exposures (smoking or not) and outcomes (LBW and mortality), failing to incorporate inter-correlations between variables and confounding effects, conceptualised by theory and DAGs, is unlikely to provide reliable causal inference.

Taking another example, understanding the association between maternal stress and lower infant cognitive outcome [11] warrants pertinent exploration into the relative contributions of other exposures concomitant to maternal stress, such as under- or overnutrition, infections and toxicants, and their interrelationships. Here, modelling methods should integrate observed variables, latent variables (not directly observed but derived from questionnaires or other observed variables, i.e. stress), and their measurement errors, alongside time indicators. Moreover, the mediating mechanisms proposed in the literature, such as epigenetic modulation, the microbiome, metabolism, and (offspring) endogenous immunity, would also have to be incorporated. In practice, a single model that simultaneously incorporates multiple predictive pathways and associations will more accurately capture the causal relationships of interest between the exposure and outcome of interest [12, 13]. Of translational value, such epidemiological modelling would eventually result in developing better targeted interventions.

25.2.1 Data: What Are We Collecting, What Are We Measuring?

High-quality data that are fit for purpose and meet the criteria of accuracy, validity, completeness, and consistency are a cornerstone of empirical science. Data quality may be affected at the stages of data collection, cleaning, or the numerical transformation that is often used to meet required assumptions such as the normal distribution in statistics. Measurement errors, whether systematic or random, are present in all observational studies. While these errors impact the validity and reliability of data and introduce biases, they are rarely acknowledged or accounted for in the epidemiological literature. Makin and de Xivry address common statistical mistakes [14], and Wagenmakers et al. [15] present guidelines on how to report statistical analyses transparently based on four scientific norms of 'communalism, universalism, disinterestedness and organised skepticism'.

Since we allude above to the notion of variable choice and availability, next, we discuss the importance of clear terminology and data quality in DOHaD research methods. How we define and measure exposures and outcomes impacts inferences, findings, and subsequent interventions and policies. One example of this is the work of researchers who rely on clinically defined groupings based on dichotomisation, such as diabetes diagnosis, or the classification of body mass index (BMI) as obese/overweight/normal-weight/underweight. One obvious risk of using a strict classification of body morphology by BMI alone is undermining the field's knowledge about fat distribution being a strong determinant for metabolism and cardiovascular health, especially fat within the abdomen (visceral adiposity). Without other markers to corroborate metabolic health risks (blood pressure, cholesterol, visceral fat mass, etc.), some individuals with normal weight, categorised as 'controls', may be metabolically unhealthy and 'at-risk' of physiological phenotypes. In fact, this group represents 35 per cent of normal-weight individuals [16]. This problem extends to gestational diabetes screening in pregnancy, which is provided to women meeting the BMI > 30 kg/m^2 criteria in the UK, while those under 30 are assumed to be void of any hyperglycaemia risks during pregnancy. The absence of evidence, however, is not evidence of absence. The consequence of such hidden (latent) subgroups of individuals within a 'control' or 'normal-weight' category is the introduction of bias into the statistical analyses that epidemiological models rely on for inference, thus leading to inaccurate conclusions.

Similarly, in psychology, the diagnosis of autism as present/absent is common, although autism spectrum disorder (ASD) is typically conceptualised by experts as a continuum (see also Azevedo et al. in this volume). Such a binary diagnosis of ASD ignores potential distinct mechanisms of importance for the DOHaD of autism subtypes, which could possibly relate to the timing of any 'disruption' in brain development and could be informative for mechanistic studies and prognosis [17].

Overall, what we suggest above is that DOHaD researchers must be conscious of relying on clinical data alone such as those retrieved from EHRs without clarifying sources of biases, the caveats of present/absent dichotomised diagnoses [18], and the local clinical guidelines from which they derive. We suggest, however, that some classification approaches are available to limit some of these caveats such as collating multiple variables and produce profiles based on similarities of exposure and/or outcomes at one time point (e.g. latent class modelling) or many time points over time to uncover trajectories (latent class growth analysis and piecewise modelling). This could mean, for example, retrieving glucose measures sampled throughout pregnancy and establishing the likely glycaemic status rather than relying only on a single GDM diagnosis. These approaches also help identify profiles of individual responses to interventions and can therefore improve tailored treatment allocation.

Additionally, missing data, either by design (e.g. unmeasured exposures/outcomes) or attrition, negatively impact data quality and challenge causal inference. This can be addressed by powerful analytical tools that recognise data complexity and the impact of missing data [19, 20]. Several methods are available to address missing data, including maximum likelihood, multiple imputation, and Bayesian methods. Complete case analysis leads to loss of data and statistical power but is widely used, while other complex but more justifiable methods are not often attempted [21]. Assumptions about the properties of missing data, whether these are missing completely at random or not, must be made. With the emergence of Big Data and EHRs that tend to have a high prevalence of missing information, appropriate techniques that deal with missing data need to be carefully applied.

25.3 Big Data: Challenges and Opportunities

As referenced above, Big Data refers to data large in volume, collected at high velocity, and comes in a variety of sources, formats, and dimensions, such as from birth cohort and longitudinal studies, medical records, or wearable/phone devices. Birth cohort studies, such as the Avon Longitudinal Study of Parents and Children study, have supported the DOHaD hypothesis by in-depth prospective sampling and large multidimensional data collection from human participants. While integral to the DOHaD evidence base, standard cohort studies are costly and may be of limited size. EHRs, a source of Big Data, can be obtained from centralised systems, while large omics data sets (genomics, transcriptomics, metabolomics, etc.) are often sourced from biobanks and can be added to increasingly available personal and external 'exposome' data (e.g. lifestyle and environmental). Among the benefits of EHRs is their level of comprehensiveness, and so with larger samples, this also improves the statistical power required to provide accurate estimates of effect size. The availability of such data means that if taken up in DOHaD research, the scope for such studies would no longer be limited by small sample sizes due to funding and/or the restrictive protocols of conventional longitudinal birth cohorts [22]. In practice already, linkage study designs join primary- and secondary-care databases or merge multiple EHR databases and registries, potentially offering new insight into disease pathways. For example, the UK-based CALIBER study drew on EHR sources to investigate the cumulative incidence and period prevalence of diseases over the lifecourse. Results were presented in the form of a chronological map of 308 physical and mental health conditions from four million individuals, from infants to the elderly [23]. The role of universal medical coverage and centralised digital health records, such as the English National Health Service, in enabling such exploration in this particular study cannot be underestimated.

More recently, data acquired from real-time biosensors measuring pollution exposure, blood glucose levels, or heart rate from wearable devices have become available. Data involving behaviour and social networks can also be retrieved from open social media platforms at high speed. The past three years, especially during the COVID-19 pandemic, have seen a surge of software developments intended to meet the needs of monitoring health markers and well-being remotely. The uptake of telemedicine was enabled, for example, by digital platforms used by clinicians to manage antenatal hyperglycaemia [24] and the self-report of glucose levels by pregnant women on their phones [25]. These tools could be employed in future DOHaD studies. However, key ethical issues related to privacy, rights, and moral code of conduct when retrieving these data require careful considerations in this changing research landscape.

25.3.1 Limitations of Current Big Data Sources and Applications

One first potential caveat of relying on Big Data sources it that DOHaD researchers wanting to use Big Data may be obliged to formulate research questions based on data availability or including data not necessarily designed primarily for DOHaD research. These researchers will have less control over data quality because of the larger distance from data collection, that is the inputting user (clinician for EHR / hospitals, or user of a phone app), and from the decisions made in defining and measuring the variables in these data sets. Overall, sources of error need to be considered when evidence from Big Data is evaluated. Without researchers' involvement in data collection, it may be impossible to subsequently correct or even identify these errors.

The task of comparing and validating DOHaD models across populations may be further hindered by the heterogeneity in data architectures across national and international sources. Before the term Big Data surfaced, omics-derived data alone (e.g. genomics, transcriptomics, and proteomics) already inferred the outputs of millions of data points [3]. Formulating a cascading model of these omics layers, which follow biologically downstream from one another, is both necessary and extremely complex. Further, linking biologically derived material to clinical data of different formats, and based on a variety of measurements, including imaging, questionnaires, and diagnoses, requires technologies that facilitate multidimensional integration. Thereafter, powerful methods that support analysis are necessary.

Larger sample sizes improve the power to detect effects, and clearly the whole DOHaD framework requires both large samples and a comprehensive set of exposures and events to be modelled. However, the primary issue is that complex models are more difficult to explain and thus could complicate their practical translation into actionable policies. Users and clinicians equally need to be versed in their use and interpretation.

The use of Big Data also raises issues of data security and representation, particularly data obtained outside conventional academic institutions, in contexts where systems and resources are not fit for this purpose, such as in low- and middle-income countries (LMICs). Users of both healthcare services and digital platforms, such as social media, may represent distinct groups with possibly little overlap in demography, risks, and healthcare needs [22]. It is plausible to assume that LMICs are unlikely to have population-wide health records or access to digital data collection and remote health monitoring from which DOHaD modelling could be done. Here, validation and reproducibility of DOHaD models are less feasible and highlight the lack of representation through their exclusion.

25.4 Artificial Intelligence: Challenges and Opportunities

When Big Data is considered, the word AI is not far behind. Pattern recognition, similarity profiling, and predictions are tasks for which AI methods such as machine learning (ML) have been developed, and these have potential applications to DOHaD research. It should be noted that ML and conventional statistical methods may be seen as a continuum since the algorithms behind ML, including linear and logistic regression, and several dimensionality reduction techniques have existed for decades. (For a contrast between ML and conventional statistics, see [26].) However, the real advantage of AI is that it supports the analysis of large data volumes alongside multidimensionality (i.e. where the number of variables is larger than the subjects).

AI is already being tested and implemented in the clinical domain, including to improve the efficiency of hospital administration. AI is also being used to predict medication side effects and patient outcomes from radiological imaging and thereby promote patient-tailored medicine and interventions. In DOHaD, ML approaches would subserve exploratory designs to identify biological pathways, which appear more frequently in the mosaic of data, in the form of associations, including from DNA sequences and omics data, and those obtained from EHRs [26]. Certain applications require user input from which the ML 'learns' to classify new data from sets of rules from previous data (supervised learning) or is completely unsupervised in detecting patterns. This is similar to the latent modelling techniques mentioned earlier that derive from the 'classical' statistics and the structural equation modelling framework. Other subfields of AI associated with ML include deep learning, rooted in multi-layered neural networks, which also allow computers to identify relations between concepts/features and characterise these associations from complex to simpler concepts [27]. ML methods to date could also assist in the processing of single modalities or data collection methods, such as magnetic resonance imaging of the brain, heart rate variability in the fetus, and DNA methylation patterns in disease [28], all of which are relevant for DOHaD research.

Despite the potential of ML for DOHaD described, very few ML studies have so far transitioned from single data type and scale to 'fusing' several dimensions, or and towards the integration of additional outcome measures retrieved from EHRs, medical imaging, and biospecimens. Data harmonising and deployment of ML is an ongoing endeavour, but some attempts have been made in relation to cardiovascular medicine (reviewed by [29]). The issue to date is that these algorithms exploit two modalities at most (e.g. radiological imaging and free text from clinical reports). (For an in-depth review of the current landscape of AI for multi-modal integration, see [30]).

In our previous section, we discussed the necessity to characterise accurately DOHaD prediction models. It is at present the case that the several competing ML approaches and the rapidly evolving demands of AI have yet to produce a consensus regarding how to develop or validate a prediction model relying on these novel tools. For example, in predicting Type 2 diabetes and cardiovascular disease, Dalakleidi et al. reported the best performance to have been achieved by groups of artificial neural networks. However, the so-called decision trees, random forest algorithm, and support vector machines were said to provide the best accuracy measures by Zheng et al. [31]. Furthermore, AI methods do not necessarily outperform conventional statistical regression applications and are not free of methodological biases [32]. Additionally, scholars warn that ML studies are often computationally demanding on resources (e.g. support vector machines, logistic regression, random forests, gradient-boosted machines, and neural networks) [33].

25.4.1 Issues of Interpretation and Reporting

Concerns are often raised about the scope, complexity, transparency, reproducibility across different scientific teams and different populations, and the interpretability of prediction models. While AI operates from a 'black box' within deep neural networks and unsupervised learning, the biological plausibility and meanings of the output are generated by researchers. Given that so far only a few published prediction models have found utility in clinical practice, the utility of AI when compared to conventional methods remains an open question. It is unclear whether AI can address the questions of causality most pertinent in DOHaD, when DOHaD draws from interpretability and theory and is moving towards the integration of social science and ethnography. (See Richardson, in this volume for a discussion of how DOHaD is characterised by 'cryptic causality'.)

Guidelines regarding AI are developing rapidly. For example, following a quality assessment of the conduct and reporting of multi-variable prediction models, a 22-item checklist (TRIPOD) was developed [34]. The risk of bias tool (PROBAST-AI) for diagnostic and prognostic prediction model studies based on AI has also emerged to ensure that users have key information about the design, conduct, and analysis, alongside a robust standardised tool for bias evaluation that would allow a fair judgement on the utility of these models [31, 35, 36]. Guidelines should be consulted by authors, reviewers, and editors, to ensure reproducibility, reliability, and validity, and hence safe implementation. Again, even prior to applying AI-derived analytics, the uncertainty of measurements in Big Data and its sources of error must be accounted for and possibly identified systematically, and the data quality validated.

25.6 Ethical Questions about Big Data and AI

The rapid expansion of Big Data and AI raises a range of ethical concerns. First, the question of who audits and protects data including EHRs (which can also be used as testing data by commercial parties) is central to ensuring ethical research in the DOHaD field and is currently insufficiently addressed [22, 37]. The lack of standardisation of data protection laws between countries adds to this issue.

Additionally, the most powerful AI pipelines are deployed from within the very few corporations with the computational and financial resources. The commercialisation of both healthcare software or AI tools and their findings within the private sector is another challenge that research institutions must navigate if the potential of such data is to be realised. Such a feat would require more transparency and possibly a move to open sources of data. (For an example of Google's DeepMind approach to open data, see [38].)

Nevertheless, open and public data collection is also likely to introduce other ethical issues that need to be carefully considered [39]. Big Data collection and usage may move the position of the individual (the unique data provider) from the one fulfilling the 'social vision' of the healthcare system and science into the 'economic vision' of the commercial enterprise [22]. Participants recruited through academic institutions consciously engage with the scientific community with consent and pledge their time voluntarily. This contrasts with the passive and often unwitting involvement in Big Data collection via the data generated by medical records and phone devices. The use of such data without consent raises concerns regarding data ownership, privacy, and the circulation of profits. Data protection in secondary research by academic institutions using public data is enforced by the institutions themselves through university and institutional ethics boards, but enforcing consent and data protection may be less clear when third-party commercial and private bodies are concerned.

Rarely mentioned in the discussion of AI-derived methods are the risks introduced or heightened to certain populations because of their implementation. Experts such as Professor Kate Crawford at the AI Now Institute are re-evaluating the societal burden of AI. She states AI is not 'artificial' since it requires the same earthly resources and labour to mine the power and hardware sustaining it. Consequently, this is also becoming a source of disparity and power imbalance on the ground, within and between populations who compete to mine these resources [40]. Such ramifications would be the real irony for an AI integration into DOHaD research and the long-term agenda of the scientific community.

25.7 Conclusion

There is a strong anticipation that in the future, DOHaD researchers will benefit from innovative methodological designs. This could build on the best of current biostatistical methods and soon include AI technologies where the multidimensionality of data sources and a longitudinal format can be integrated, and the outputs shown to be interpretable. Current and novel 'mega' projects may push this progress forward. An example is the protocol implemented in the EarlyCause project [41] that will explore the causal mechanisms between early-life adversity (antenatal and postnatal) and future psycho-cardio-metabolic multi-morbidity. It will involve the participation of 14 European institutions and include three complementary and sequential phases that integrate longitudinal population data sets (e.g. ALSPAC and UK BIOBANK), animal studies, and cellular models with analytical tools from structural equation modelling and machine learning. It also aims to offer a web-based platform for data access and information on research standards and best practices to support future study designs and exploration. Such a mix of granular data collection and Big Data sources in open access, along with AI and conventional statistical approaches, holds great potential for DOHaD research.

The DOHaD research community may look to other fields and consider how to train their own data and solution architects in the newest technologies and Big Data usage. Interdisciplinary teamwork will be crucial in ensuring both robust management and use of data as well as anticipating ethical and governance issues [42]. It is crucial to assess whether certain limitations are inevitable or can be remedied to create the necessary, transparent, and reliable evidence base. Collaborations in data collection could be expanded more frequently to 'crowdsourcing' in data analysis and interpretation. Of course, teamwork does not come without caveats when studying complex and dynamic modelling, such as leading to further heterogeneity in findings and conclusions [43]. Nevertheless, we reiterate that attention to operationalisation of exposures and outcomes, reducing bias in data collection and analysis, and the necessity for interpretability should be at the forefront of the DOHaD agenda in the era of Big Data and AI.

References

1. Johnson W, Kuh D, Hardy R. A life course perspective on body size and cardio-metabolic health. In: Burton-Jeangros C, Cullati S, Sacker A, Blane D, editors. A Life Course Perspective on Health Trajectories and Transitions. Cham: Springer; 2016.

2. Zolitschka KA, Razum O, Breckenkamp J, Sauzet O. Social mechanisms in epidemiological publications on small-area health inequalities – A scoping review [Internet]. Front Public Health. 2019; 7. Available from: http://dx.doi.org/10.3389/fpubh.2019.00393

3. Lapehn S, Paquette AG. The placental epigenome as a molecular link between prenatal exposures and fetal health outcomes through the DOHaD hypothesis. Curr Environ Health Rep [Internet]. 2022 29 Apr:490–50. Available from: http://dx.doi.org/10.1007/s40572–022-00354-8

4. Bowman CE, Arany Z, Wolfgang MJ. Regulation of maternal-fetal metabolic communication. Cell Mol Life Sci. 2021 Feb;78(4):1455–86.

5. Huynh J, Dawson D, Roberts D, Bentley-Lewis R. A systematic review of placental pathology in maternal diabetes mellitus. Placenta. 2015 Feb;36(2):101–14.

6. Brandlistuen RE, Ystrom E, Nulman I, Koren G, Nordeng H. Prenatal paracetamol exposure and child neurodevelopment: A sibling-controlled cohort study. Int J Epidemiol. 2013 Dec;42(6):1702–13.

7. Abdul-Hussein A, Kareem A, Tewari S, Bergeron J, Briollais L, Challis JRG, et al. Early life risk and resiliency factors and their influences on developmental outcomes and disease pathways: A rapid evidence review of systematic reviews and meta-analyses. J Dev Orig Health Dis. 2021 Jun;12(3):357–72.

8. Berkson J. Limitations of the application of fourfold table analysis to hospital data. Int J Epidemiol. 2014 Apr;43(2):511–15.

9. Whitcomb BW, Schisterman EF, Perkins NJ, Platt RW. Quantification of collider-stratification bias and the birthweight paradox. Paediatr Perinat Epidemiol. 2009 Sep;23(5):394–402.

10. Greenland S, Pearl J, Robins JM. Causal diagrams for epidemiologic research [Internet]. Epidemiology. 1999; 10:37–48. Available from: http://dx.doi.org/10.1097/00001648-199901000-00008

11. Wu Y, Espinosa KM, Barnett SD, Kapse A, Quistorff JL, Lopez C, et al. Association of elevated maternal psychological distress, altered fetal brain, and offspring cognitive and social-emotional outcomes at 18 months. JAMA Netw Open. 2022 Apr 1;5(4):e229244.

12. Monk C, Fernández CR. Neuroscience advances and the developmental origins of health and disease research. JAMA Netw Open. 2022 1 Apr;5(4):e229251.

13. Sigurdardottir JN, White S, Flynn A, Singh C, Briley A, Rutherford M, et al. Longitudinal phenotyping of maternal antenatal depression in obese pregnant women supports multiple-hit hypothesis for fetal brain development, a secondary analysis of the UPBEAT study. EClinicalMed. 2022 Aug;50:101512.

14. Makin TR, de Xivry JJO. Ten common statistical mistakes to watch out for when writing or reviewing a manuscript [Internet]. eLife. 2019; 8:e48175. Available from: http://dx.doi.org/10.7554/elife.48175

15. Wagenmakers EJ, Sarafoglou A, Aarts S, Albers C, Algermissen J, Bahník Š, et al. Seven steps toward more transparency in statistical practice. Nat Hum Behav. 2021 Nov;5(11):1473–80.

16. Fan L, Qiu J, Zhao Y, Yin T, Li X, Wang Q, et al. The association between body composition and metabolically unhealthy profile of adults with normal weight in Northwest China. PLoS One. 2021 25 Mar;16(3):e0248782.

17. Lai MC, Kassee C, Besney R, Bonato S, Hull L, Mandy W, et al. Prevalence of co-occurring mental health diagnoses in the autism population: A systematic review and meta-analysis. Lancet Psychiatry. 2019 Oct;6(10):819–29.

18. Altman DG, Bland JM. Statistics notes: Absence of evidence is not evidence of absence [Internet]. BMJ. 1995; 311:485–485. Available from: http://dx.doi.org/10.1136/bmj.311.7003.485

19. Stavola BLD, De Stavola BL, Nitsch D, dos Santos Silva I, McCormack V, Hardy R, et al. Statistical issues in life course epidemiology [Internet]. Am J Epidemiol. 2006; 163: 84–96. Available from: http://dx.doi.org/10.1093/aje/kwj003

20. Johnson W. Analytical strategies in human growth research [Internet]. Am J Hum Biol. 2015; 27: 69–83. Available from: http://dx.doi.org/10.1002/ajhb.22589

21. Bell ML, Fiero M, Horton NJ, Hsu CH. Handling missing data in RCTs; a review of the top medical journals. BMC Med Res Methodol. 2014 19 Nov;14:118.

22. Delpierre C, Kelly-Irving M. Big data and the study of social inequalities in health: Expectations and issues [Internet]. Front Public Health. 2018; 6:1–5. Available from: http://dx.doi.org/10.3389/fpubh.2018.00312

23. Kuan V, Denaxas S, Gonzalez-Izquierdo A, Direk K, Bhatti O, Husain S, et al. A chronological map of 308 physical and mental health conditions from 4 million individuals in the English National Health Service. Lancet Digit Health. 2019 Jun;1(2):e63–77.

24. Jardine J, Relph S, Magee LA, von Dadelszen P, Morris E, Ross-Davie M, et al. Maternity services in the UK during the coronavirus disease 2019 pandemic: A national survey of modifications to standard care. BJOG. 2021 Apr;128(5):880–9.

25. Mackillop L, Hirst JE, Bartlett KJ, Birks JS, Clifton L, Farmer AJ, et al. Comparing the efficacy of a mobile phone-based blood glucose management system with standard clinic care in women with gestational diabetes: Randomized Controlled Trial. JMIR Mhealth Uhealth. 2018 20 Mar;6(3):e71.

26. Bzdok D, Altman N, Krzywinski M. Statistics versus machine learning [Internet]. Nat Methods. 2018; 15: 233–34. Available from: http://dx.doi.org/10.1038/nmeth.4642

27. Richards BA, Lillicrap TP, Beaudoin P, Bengio Y, Bogacz R, Christensen A, et al. A deep learning framework for neuroscience. Nat Neurosci. 2019 Nov;22(11):1761–70.

28. Rauschert S, Raubenheimer K, Melton PE, Huang RC. Machine learning and clinical epigenetics: A review of challenges for diagnosis and classification. Clin Epigenetics. 2020 3 Apr;12(1):1–11.

29. Amal S, Safarnejad L, Omiye JA, Ghanzouri I, Cabot JH, Ross EG. Use of multi-modal data and machine learning to improve cardiovascular disease care. Front Cardiovasc Med [Internet]. 2022 [cited 19 Oct 2022];9:1–11. Available from: http://dx.doi.org/10.3389/fcvm.2022.840262

30. Acosta JN, Falcone GJ, Rajpurkar P, Topol EJ. Multimodal biomedical AI. Nat Med. 2022 15 Sep;28(9):1773–84.

31. Zheng T, Xie W, Xu L, He X, Zhang Y, You M, et al. A machine learning-based framework to identify type 2 diabetes through electronic health records. Int J Med Inform. 2017 Jan;97:120–7.

32. Collins GS, Mallett S, Omar O, Yu LM. Developing risk prediction models for type 2 diabetes: A systematic review of methodology and reporting. BMC Med. 2011 8 Sep;9:103.

33. Christodoulou E, Ma J, Collins GS, Steyerberg EW, Verbakel JY, Van Calster B. A systematic review shows no performance benefit of machine learning over logistic regression for clinical prediction models. J Clin Epidemiol. 2019 Jun;110:12–22.

34. Collins GS, Reitsma JB, Altman DG, Moons KGM. Transparent reporting of a multivariable prediction model for individual prognosis or diagnosis (TRIPOD): The TRIPOD Statement [Internet]. Eur Urol. 2015; 67:1142–51. Available from: http://dx.doi.org/10.1016/j.eururo.2014.11.025

35. Sounderajah V, Ashrafian H, Golub RM, Shetty S, De Fauw J, Hooft L, et al.

Developing a reporting guideline for artificial intelligence-centred diagnostic test accuracy studies: the STARD-AI protocol. BMJ Open. 2021 28 Jun;11(6):e047709.

36. Collins GS, Dhiman P, Andaur Navarro CL, Ma J, Hooft L, Reitsma JB, et al. Protocol for development of a reporting guideline (TRIPOD-AI) and risk of bias tool (PROBAST-AI) for diagnostic and prognostic prediction model studies based on artificial intelligence. BMJ Open. 2021 9 Jul;11(7):e048008.

37. Ruckenstein M, Schüll ND. The datafication of health [Internet]. Ann Rev Anthropol. 2017; 46:261–78. Available from: http://dx.doi.org/10.1146/annurev-anthro-102116-041244

38. Jumper J, Evans R, Pritzel A, Green T, Figurnov M, Ronneberger O, et al. Highly accurate protein structure prediction with AlphaFold. Nature. 2021 Aug;596 (7873):583–9.

39. de Laat PB. Algorithmic decision-making based on machine learning from Big Data: Can transparency restore accountability? Philos Technol. 2018;31 (4):525–41.

40. Campolo A, Crawford K. Enchanted determinism: Power without responsibility in artificial intelligence [Internet]. Engaging Sci Technol Soc. 2020; 6:1–19. Available from: http://dx.doi.org/10.17351/ests2020.277

41. Mariani N, Borsini A, Cecil CAM, Felix JF, Sebert S, Cattaneo A, et al. Identifying causative mechanisms linking early-life stress to psycho-cardio-metabolic multi-morbidity: The EarlyCause project. PLoS One. 2021 21 Jan;16(1):e0245475.

42. O'Doherty KC, Shabani M, Dove ES, Bentzen HB, Borry P, Burgess MM, et al. Toward better governance of human genomic data. Nat Genet. 2021 Jan;53 (1):2–8.

43. Silberzahn R, Uhlmann EL. Crowdsourced research: Many hands make tight work. Nature. 2015 8 Oct;526 (7572):189–91.

Chapter

26

The Promise of Reversibility in Neuroepigenetics Research on Traumatic Memories

Stephanie Lloyd, Pierre-Eric Lutz, and Chani Bonventre

26.1 Introduction

Just over 20 years ago, molecular biologists Leonie Ringrose and Renato Paro published an article with a provocative title: 'Remembering Silence' [1]. The article focused on how epigenetic elements, modified through a variety of means, could subsequently return to their silent state. Silencing is operationally defined as their epigenetic status before modulation by experimental or environmental factors. Ringrose and Paro's article described research on fruit flies and factors affecting embryological growth. Yet it asked a question of considerable importance to parallel and rapidly expanding research in human neuroepigenetics, that of *reversibility* of the molecular impact of the environment on an individual's biological profile. In the case of epigenetic modifications that are thought to be mediators between life trauma and the risk of psychopathology, this question would be translated as follows: if you experience a traumatic event and, as a result, acquire an epigenetic state considered to place you at higher risk, can you free yourself of that state? Through a critical assessment of contemporary neuroepigenetics research, in this chapter we consider researchers' ambitions to account for the indeterminacy of life and the speculative possibility of reversing acquired epigenetic states. Bringing together the perspectives of medical anthropology and molecular biology, we are interested in clarifying how reversibility – a return to silence – is envisioned, how therapeutic interventions purported to bring about that silence might function, and what this might mean for the mental health of people who live in the aftermath of trauma.

The question of reversibility is compelling for a wide range of research agendas in epigenetics, a science that has produced an evidentiary base of significant importance for the field of Developmental Origins of Health and Disease (DOHaD). Indeed, epigenetics research has provided insights into the molecular means by which life experiences might be associated with risk and resilience for the subsequent development of pathology. While the concepts of risk and resilience have received increasing attention in developmental research in recent years, little is known about their purportedly associated epigenetic states, such as their durability. In neuroepigenetics research, resilience is conceived of as a mechanism that may recruit different biological pathways than those triggered by adversity. It is often assessed in two ways: behaviourally and molecularly. Behavioural resilience has been conceived of as the possibility of not being affected by a negative experience at psychological and clinical levels; in other words, as being able to actively counteract what are considered pathological molecular states. Molecular resilience has been studied as the

Lloyd S, Lutz PE, Bonventre C. Can you remember silence? Epigenetic memory and reversibility as a site of intervention. BioEssays. 2023 Jul;45(7):2300019.

failure to be negatively affected, in terms of acquired epigenetic states, by adverse circumstances. The two conceptualisations of resilience are drawn together in experimental contexts, most often with model organisms, in which molecular profiles are sought to explain why different animals might exhibit what are seen as at-risk or resilient states. Risk, for its part, has been framed as the development of an epigenetic state associated with psychopathology, following a traumatic event; in effect, a molecular memory of that event.

Yet neuroepigenetics researchers only have speculative models to guide studies of the type or number of epigenetic states considered sufficient to confer risk or resilience in the face of adverse experiences, alongside the means by which one might reverse acquired risk. Efforts at reversibility – or remembering silence – by necessity include considerations of the relationship between subjective states, past events, and memories of those events. Since past events cannot change, it is the memory of these experiences that may be the target of a panoply of clinical evaluations and interventions (whether pharmaco- or psychotherapy). Neuroepigeneticists consider mapping these processes an urgent priority given the prevalence of trauma; for instance, approximately 80 per cent of the American population is thought to have experienced trauma-level events [2]. These statistics are deemed particularly worrying given research that suggests that the epigenetic effects of traumatic events may contribute to a variety of pathologies, from cardiovascular to suicide risk, including anxiety and depressive disorders, addiction, and more [3].

Researchers hope that a greater understanding of molecular memories (i.e. epigenetic states) thought to be acquired through the experience of traumatic events, and their relationship to subsequent risk of psychopathology, might allow the development of targeted interventions to help people 'remember silence': to reverse the effects of presumably acquired pathological traits. While pre-existing and emerging models alike tend to presume the durability of epigenetic states acquired during early life, Ringrose and Paro's evaluation of epigenetics research remains productively provocative as it conceptually fuels the hypothesis of the potential for epigenetic reversibility. It also foreshadows more recent shifts in some DOHaD research agendas that are moving away from deterministic models of early-life experiences leading to diseases later in life and are instead focused on conditioning, which implies the possibility for change [4].

Through the following sections, we discuss polysemic understandings of memory and how research on reversibility is entangled with metaphors of silence as a subjectively untroubled or unaffected state. We begin with a consideration of the tensions between narratives of reversibility and persistence in epigenetics research to sketch out what is currently known and unknown about these processes.

26.2 Persistence and Reversibility in Epigenetics Research

In 2001, biologists Ringrose and Paro evaluated emerging research, indicating that, in *Drosophila*, regulatory elements that are experimentally switched to their active state can '"remember" and restore their previous [silent] state'. These 'regulatory elements' are defined as regions within genes where, under epigenetic control, proteins that regulate gene activity may have different functional impacts. The authors noted that silenced states can be remembered after several cell generations during which those elements were active, though they could only hypothesise as to how or why regulatory factors would return to silence. This article dates from the early days of epigenetics research, yet Ringrose and Paro's interests in how epigenetic elements change, with what effects, and whether they are reversible persist. In their contemporary version, they might be:

how might epigenetic states acquired through exposures contribute to health and disease? And are the molecular traces of those experiences reversible?

The research discussed by Ringrose and Paro yielded findings on the varying effects of single epigenetic alterations depending on the type and timing of the modification. Each of the studies raised questions about the stability and reversibility of epigenetic states and their developmental effects. For instance, even if an epigenetic state is only modified for a limited period of time, it will nonetheless affect downstream biological processes, which may have longer term consequences than the bout of epigenetic plasticity itself. Ringrose and Paro also observed that while certain experimental data suggested that the restoration of silence was not possible after a significant period of activation, other results pointed to the possibility of silencing even after cell division [1]. Moreover, genes implicated in molecular memories may switch status surprisingly late in development or switch dynamically and have regulatory patterns that are far more complex than a single transition between on or off states [1]. Thus, there was a trend towards stable effects of epigenetic states on development, but with significant variability.

Research on the reversibility of epigenetic states has since moved beyond fruit flies, and spans multiple types of in vitro models, model organisms, and work on human tissues, in situations of both health and disease. Key areas of research include the determination of cellular identity during embryological development, modelled using induced pluripotent stem cells (iPSCs). iPSCs rely on a method whereby differentiated cells – such as a fully developed skin cell – can be reprogrammed to an undetermined state and then redirected to a new developmental path. Part of the enthusiasm for these cells comes from the fact that reprogramming to the undifferentiated state does not implicate any manipulation of the genome but relies on triggering epigenetic plasticity at regulatory elements implicated in cellular identity. In other words, interventions targeting the epigenome [5] may potentially rewrite cell fates by erasing or reversing memories of their pasts to produce cells perfectly identical to 'true' stem cells, which would amount to a process of full reversibility. However, it is now clear that iPSCs retain epigenetic traces of their previous differentiated state [6], suggesting an only partial reversal. Therefore, what scientists have referred to as silence (i.e. the return to undifferentiation), in these experiments, is only partially restored. This molecular plasticity underlying cellular identity over the cell lifespan argues against a binary model (e.g. with an epigenetic landscape as either mature or immature) and instead supports a gradual, context-dependent balance between persistence and reversibility. This emerging research echoes findings discussed by Ringrose and Paro regarding highly dynamic shifts or epigenetic traces of a cell's history that resist experimental erasure.

Researchers working at the scale of the human lifespan do not necessarily depict such nuanced portraits of the dynamics of epigenetic states. Instead, they have argued that durable epigenetic states result from traumatic events [3]. (See also Keaney et al. in this volume, Chapter 14.) These epigenetic states are described as setting off brain alterations that contribute to psychological traits – such as impulsivity, interpersonal difficulties, or emotional lability – that ultimately potentiate the risk of mental illness. Research on reversibility – on a variety of species and scales – provides critical insights into human lifespan and DOHaD researchers. A careful review of this work reveals the considerable uncertainty about the dynamics of these processes. Yet it is only through a fine-grained understanding of such processes that scientists may conceive of how reversibility of epigenetic states may occur and how therapeutic interventions might silence molecular traces of past adverse events.

26.3 The Epigenetics of Memory Formation and Its Effects

Recent neuroepigenetics research advances that traumatic experiences may increase the risk of psychopathology through acquired molecular states etched into memories. The use of the term 'memory' in neuroscience research is polysemic, referring to a range of processes at different scales. In particular, it is often evoked in ways that are consistent with its common sense description, which roughly overlaps with the concept of episodic memory. Episodic memory, formally, refers to the ability to encode one's life events and includes a range of cognitive functions that rely on interacting brain structures. The term molecular memory, by contrast, refers to molecular mechanisms correlated with any event leading to lasting cellular changes, whatever their implication in episodic memory, or any other brain property.

In this chapter, we are interested in epigenetic states as they are thought to correlate with the experience of past adversity (regardless of whether they may affect episodic memory or other physiological systems, for example reactivity to stress), and how they are believed to maintain – or not – a molecular modulation of gene activity: in effect, producing at-risk states. In order to determine which notions of memory are implicit or explicit in researchers' hypotheses about whether molecular memories and their effects might be silenced, it is necessary to examine the uses of the concept of memory in epigenetics research.

A subset of researchers interested in memory and epigenetics have explored the so-called '"epigenetic code" in the central nervous system that mediates synaptic plasticity, learning, and memory' [7]. In their models, neuroscientists Jeremy Day and David Sweatt evoke 'the controversial theory of the "engram" – a (hypothetical) biophysical change in the brain that accounts for the material existence of memory (Josselyn et al., 2015: 201) . . . [and] suggest that epigenetic mechanisms, such as DNA methylation, may be a window into the brain's memory' [8]. They and other researchers became interested in how memory can be traced through epigenetic mechanisms in the brain, at a molecular level. Drawing mostly on research on model organisms, Day and Sweatt further argue that:

> An interesting new understanding has emerged: developmental regulation of cell division and cell terminal differentiation involve many of the same molecular signalling cascades that are employed in learning and memory storage. Therefore, cellular development and cognitive memory processes are not just analogous but homologous at the molecular level. [7]

Their research presents cellular epigenetic and developmental mechanisms, and cognitive memory processes, as intertwined, and thus potentially actionable on a molecular level. In this understanding of molecular memory, the epigenome is 'a crucial 'missing link' between life experiences and gene expression, which in turn will influence the ways in which neuronal circuitry and brain structures develop' [8].

In these models, two characteristics of epigenetics are advanced, both of which we suggest should be approached with caution. First, that molecular memory may be homologous to episodic memory, and second, that epigenetics makes an exceptional contribution to the chain of events leading from life experience to the molecular memories of these events and their subsequent effects. Any proposition to silence memories of traumatic events would hinge on these relationships and the possibility of an intervention acting specifically on them. While Day and Sweatt put these ideas forward most explicitly, they implicitly inform many other researchers' models of epigenetic memory and its potential reversal [9].

Day and Sweatt's first proposition may be particularly misleading. Recent research indicates that every physiological function of the nervous system – such as feeding, sleep, or nociception – may implicate molecular mechanisms occurring in part through gene expression changes, under epigenetic regulation [10, 11]. In these studies, the role of molecular and epigenetic processes in the emergence and long-term regulation of those states appears similar to what has been identified in relation to the physiological function of episodic memory. This complicates any assertions of *specificity* or *homology* (besides the use of a common word) in the relationship between *epigenetic* and *episodic memories*. Episodic memory, instead, might be seen as affected by gene expression changes and epigenetic plasticity, much as the aforementioned other physiological functions, without necessarily being homologous to them.

The second proposition is similarly debatable. Responses to life experiences are complex and multi-scalar. In the case of trauma, their perception and encoding start with sensory processing of, for instance, sounds or movements, which are then cognitively apprehended by devoted brain areas, triggering negative emotions. Each of these operations relies on specialised cellular processes. At the sensory level, they include chemical (e.g. release of neurotransmitters in activated brain regions), physical (e.g. light sensing in the retina), or mechanical (e.g. transduction of sound waves by the tympanum) properties that act on temporal and spatial scales not necessarily compatible with or dependent upon any epigenetic plasticity. Moreover, it is the overall psychological impact of adversity, downstream of these multi-scalar processes, that is considered to trigger epigenetic changes.

Neuroepigenetic mechanisms are nonetheless widely considered to be implicated, to some extent, in the formation of molecular memories. Most of this research investigates DNA methylation, which we will focus on below. Changes in DNA methylation are considered not only to reflect past experiences but also to contribute to behavioural changes through, for example, the modulation of neuronal processes, heightened sensitivity to stress, and increased psychopathological risk. In terms of experimental designs, research on these processes is grounded in the triangulation of incongruent experimental designs. On the one hand, animal studies document how embodied epigenetic memories of early adversity may manifest in adulthood in controlled settings that limit confounding factors. Even in these studies, causal attribution of abnormal behaviour to epigenetic changes would require dedicated experiments that manipulate the proposed epigenetic substrate to prevent or reverse the abnormal behaviour (see next section). In humans, on the other hand, associations between adversity, epigenetic alterations, and later psychopathology are even more questionable. Sources of unaccounted variability over the lifespan, following trauma, are incomparably higher as studies typically analyse postmortem brains of people who often die decades after experiencing adversity. Alternatively, peripheral 'liquid' biopsies (blood and saliva) that can be taken throughout life are more accessible but are less relevant for understandings of brain epigenetics. Thus, there is only a tenuous, associative relationship in animal and human studies between early adversity, epigenetic memories of these experiences, and drivers of later behaviours.

Ultimately, based on existing evidence, any delayed or long-lasting embodied memories are likely associated with multi-scalar adaptations, which include but are not exclusively encoded by epigenetic changes. Therefore, while epigenetic processes are plausibly recruited over the lifespan, during early adversity, and later when a host of related biological consequences mediate the impact of more recent life events, they do not operate in isolation. In this context, influential conceptualisations of epigenetic processes as exceptional contributors to molecular memories of past experiences appear to reflect an inability to place them in these long chains of back-and-forth, across temporal and spatial biological scales [12]. These limitations suggest caution when postulating relationships between life experiences, epigenetic modifications, and memory, particularly in the context of human adversity and psychopathology. Moreover, current understandings of this relationship might encourage attentiveness to the ways in which slippage between different types of memory explicitly or implicitly populates research on epigenetic plasticity and its potential silencing. This slippage contributes to conclusions that too easily conflate behavioural and molecular risk or resilience.

26.4 Experiments in Reversibility

In addition to efforts to understand the molecular mechanisms that may be associated with the experience of trauma and subsequent psychopathology, researchers are attempting to identify interventions that might reverse or modify epigenetic states and the psychopathology correlated with them. The most targeted epigenetic editing interventions aspire to modify the fundamental molecular processes associated with past experiences of trauma. Researchers hope that these modifications will affect neurobiological processes and, as a consequence, behavioural traits and reactivity to stress (e.g. as in the case of PTSD). The primary target of these interventions is not considered to be the factual or emotional content of an episodic memory such as the emotional relationship between the person and a specific object/event, but rather an affective state thought to be related to behaviour associated with past experiences of trauma. Affective states, in this perspective, are conceived as triggered neurobiological dispositions 'operating outside the domain of consciousness and intentional action' [13]. In this conceptualisation of neuropsychiatric risk, triggers are considered both devoid of exceptional qualities and sufficient to set into motion pathological responses. At their extreme, in certain neuroepigenetic research agendas, affective responses to triggers are thought to be sufficient to lead to suicidal acts [14].

Some of the research on the reversal or modification of epigenetic states focuses on well-established interventions such as antidepressants and psychotherapy. These therapies seek to mitigate the effects of past traumas through the alleviation of symptoms in the present (e.g. anxiety) and are now also studied for their effects on epigenetic mechanisms. This involves a reconceptualisation of these interventions as modulating basic affective states underlying clinically measured symptoms. Concerning antidepressants, researchers have associated several different epigenetic modifications (in the aforementioned peripheral samples, not the brain) with a positive response to antidepressants and are attempting to identify which epigenetic states might be able to predict responsiveness to these medications [15]. In a similar line of reasoning, researchers have suggested that epigenetic mechanisms may constitute 'dynamic biological correlates of [psychotherapeutic] interventions' [16]. However, the processes, directionality, or interactions linking symptom alleviation, intervention, and epigenetic states are far from comprehensively understood. For example, such research does not demonstrate whether (1) it is the intervention that reduces a person's symptoms and this reduction subsequently impacts epigenetic profiles, (2) the intervention directly influences epigenetic plasticity, thereby modifying symptoms, or (3) some combination of the two. Therefore, at present, reasoning about the reversibility of behavioural and molecular states – and how they might relate to states of risk or resilience – remains muddled. This raises important questions about the inference of causality, as distinguishing between these possibilities would require direct and specific manipulation, or 'editing', of the epigenome.

Experimental approaches are being developed in rodent models to address the challenge of causal inference. Researchers such as Elizabeth Heller and Eric Nestler are attempting to carry out locus-specific epigenetic editing (i.e. affecting only a specific location in the genome [17]). Using this method, Heller and collaborators epigenetically reprogrammed a gene in a specific brain region to modify behavioural responses to *later* stress exposure, promoting susceptibility, or alternatively resilience, to this experience. They argue that the specificity of their approach allows them to understand how locus-specific epigenetic states may be causally implicated in the modulation of stress responses. The extent to which such manipulations are truly specific – affecting the targeted gene only – is unclear, with difficult technical and experimental challenges ahead. Nonetheless, these findings demonstrate the potential feasibility of intervening in targeted ways on the molecular processes implicated in stress or trauma responses to potentially silence molecular memories of past experiences.

Other researchers are drawing on different approaches to target the molecular machinery that may mediate epigenetic reprogramming. A team led by Moshe Szyf and Gal Yadid recently investigated a rat model of post-traumatic stress disorder (PTSD), in which they identified changes in DNA methylation [18]. In an attempt to undo PTSD-like behaviours, they manipulated the expression of one of the two enzymes responsible for methylating DNA in the mammalian brain (Dnmt3a). While the results offer support for the hypothesis that DNA methylation changes may contribute to PTSD-like behaviours, the evidence of causality through epigenetic reversibility may be considered more indirect than in the previous study by Heller et al. For instance, they did not identify if or how their manipulation of the enzyme directly affected the DNA methylation states that were triggered in the model, but instead reasoned by inference that the enzyme must have affected them. Despite these limitations, Yadid et al. suggest that it may be possible to translate their intervention to humans using a systemic therapy rather than direct manipulation in the brain [18]. They propose the addition of a chemical donor for methyl groups to our diets, which raises further questions about the specificity of the intervention. Indeed, systemic therapy would likely affect every cell in the whole body in which methylation of DNA affects their activities. Such an induction of epigenetic plasticity may have broad and potentially detrimental effects throughout the body.

Together, these approaches bypass existing symptom-oriented therapeutic interventions that are aimed at alleviating the emotional impact of distressing and presumably durable memories, and instead aim to directly reverse the molecular imprints of traumatic memories. In theory, they are more akin to an intervention targeting the aetiology of post-traumatic states, returning a person to the affective silence of an epigenetic landscape unmarred by (mal)adaptive shifts brought on by adversity. Such interventions would hypothetically target a range of regulatory elements. Systemic global methyl donor treatments, for instance, may have the potential – to use an analogy – to reopen critical windows of neuroplasticity among people who are biologically beyond the developmental period associated with early-life plasticity, when the effects of negative experiences are considered to be particularly harmful (Reh et al. 2020). In other words, the treatment is conceived of as affecting the canalisation that presumably takes place in a person's life and sets them on a particular life trajectory [12].

It should be underscored that any judgement of a *return* to silence in this research might be considered arbitrary. At the extreme end of wiping cellular memories clean, as in the case of iPSCs, even efforts to epigenetically reprogramme cells back to stem cell states are unable to completely remove molecular traces of their past differentiated identity. In addition, it is clear that epigenetics is only one part of multi-scalar responses to life experiences, and whether the latter would be able to return to silence upon epigenetic editing is unknown. In terms of particular interventions, systemic therapies that aspire to modulate epigenetic processes come with the potential for sweeping effects on our bodily processes. Even targeted epigenetic editing interventions may either miss their mark (being unable to remove the molecular memories associated with past trauma) or destabilise people's affective identities in unforeseen ways. The limitations of these interventions place the appraisal of a return to silence in a relative framework.

In addition, epigenetics research on the effects of trauma is grounded in the comparison of model organisms that were exposed or not. Yet the animals are not tested prior to exposure and interventions, an assessment that would be necessary to provide a glimpse of 'before', which would hypothetically reflect a state of silence. In humans, these before states are not tested either, given that brain tissue can only be studied post-mortem. Further complicating judgements of before, after, or a return to a previous unaffected state, research on inter- and transgenerational effects of trauma and long-term evolutionary inheritance of epigenetic states raises additional questions of whether before should be considered a state during an individual's life or whether it should include in utero or preconception experiences, including potentially those of parents, or even longer time scales [19]. Thus, the before state to which a person would return is rarely assessed in this research, and questions remain as to when before should be identified in a person's or a lineage's trajectory. In the light of current understanding of molecular memories, it might one day be possible to reverse a single epigenetic state with a richer understanding of the processes involved, but we are not there yet. These understandings would necessarily include the kinetics, particularities, and potential reversibility of epigenetic processes in the brain; their reciprocal interactions with other levels of biological organisation; and, finally, the development of more precise interventions, targeting pathophysiological substrates only.

Limitations notwithstanding, the silence envisioned in these interventions for stress or PTSD spans ideas about memories and silencing through interventions targeting reversibility and plasticity, with epigenetic manipulations proposed as the key means of undoing the effects of past adversity. These perspectives integrate beliefs about the tendency towards stability of epigenetic states, as discussed by Ringrose and Paro over 20 years ago. They presume that molecular profiles are fixed and in need of molecular interventions to be righted. What is set aside, in terms of Ringrose and Paro's analysis, is indeterminacy and the context and variability of epigenetic states: whether, and under what conditions, acquired epigenetic states may be reversed and with what effect.

26.5 Conclusion

The interventions described in this chapter aim to silence memories of the past to create an unencumbered present and future: by wiping a person's past slate clean – whether in a targeted or more generalised way, depending on the intervention – it is assumed that the problem lies in the individual and only in their past as an isolated event/biomarker. Our goal has been to assess the state of knowledge about memories and their silencing and to consider the complexity of reasoning between molecular and experiential levels. We contend that researchers who aim to help people 'remember silence' should carefully reflect on the tenuous relationship between potential epigenetic and behavioural states of risk or resilience. We also argue for closer attention to the multi-scalar processes that may affect this relationship. Indeed, even if the trauma occurred in the past and a therapy was able to reverse an epigenetic state correlated with it at a later date, this does not mean that the multitude of multi-scalar processes associated with the traumatic event would also be silenced. Moreover, for many people who experience early-life adversity, ongoing trauma is as much an experience of the present as of the past [20, 21].

Ultimately, Ringrose and Paro's essential provocation concerning the indeterminacy of epigenetic states remains a powerful reminder for research that frames epigenetic trajectories as linear and fixed. While we may seem closer to the possibility of remembering silence based on claims in emerging research about epigenetic reversibility, there remains a chasm between understandings of epigenetic reversibility and the emotional and affective states associated with what are considered states of neuropsychiatric risk or resilience.

References

1. Ringrose L, Paro R. Remembering silence. Bioessays. 2001;23:566–70.

2. Breslau N. The epidemiology of trauma, PTSD, and other posttrauma disorders. Trauma Violence Abuse. 2009;10:198–210.

3. Nemeroff CB. Paradise lost: The neurobiological and clinical consequences of child abuse and neglect. Neuron. 2016;89:892–909.

4. Hanson M, Gluckman PD. Early developmental conditioning of later health and disease: Physiology or pathophysiology? Physiol Rev. 2014;94:1027–1076.

5. Guan J, Wang G, Wang J, Zhang Z, Fu Y, Cheng L, et al. Chemical reprogramming of human somatic cells to pluripotent stem cells. Nature. 2022;605:325–31.

6. Lister R, Pelizzola M, Kida YS, Hawkins RD, Nery JR, Hon G, et al. Hotspots of aberrant epigenomic reprogramming in human induced pluripotent stem cells. Nature. 2011;471:68–73.

7. Day JJ, Sweatt JD. Epigenetic mechanisms in cognition. Neuron. 2011;70:813–29.

8. Lawson-Boyd E, Meloni M. Gender beneath the skull: Agency, trauma and persisting stereotypes in neuroepigenetics. Front Hum Neurosci. 2021;15:280.

9. Thumfart KM, Jawaid A, Bright K, Flachsmann M, Mansuy IM. Epigenetics of childhood trauma: Long term sequelae and potential for treatment. Neurosci Biobehav Rev. 2022;132:1049–1066.

10. Guo L, Li P, Li H, Colicino E, Colicino S, Wen Y, et al. Effects of environmental noise exposure on DNA methylation in the brain and metabolic health. Environ Res. 2017;153:73–82.

11. Richard MA, Huan T, Ligthart S, Gondalia R, Jhun MA, Brody JA, et al. DNA methylation analysis identifies loci for blood pressure regulation. Am J Hum Genet. 2017;101:888–902.

12. Lloyd S, Larivée A, Lutz P-E. Homeorhesis: Envisaging the logic of life trajectories in molecular research on trauma and its effects. Hist Philos Life Sci. 2022;44:1–29.

13. Leys R. The turn to affect: A critique. Crit Inq. 2011;37:434–72.

14. Lloyd S, Larivée A. Time, trauma, and the brain: How suicide came to have no significant precipitating event. Sci Context. 2020;33:299–327.

15. Menke A, Binder EB. Epigenetic alterations in depression and antidepressant treatment. Dialogues Clin Neurosci. 2022;16:395–404.

16. Ziegler M, Richter J, Mahr M, Gajewska A, Schiele MA, Gehrmann A, et al. MAOA gene hypomethylation in panic disorder – reversibility of an epigenetic risk pattern by psychotherapy. Transl Psychiatry. 2016;6:e773.

17. Hamilton PJ, Burek DJ, Lombroso SI, Neve RL, Robison AJ, Nestler EJ, et al. Cell-type-specific epigenetic editing at the Fosb gene controls susceptibility to social defeat stress. Neuropsychopharmacology. 2018;43:272–84.

18. Warhaftig G, Zifman N, Sokolik CM, Massart R, Gabay O, Sapozhnikov D, et al. Reduction of DNMT3a and RORA in the nucleus accumbens plays a causal role in post-traumatic stress disorder-like behavior: Reversal by combinatorial epigenetic therapy. Mol Psychiatry. 2021;26:7481–97.

19. Pentecost M, Meloni M. 'It's Never Too Early': Preconception care and postgenomic models of life. Front Sociol. 2020;5:21.

20. Lloyd S, Larivée A. Shared relations: Trauma and kinship in the afterlife of death. Med Anthropol Q. 2021;35:476–92.

21. Bloom BE, Alcalá HE, Delva J. Early life adversity, use of specialist care and unmet specialist care need among children. J Child Health Care. 2019;23:392–402.

27

Disability in DOHaD and Epigenetics
Towards Inclusive Practice

Kaleb Saulnier, Lara Azevedo, Neera Bhatia, Lillian Dipnall, Evie Kendal, Garth Stephenson, and Jeffrey M. Craig

27.1 Introduction

Developmental Origins of Health and Disease (DOHaD) and epigenetic research that investigate causal mechanisms and predictive biomarkers have often occurred in the absence of discussion of ethical, legal, and social implications or engagement with disability communities. This has often led to maternal blaming, labelling, stigmatisation, and ableism. Considering the debate on different models of disability by disability activists and social scientists, this is a timely opportunity to optimise the design of epigenetic research into conditions labelled as disabilities. Research aims should address the needs of disability communities, acknowledge diversity, and move away from medical to social models of disability.

Our chapter considers the implications of epigenetics research, as a mediator of DoHAD, for people with autism, an example of a condition some label a disability. We discuss how views on epigenetics and autism have changed over time, including how research can enhance the lived experience of autistic people through contributions to understanding how autism develops and how the strengths and needs of autistic people can best be identified and supported. We argue there is a need for researchers, including those with autism, to work with autistic people and their supporters to co-design studies promoting this understanding, centring autonomy and the provision of information to autistic individuals, including whether to engage with current and future epigenetic tests, particularly those available direct to consumers. In summary, we urge researchers planning such studies to first engage meaningfully and non-tokenistically with disability communities and continue to engage through to the writing and dissemination phases of their research.

27.1.1 On Terminology

Genetics research and autism studies have a complicated history, so we begin by establishing our choice of terminology and rationale for this. We acknowledge that there are strong and often polarising views about the issues presented in this chapter; however, we hope that we can contribute to meaningful discussion.

At the time of writing, Mx Saulnier was professionally affiliated with a federal agency tied to Canadian research funding and management. The contents of this article are reflective of their own views and those of the other chapter authors only.

The principle 'nothing about us without us' communicates that decision-making that impacts a particular group should not take place without the full and direct participation of its members [1]. Thus, it is crucial that individuals be referred to using their preferred terminology. Person-first language evolved in the 1970s to separate the person from the descriptive trait, for example 'a person with autism' rather than 'an autistic person', and to give primacy to their identity as a person. Although this is well-intentioned, some disability activists have noted that this forced separation between person and trait reinforces the idea that disability is inherently negative and ignores the integral role that disability plays in shaping a person's character and experience. As such, there has been a move towards identity-first language.

This terminology is by no means ubiquitous. A person-centred approach to language recommends that on an individual level, words that people use to self-describe should be prioritised.[1] For coherence, we have chosen to use 'autistic person' here, except where a direct quote incorporates other terminology. This is reflective of the preferred language identified by many autistic individuals and autism self-advocacy organisations [2].

27.2 Disability Politics in the Framing of Health

Disability studies emerged in the 1980s and engage with the concepts and consequences of disability, exploring, among other topics, what it means to be disabled in relation to the self and society [3]. Critical disability theory, which focuses on analysing and dismantling systems of ableist oppression, sits at the intersection of academia and activism [4]. Systems that privilege able-bodied people over those with disabilities are not only concerned with understanding the impacts of pathologisation but also undoing them. While there is no single approach to disability studies or politics, both consider the importance of centring and uplifting the stories, voices, and perspectives of disabled individuals in all disability work [1].

27.2.1 Models of Disability

Two dominant models of disability are often contrasted in literature and practice. The medical model ties disability directly to the body, focusing on possible interventions to bring it to a particular type of functioning [5]. The social model situates disability in the social context and physical environment of the individual and is focused on identifying barriers that prevent full participation in society. The latter model differentiates between impairments – attributes impacting how the body and brain operate – and disabilities – restrictions imposed by societal standards that reflect normative ideas of how bodies *should* function. A third model is 'neurodiversity', a term first coined by autistic sociologist Judy Singer and popularised by Steven Silberman in his book, *Neurotribes*, in which he defines it as follows:

> the notion that conditions like autism, dyslexia, and attention-deficit/hyperactivity disorder (ADHD) should be regarded as naturally occurring cognitive variations with distinctive strengths that have contributed to the evolution of technology and culture rather than mere checklists of deficits and dysfunctions. [6]

---

[1] Of relevance here to this topic that this might include a wide-ranging list of terms, including 'autistic person', 'person with autism', 'Autie', 'Aspie', 'person with Asperger's', 'person on the spectrum', and many more.

Like the social model of disability, neurodiversity emphasises the disabling nature of stigmatisation and the prioritisation of brains classified as 'normal'.

27.2.2 Disability in Research

To de-pathologise disability requires engagement with disability communities and scholars in developing frameworks from research design to knowledge translation. Sometimes referred to as participatory or community-engaged research [7], evidence indicates this approach contributes to better health and social outcomes. It is critical to respect the contributions of disabled scholars, activists, and organisations and promote collaboration between disabled and non-disabled researchers, and disabled participants and their advocates. Participatory research means an increasing understanding of disabled individuals as co-creators of scientific knowledge, rather than passive subjects.

There is, understandably, hesitation in disability communities regarding participation in medical research. As with many vulnerable communities, the history of unconsented research and other research harms is long and fraught [8]. Community members are quick to spot ableist rhetoric and stigmatisation in research documentation and are reluctant to participate if their bodies, lives, and experiences may be used to pursue goals not aligned with the expressed needs of disabled individuals. Thus, participatory research does not begin with inviting disabled individuals as research subjects, but rather, with listening, learning, humility, and trust-building on the part of non-disabled researchers, using the principle of co-design and through participant advisory groups.

27.3 Mapping Disability onto DOHaD and Epigenetics

As discourse shifts from the medical model, bioethicists and clinicians have begun to recognise how social factors play a primary role in the treatment of disabled individuals. The DOHaD model represents a particularly fruitful opportunity for this shift, focused on a bio-psycho-social model of health and disease [16]. Similarly, epigenetics' attention to the role of environment, exposures, and stress moves away from the biological determinism of the genomics era [17] towards a more holistic understanding of health. Nonetheless, researchers in DOHaD and epigenetics should refrain from importing potentially harmful presumptions into these emerging fields, with bioethicists and disability scholars already expressing concerns that applying the medical model to these areas risks intensifying rhetoric around responsibility and blame for social and environmental exposures, particularly when associating maternal exposures with future disability [18, 19].

The DOHaD phenomenon is supported by ample animal and human evidence but has an intrinsic focus on 'health vs disease'. This neglects natural variations not classified as 'health' or 'disease', including a wide range of ongoing or recurring behaviours, cognitions, and health conditions that are multidimensional. These include neurodiverse conditions such as autism, whose communities refute the labels of 'disease' and 'disability', similarly to the deaf community. This is relevant when attempting to apply epigenetic models of disabilities to traits that cannot reasonably be classified as 'disease symptoms'. Therefore, we have a responsibility to be careful with terminology when engaging with participants from the disability community, including when planning and reporting epigenetics research.

27.4 The Case of Autism

Autism presents a valuable case study to explore the intersection of disability, DOHaD, and epigenetics, as a condition that has long oscillated in medical and public imagination between having social, environmental, or biological origins. DOHaD research has shown that early-life exposures to social, biological, and environmental factors can influence fetal development. Influential biological factors include maternal infection and inflammation, which can lead to a state of maternal immune activation where immune regulatory mediators are expressed in higher-than-normal ranges, a possible risk factor for autism and other neurodevelopmental and psychiatric conditions [20, 21]. Suboptimal nutrition before or during pregnancy, particularly vitamin B9 (folic acid), has also been implicated [22], as well as prenatal exposure to traffic-related air pollution and some insecticides [23]. Factors that cannot be explained by shared genetics and environment have also been associated with autistic traits, for example in one twin from a genetically identical pair.

Despite a strong genetic influence, there is considerable genetic heterogeneity across autistic individuals [24]. Around 5 per cent are also diagnosed with a clinically and genetically diagnosable syndrome, and around 15 per cent can be attributed to simple genetic changes such as single gene mutations or copy number variations. For the remaining individuals, evidence points to autism as a polygenic condition, that is resulting from genetic differences spread across hundreds, possibly thousands of genes [24]. These genes appear commonly involved in brain development, epigenetic regulation of gene activity, and metabolism, suggesting possible causal mechanisms for autism. Since the early 2020s, autism-associated variants have been grouped together to form a 'polygenic risk score', with a higher score theoretically indicating a higher likelihood of autism [25].

There are more genetic differences in genes encoding components of epigenetic mechanisms in autistic people as a group compared to non-autistic people. As their gene products are likely to act at multiple genomic regions, some autism-specific epigenetic differences will likely have strong genetic components, [26] increasing their likelihood of being stable over time and therefore useful as diagnostic and prognostic biomarkers. Associations between epigenetic states in the sperm of fathers of autistic children compared to those with neurotypical children [27] are more likely to be explained by genetic factors, unless genetics are controlled for, for example, in identical twin studies.

Epigenetic studies of autism have identified similar genes and gene functions to genetic studies, including those involved in epigenetic regulation and synaptic function. However, far more immune system genes have been identified in epigenetic studies of autism diagnoses [34]. Epigenetic studies have also investigated specific dimensions of autism, for example social communication [28], potentially predicting biomarkers at birth [29], and risk scores [30]. However, these findings have yet to be replicated.

27.4.1 The Social Construction of Autism

Criteria for autism in the Diagnostic and Statistical Manual (version 5) include but are not limited to 'persistent deficits in each of three areas of social communication and interaction plus at least two of four types of restricted, repetitive behaviours' [31]. This deficit model, at times focused on the external viewer's perception of autistic experiences, typically shapes research seeking to minimise these behaviours and accompanied distress. By contrast, neurodiversity-focused groups frame autism as a constellation of strengths and challenges across social and sensory spectra and focus on research and resources to support autistic individuals in achieving their best quality of life [32].

Another current view considers autism as a potentially disabling condition that nevertheless may confer various positive traits [33]. However, in many cases this view has merely re-circumscribed capitalist values of productivity, for example celebrating those autistic traits, such as hyperfocus, that can be exploited by employers to improve work output. While this view has partly enhanced our understanding of neurodiversity and the need for better neuroergonomics in the workplace, the ultimate focus has not been on promoting quality of life for autistic people. Moreover, other autistic traits that are considered neutral or positive within the autism community, such as stimming to self-soothe and express emotions, are still misunderstood as negatives or viewed with discomfort.

The experiences of autistic individuals in healthcare provide an opportunity for examining pathologisation of their condition via scientific research into DOHaD and epigenetics. These research areas rely heavily on the interpretation of links between social and other environmental factors with biological outcomes. Perhaps the most widely recognised image of the autistic individual is that of a white, masculine-presenting child with an inability to make eye contact, limited or stilted speech, and a fascination with patterns or trains. This perception has recently begun to shift, prompted in part by an increase in later-in-life diagnoses in cisgender women as well as non-binary individuals and transgender men and women, who may present differently from this stereotype.[2]

Autism and diversity of gender identities and experiences overlap substantially, further impacting access to appropriate support and care. Gendered differences in presentation have led autistic girls and women to be underdiagnosed, misdiagnosed, or diagnosed at a later age, sometimes only after their own child's diagnosis [34]. This discrepancy has contributed to a lack of understanding of key mental health conditions that co-occur alongside autism, including eating disorders, depression, anxiety, and suicidality. Similarly, disparities in the impact of race and ethnicity on the timing and frequency of diagnosis have led to a paucity of resources and support for racialised/ethnic minority autistic youth, who at the same time experience increased risks and rates of police and other state-sanctioned violence and incarceration [35]. There is an urgent need for an intersectional approach to all disability research, but particularly epigenetic studies examining the social and environmental contexts for the lived experiences of autistic and other disabled individuals.[3]

---

[2] Cisgender refers to the experience of having a gender identity that aligns with the sex that is assigned at birth, whereas transgender refers very broadly to the experience of these elements not aligning in some way.

[3] Intersectionality is a term coined by Black critical theorist Kimberlé Crenshaw to describe how oppressive institutions (e.g. racism, sexism, homophobia, ableism, etc.) are interconnected and cannot be examined separately from one another.

27.5 Reframing Epigenetics Research to Address the Needs of People with Disabilities

27.5.1 Biomarker Development for Conditions Classed as Disabilities

We are still far from having reliable predictive or diagnostic genetic or epigenetic biomarkers for conditions such as autism. One major factor that clouds the interpretation of such research is study design. Most classify autism as one entity, whereas it is a highly heterogeneous condition. Furthermore, co-occurring conditions such as ADHD are largely ignored in such studies. Some researchers have turned away from a categorical to a dimensional approach to the origins of autism, using continuously variable dimensions such as anxiety, attention, sensory processing, specific interests, repetition, social interaction, and communication [36]. We suggest that this method is preferred because it targets traits that can be clinically defined and can identify areas of strength as well as areas in which autistic individuals may require understanding and assistance. This approach also captures intersecting dimensions of co-occurrences, such as ADHD, for example, sustained attention.

We suggest that future studies be based on dimensions of autism with a view to meeting the self-determined needs of autistic individuals and the autism community. A dimensional approach also reflects the spectrum of neurodiversity within and outside the autism community and the reality of the social model of autism rather than the medical model.

As the field of epigenetics moves towards identifying more biomarkers for conditions and associating these with developmental, social, and environmental correlates, the rhetoric surrounding curative approaches to disability could increase. This rhetoric is closely tied to medical and deficit models of disability, with their foundational assumptions that people with disabilities wish to be rid of the disabled parts of themselves. For some, this may be true; the existence of the social and neurodiversity models does not detract from the struggles precipitated by certain features associated with disability, such as chronic pain, anxiety, loss of quality of life, or early mortality. Rather than attempting to categorise disabilities wholesale as 'bad' (e.g. where we may aim to repair or alter the body or brain) or 'good' (where we may instead target disabling factors in the society or environment), a more useful account would examine components of disability that are *unwanted by the individual who experiences them*. Again, following the principle of 'nothing about us without us', it is important to differentiate between calls for prevention and cure that come from researchers and healthcare providers, and policies based on the lived experiences of disabled individuals and their advocates. In doing so, a stark divide can appear between the expectation of the disabled experience and the reality.

It has long been argued that health economic metrics, such as the quality-adjusted life year (QALY) or disability-adjusted life year (DALY), are not sensitive to the real experiences of disabled people and ignore the significant adaptive ability of individuals [37]. Inviting more conscious consideration of disabled peoples' own experiences of their disability can also avoid the tendency to objectify disabled persons' bodies and view them as separate from the disabled experience. This helps avoid the risk of ignoring meaningful needs assessments conducted by the community. In other words, embracing a neurodiversity model does not mean neglecting to provide support for autistic individuals who consider certain traits to be personally disabling or undesirable. Ethically, it is important to remember another classic phrase in the disability community, coined by autism advocate Dr Stephen Shore: 'If you've met one person with autism, you've met one person with autism' [38]. Again, the diversity of manifestations and personal experiences can only be incorporated effectively into epigenetics and genetics research if studies are co-designed and guided by diverse members of the autism community.

27.5.2 Direct-to-Consumer (DTC) Epigenetic Tests

In the past five years, there has been a growing number of companies selling epigenetic tests directly to consumers, that is without the need for a referral from a healthcare practitioner [39]. Despite being unable to define a 'healthy' epigenome, DTC companies focus on identifying epigenetic biomarkers in consumers' blood or saliva samples with the promise of enabling consumers to improve their health outcomes. An 'altered' epigenetic status could indicate early-life exposures that increase the likelihood of developing certain conditions, which could be targeted for intervention due to the potential reversibility of epigenetic changes. Identifying environmental risks for the development of a condition also means that prevention strategies could be adopted to reduce the chance of its development, for example, via diet and exercise changes. In the case of autism, there are currently tests being developed to facilitate diagnosis in children as young as 18 months old [40]. Here, the promise is to provide biological data to complement more subjective analyses to expedite autism diagnoses and access to early intervention and resources.

However, DTC epigenetic testing raises various ethico-legal issues, related to the core technical issue surrounding the precision of epigenetic biomarkers for diagnosing complex conditions. Marketing that overestimates the reliability of epigenetic test results could exploit consumer trust in science to sell a product that falls short of its promises. Test results could also affect an individual's access to insurance policies, particularly life insurance, as the reporting of test results is often a legal obligation of the applicant. With a focus on environmental risks, there is also a tendency to blame individuals for the development of associated conditions. Here we acknowledge the long history of blaming mothers for autism, a fact well demonstrated by the term 'refrigerator mothers'[4] often used to describe them [19]. While parents of children with autism seem to support the development of epigenetic testing for improvement of the diagnosis process [41], there is a need for clear regulations of the DTC market to protect consumers, especially vulnerable populations.

27.5.3 Ethical, Legal, and Social Implications of DoHAD Research for People with Disabilities

From an ethical perspective 'respect for persons' is one of the fundamental tenets of Western biomedical ethics. Its application in DOHaD research is often more complex than in standard clinical care [42]. Core ethico-legal issues here include maintaining confidentiality and privacy, and gaining informed consent for medical interventions, which work together to promote autonomy. While protecting sensitive information such

---

[4] "Refrigerator mothers" refers to a discredited mid-20th-century theory that cold and unemotional parenting, particularly by mothers, was the cause of autism.

as medical diagnoses and treatment decisions may be relatively simple within the practitioner–client communication paradigm, genetic information, for example, might be problematic for the individualistic Western ethico-legal model. (See Karpin in this volume.) From a DOHaD perspective, genetic and epigenetic information might best be conceived of as *family* information, making privacy concerns more complex. However, the rationale behind protecting this information remains the same: promoting autonomy, including through avoiding potential coercion from those who would misuse sensitive information to discriminate against individuals. The latter is relevant for accessing employment, health and life insurance, and healthcare services. Whether DOHaD and epigenetics research should aim for family or community, rather than individual consent, falls beyond our scope here, but we recognise that when a test impacts more than the individual, there is potential for social harm against others who are impacted by the results. For research on communities with disabilities, especially those with a potential genetic contribution, this suggests the co-design of research studies is important to ensure knowledge about inheritance is not weaponised against the community or used to engage in blaming or labelling of parents or offspring.

Confidentiality is a key pillar in the doctor–patient relationship protected under common law and statutory regulation. For example, privacy laws in Australia governed under the *Privacy Act 1988* (Cth) have a broad reach, protecting a range of information, including health information. According to the 'For your information: Australian Privacy Law and Practice' ALRC Report No 108) [43], 'privacy' covers several aspects, including data protection, such as medical and government records; bodily privacy, such as invasive procedures that may include genetic and epigenetic tests; and communication, such as emails.

The disclosure or privacy of sensitive genetic information in some instances might be problematic. For the disability community, it is possible that epigenetic data collected from one consenting individual or family may have immediate relevance to other community members. For this, the right 'not to know' might be as important as the right to know the genetic factors involved in the development of autism. Importantly, once these data exist, they may have wide-ranging impacts on members of the community who did not consent to the research.

27.5.4 Incorporating Perspectives from Multiple Stakeholders

A goal of disability activists has been to reframe conversations about disability, health, and disease away from views that centre concepts of 'normalcy' and 'functionality' and to instead centre the disabled individual as the core stakeholder in the discussion of their own body and experience. Throughout the twentieth century in particular, the concept of 'wellness' came to be equated with 'virtue', situating the body as a 'site for moral action' [44] with regard to the pursuit of health. The medical model, in addition to enforcing the idea of a 'normal' state of the body to which its owner should aspire [45], increasingly pushed a 'functionality' argument that privileged a body's capacity to contribute to labour [46], and disdained disability precisely because of the implication that the disabled individual is of inherently reduced worth under capitalism.

The term 'stakeholders' is suggestive of a consumer-driven approach to health and well-being that places disabled individuals immediately at a disadvantage [47]. As a result, the stakeholders most often centred on disability research have been medical practitioners and families of disabled individuals. While both caregivers and practitioners have a significant interest in the disability conversation and valuable experiences to contribute, at times, this has come at the expense of the voices and narratives from disability communities and their advocates. In autism research, this has contributed to frustration and conflict. As this research moves forward, it must include autistic individuals and their caregivers where necessary (as participants, researchers, and scholars) at the centre of the conversation from research development to knowledge translation.

27.6 Conclusion: Recommendations for Engagement with Disability Communities in DOHaD and Epigenetic Studies

It is essential to engage with disability communities and their supporters at every step from research design to knowledge translation. Previous experiences within these communities highlight the risks that genetic research can lead to discrimination and stigmatisation, and in the case of DOHaD, this extends not only to individuals with the condition of interest but also to their parents [48]. For this reason, we advocate for more inclusive research practices that build trust with disability communities, listen to their needs, and promote support, while maximising autonomy, dignity, and respect for all members of the community.

In the case of autism, we call on researchers to reflect on their motivations when planning epigenetic studies of autism, considering whether predictive testing prior to the typical onset of symptoms would allow for early modes of support [49]. We urge researchers to seek advice from the autistic community when studying environmental contributions to autism to consider structural frames aimed at policy change in addition to those focused on the agency of individuals. Researchers should also be mindful of the language they use in planning and reporting research findings and of adopting a dimensional framework for cognitive assessment.

Future studies may look at the ethical implications of handling and releasing wide-scale epigenetics research data on autistic communities to ensure knowledge is used to meet the needs of this community and improve the quality of life. In summary, we urge researchers planning DOHaD and epigenetics research to listen to and engage with disability communities when they say, 'nothing about us without us'.

References

1. Charlton JI. Nothing about Us without Us, Disability Oppression and Empowerment. Berkeley: University of California Press; 1998.

2. Dwyer P. Stigma, Incommensurability, or Both? Pathology-First, Person-First, and Identity-First Language and the Challenges of Discourse in Divided Autism Communities. J Dev Behav Pediatr. 2022;43(2):111–13.

3. Ferguson PM, Nusbaum E. Disability Studies: What Is It and What Difference Does It Make? Research and Practice for Persons with Severe Disabilities. 2012;37(2):70–80.

4. Oliver M, Barnes C. Disability Studies, Disabled People and the Struggle for Inclusion. British Journal of Sociology of Education. 2010;31(5):547–60.

5. Shyman E. The Reinforcement of Ableism: Normality, the Medical Model of Disability, and Humanism in Applied Behavior Analysis and ASD. Intellectual and Developmental Disabilities. 2016;54(5):366–76.

6. Silberman S. Neurotribes : The Legacy of Autism and the Future of Neurodiversity.

New York: Penguin Random House; 2015.

7. Wallerstein N, Oetzel JG, Sanchez-Youngman S, Boursaw B, Dickson E, Kastelic S, et al. Engage for Equity: A Long-Term Study of Community-Based Participatory Research and Community-Engaged Research Practices and Outcomes. Health Educational Behavior. 2020;47(3):380–90.

8. Bhambra S. The Montreal Experiments: Brainwashing and the Ethics of Psychiatric Experimentation. Hektoen International Journal [Internet]. 2009 [cited 29 July 2022]. Available from: https://hekint.org/2019/04/30/the-montreal-experiments-brainwashing-and-the-ethics-of-psychiatric-experimentation/.

9. Hagemann E, Silva DT, Davis JA, Gibson LY, Prescott SL. Developmental Origins of Health and Disease (DOHaD): The Importance of Life-course and Transgenerational Approaches. Paediatric Respiratory Reviews. 2021;40:3–9.

10. Tronick E, Hunter RG. Waddington, Dynamic Systems, and Epigenetics. Frontier in Behavioural Neurosciences. 2016;10:107.

11. Felix JF, Cecil CAM. Population DNA Methylation Studies in the Developmental Origins of Health and Disease (DOHaD) Framework. Journal of Developmental Origins of Health and Disease. 2019;10(3):306–13.

12. Ollikainen M, Smith KR, Joo EJ, Ng HK, Andronikos R, Novakovic B, et al. DNA Methylation Analysis of Multiple Tissues from Newborn Twins Reveals Both Genetic and Intrauterine Components to Variation in the Human Neonatal Epigenome. Human Molecular Genetics. 2010;19(21):4176–88.

13. Barua S, Junaid MA. Lifestyle, Pregnancy and Epigenetic Effects. Epigenomics. 2015;7(1):85–102.

14. Baylin SB, Jones PA. Epigenetic Determinants of Cancer. Cold Spring Harbor Perspective Biology. 2016;8(9):1–35.

15. Mikeska T, Craig JM. DNA Methylation Biomarkers: Cancer and Beyond. Genes (Basel). 2014;5(3):821–64.

16. Tremblay RE, Vitaro F, Côté SM. Developmental Origins of Chronic Physical Aggression: A Bio-Psycho-Social Model for the Next Generation of Preventive Interventions. Annual Review of Psychology. 2018;69(1):383–407.

17. Graves JL. Great Is Their Sin: Biological Determinism in the Age of Genomics. The Annals of the American Academy of Political and Social Science. 2015;661(1):24–50.

18. Kenney M, Müller R. Of Rats and Women: Narratives of Motherhood in Environmental Epigenetics. In: Meloni M, Cromby J, Fitzgerald D, Lloyd S, editors. The Palgrave Handbook of Biology and Society. London: Palgrave Macmillan UK; 2018. pp. 799–830.

19. Lappé M. The Maternal Body as Environment in Autism Science. Social Studies of Science. 2016;46(5):675–700.

20. Boulanger-Bertolus J, Pancaro C, Mashour GA. Increasing Role of Maternal Immune Activation in Neurodevelopmental Disorders. Frontiers in Behavioral Neuroscience. 2018;12:230.

21. Stephenson G, Craig JM. Environmental Risk Factors for Neurodevelopmental Disorders: Evidence from Twin Studies. In: Tarnoki A, Tarnoki D, Harris J, Segal N, editors. Twin Research for Everyone. Amsterdam, The Netherlands: Academic Press; 2022. pp. 625–48.

22. Hoxha B, Hoxha M, Domi E, Gervasoni J, Persichilli S, Malaj V, et al. Folic Acid and Autism: A Systematic Review of the Current State of Knowledge. Cells. 2021;10(8):1976–1995.

23. Brown AS, Cheslack-Postava K, Rantakokko P, Kiviranta H, Hinkka-Yli-Salomäki S, McKeague IW, et al. Association of Maternal Insecticide Levels with Autism in Offspring from a National Birth Cohort. American Journal of Psychiatry. 2018;175(11):1094–101.

24. Fernandez BA, Scherer SW. Syndromic Autism Spectrum Disorders: Moving

from a Clinically Defined to a Molecularly Defined Approach. Dialogues in Clinical Neuroscience. 2017;**19**(4):353–71.

25. Antaki D, Guevara J, Maihofer AX, Klein M, Gujral M, Grove J, et al. A Phenotypic Spectrum of Autism Is Attributable to the Combined Effects of Rare Variants, Polygenic Risk and Sex. Nature Genetics. 2022;**54**:1284–92.

26. Massrali A, Brunel H, Hannon E, Wong C, Baron-Cohen S, Warrier V. Integrated Genetic and Methylomic Analyses Identify Shared Biology between Autism and Autistic Traits. Molecular Autism. 2019;**10**:31.

27. Garrido N, Cruz F, Egea RR, Simon C, Sadler-Riggleman I, Beck D, et al. Sperm DNA Methylation Epimutation Biomarker for Paternal Offspring Autism Susceptibility. Clinical Epigenetics. 2021;**13**(1):6.

28. Rijlaarsdam J, Cecil CAM, Relton CL, Barker ED. Epigenetic Profiling of Social Communication Trajectories and Co-occurring Mental Health Problems: A Prospective, Methylome-Wide Association Study. Developmental Psychopathology. 2021:**34**:854–63.

29. Mordaunt CE, Jianu JM, Laufer BI, Zhu Y, Hwang H, Dunaway KW, et al. Cord Blood DNA Methylome in Newborns Later Diagnosed with Autism Spectrum Disorder Reflects Early Dysregulation of Neurodevelopmental and X-linked Genes. Genome Medicine. 2020;**12**(1):88.

30. Hannon E, Schendel D, Ladd-Acosta C, Grove J, Hansen CS, Andrews SV, et al. Elevated Polygenic Burden for Autism Is Associated with Differential DNA Methylation at Birth. Genome Medicine. 2018;**10**(1):19.

31. Prevention, CfDCa. Diagnostic and Statistical Manual of Mental Disorders. Association AP, editor. Arlington, VA: American Psychiatric Association; 2013.

32. Autistic Women & Nonbinary Network I. Autistic Women & Nonbinary Network Lincoln, NE 68506: Autistic Women & Nonbinary Network, Inc; 2022 [updated 2022; cited 25 July 2022]. Available from: https://awnnetwork.org/.

33. Stevenson N. Autism Doesn't Have to be Viewed as a Disability or Disorder Australia: Guardian News & Media Limited; 2015 [29 July 2022]. Available from: www.theguardian.com/science/blog/2015/jul/16/autism-doesnt-have-to-be-viewed-as-a-disability-or-disorder#comments.

34. Rynkiewicz A, Janas-Kozik M, Slopien A. Girls and Women with Autism. Psychiatric Pol. 2019;**53**(4):737–52.

35. Eilenberg JS, Paff M, Harrison AJ, Long KA. Disparities Based on Race, Ethnicity, and Socioeconomic Status Over the Transition to Adulthood Among Adolescents and Young Adults on the Autism Spectrum: A Systematic Review. Current Psychiatry Reports. 2019;**21**(5):32.

36. Ure A, Rose V, Bernie C, Williams K. Autism: One or Many Spectrums? Journal of Paediatric Child Health. 2018;**54**(10):1068–72.

37. Grosse SD, Lollar DJ, Campbell VA, Chamie M. Disability and Disability-Adjusted Life Years: Not the Same. Public Health Report. 2009;**124**(2):197–202.

38. Flannery KA, Wisner-Carlson R. Autism and Education. Child and Adolescent Psychiatric Clinics of North America. 2020;**29**(2):319–43.

39. Dupras C, Beauchamp E, Joly Y. Selling Direct-to-Consumer Epigenetic Tests: Are We Ready? Nature Reviews Genetics. 2020;**21**(6):335–6.

40. Inc QB. The Clarifi Autism Saliva Test: Quadrant Biosciences Inc.; 2022 [cited 29 July 2022]. Analytical test. Available from: https://quadrantbiosciences.com/.

41. Wagner KE, McCormick JB, Barns S, Carney M, Middleton FA, Hicks SD. Parent Perspectives towards Genetic and Epigenetic Testing for Autism Spectrum Disorder. Journal of Autism Development Disorders. 2020;**50**(9):3114–25.

42. Beauchamp T, Childress J. Principles of Biomedical Ethics: Marking Its Fortieth

Anniversary. Taylor & Francis; 2019. pp. 9–12.

43. Commission TALR. Australian Privacy Law and Practice. Australia: Australian Government; 2008.

44. Conrad P. Wellness as Virtue: Morality and the Pursuit of Health. Culture, Medicine and Psychiatry. 1994;**18**(3):385–401.

45. Squier SM. So Long as They Grow Out of It: Comics, the Discourse of Developmental Normalcy, and Disability. Journal of Medical Humanities. 2008;**29**(2):71–88.

46. Mitchell DTS, S. L. Disability as Multitude: Re-working Non-Productive Labor Power. Journal of Literary &

Cultural Disability Studies. 2010;**4**(2):179–93.

47. Migliaccio G. Disabled People in the Stakeholder Theory: A Literature Analysis. Journal of the Knowledge Economy. 2019;**10**(4):1657–78.

48. Dupras C, Joly Y, Rial-Sebbag E. Human Rights in the Postgenomic Era: Challenges and Opportunities Arising with Epigenetics. Social Science Information. 2020;**59**(1):12–34.

49. Yu Y, Huang J, Chen X, Fu J, Wang X, Pu L, et al. Efficacy and Safety of Diet Therapies in Children with Autism Spectrum Disorder: A Systematic Literature Review and Meta-Analysis. Frontier in Neurology. 2022;**13**:844117.

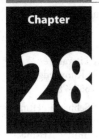

Creating Good Data Our Way
An Indigenous Lens for Epidemiology and Intergenerational Health

Sarah Bourke and Raymond Lovett

28.1 Introduction

Momentum is building for epidemiological research led by and for Indigenous peoples. Backed by a human rights agenda, this drive is gaining speed due to wider calls to decolonise the social sciences, and increased recognition of the critical importance of incorporating Indigenous expertise in the conceptualisation, development, and execution of effective health research. 'Decolonising' epidemiology may involve several processes that are best determined by the communities who contribute their data. In Australia, this has involved acknowledging the complicity of the sciences in the colonisation of Aboriginal and Torres Strait Islander lands, waters, skies, and peoples, and the need for data that reflect the ongoing impact of settler-colonial practices and ideals on our communities. This work has often been conducted within a strengths-based framework, emphasising the inherent assets and resilience of Aboriginal and Torres Strait Islander communities, and the role of culture as the foundation of our individual, social, ecological, and spiritual health and well-being. To decolonise epidemiological research about Indigenous communities, Indigenous peoples must be in control of the definition, collection, and use of their data, following Indigenous Data Sovereignty (IDS) and Indigenous Data Governance (IDG) protocols, which ensure these data serve our self-determined interests and futures.

Hoke and McDade argue that lifecourse interventions based on DOHaD research are 'rarely situated within the cultural, social, or political-economic context of the populations examined' [1, p. 190]. Further, there is a lack of research focus on intergenerational or transgenerational events impacting long-term adult health in subsequent generations:

> Rather than acknowledging the maternal body as the product of ongoing physiological, social, and political-economic processes, these influences on maternal physiology are often placed within an analytical black box and ignored. [1, p. 191]

Having a better conceptual understanding of the contexts in which people live would allow DOHaD researchers to design better measures to capture data on those concepts and then monitor any changes when interventions are put into place. We suggest that epidemiological methods that centre Indigenous lifeworlds have the potential to measure contextual influences and to identify salutogenic and protective factors that support holistic health and well-being for Indigenous peoples.

This chapter provides an overview of current discourses around centring Indigenous ontologies (ways of being), epistemologies (ways of knowing), and axiologies (ways of doing), also known as Indigenous 'lifeworlds', in epidemiology with a particular focus on Indigenous Australian (Aboriginal and Torres Strait Islander) perspectives. Mayi Kuwayu, the National Study of Aboriginal and Torres Strait Islander Wellbeing, will be used as a key example illustrating how epidemiological research may be led, owned, and governed by Indigenous peoples to produce rigorous and meaningful data that reflect Indigenous lifeworlds. Centring Indigenous perspectives may provide valuable tools for the development of the DOHaD lifecourse framework and future studies that seek to address holistic determinants of intergenerational health and well-being.

28.2 Part 1. Centring Indigenous Perspectives in Epidemiology

28.2.1 The Colonial Project as an Origin of Ill health and Disease

It is well known that colonisation and colonialism are determinants of Indigenous ill health [2]. Colonisation by nations including Britain, France, Spain, and others resulted in the mass genocide and/or displacement of Indigenous peoples across the world, and the methodical dismantling of Indigenous lifeways, undermining millennia-long connections to land, culture, and kin. Colonialism, as enacted through historical and ongoing contemporary colonial processes, encompasses a range of risk factors for health and well-being [3]. This includes interpersonal, institutional, and political processes that, at a minimum, aim to control or dominate a population and, at the extreme end of the spectrum, aim to eliminate or exterminate the population.

In Australia, it is estimated that around 90 per cent of the Aboriginal and Torres Strait Islander population lost their lives between 1788 and 1901 because of widespread colonial violence, introduced diseases, and the theft of land and water resources by British settlers [4, 5]. Those who survived were subjected to systematically racist and discriminatory programmes and policies. Many were dispossessed of their traditional lands and forced to live on Christian-run missions, which often forbade the use of any language other than English and actively suppressed important cultural practices. One particular assimilation policy enacted from 1910 to 1970 in Australia led to 11–24 per cent of all Aboriginal children being stolen from their families by government agents and held in Christian-run institutions for 're-education' and training as domestic servants for the White middle classes [6]. They are known collectively as the Stolen Generations. Colonisation has thus generated significant intergenerational trauma for Indigenous peoples, reinforced by ongoing and cumulative 'biosocial injury' inflicted by settler-colonial nation states and individuals [7].

Settler-colonialism imposes cultural values, religions, laws, and policies that often go against the rights and values of Indigenous peoples. The concept of settler-colonialism as a health risk factor is well understood within Indigenous populations [8–10]. However, in Australia there is limited ability to examine such links due to an absence of epidemiological data on settler-colonial exposures. This itself is a manifestation of racism, given the lack of research priority and attention to settler-colonialism and its impacts. White racism and discrimination against Indigenous peoples thus perpetuate colonial trauma.

A small number of studies demonstrate poorer outcomes for Aboriginal and Torres Strait Islander peoples who experience individual settler-colonial factors such as discrimination [11–15] and the Stolen Generations [16] versus those who do not. However, most, if not all, of these studies are small-scale, use measures that have not been validated, and are not population representative. In addition, there are no quantitative studies that identify factors that can act as a buffer against the negative impacts of settler-colonialism. This is critical in taking the next step past identifying associations and towards identifying practical, strengths-based solutions to guide policy and programme development.

Research conducted by Indigenous peoples, for Indigenous peoples, and with Indigenous peoples is a direct challenge to the ongoing colonisation of our lands, cultures, and communities. As Tuck and Yang [17] stated, 'Decolonization is not a metaphor'. It *unsettles* the settlers. Indigenous peoples have always conducted research, and we have always used counting as a tool for this research. This fact alone frequently unsettles non-Indigenous researchers in the field of epidemiology who often state that issues of importance to Indigenous peoples, such as culture (the practising of it or revitalisation of it), cannot be quantified. The centring of Indigenous peoples in epidemiology therefore means accounting for settler-colonial-inflicted biosocial injury and centring Indigenous definitions of health and well-being and the determinants thereof within research.

28.2.2 Indigenous Definitions of Health and Well-being

Indigenous identities and concepts of health and well-being are fundamentally connected to the land within an eco-centric relationality or kinship system that defines social and spiritual obligations to family, community, and the land [18, p. 200]. This relationality is reinforced through cultural frameworks where relationships to the past, ancestors, land, and the present are articulated through language, song, dance, storytelling, and maintaining traditional homelands, beliefs, and kinship [19]. As a result, Indigenous definitions of health and well-being are inherently holistic. The Medicine Wheel, or Sacred Hoop, has been used across Turtle Island (North America) to convey Indigenous philosophies of well-being using four quadrants (sometimes represented by the four cardinal directions – North, South, East, and West) to represent the connectedness between the physical, emotional, mental, and spiritual elements of life and the need for balance across these four areas. In Aotearoa (New Zealand), Māori holistic health and well-being also relies on a balance across four fundamentally interconnected elements – *wairua* (spiritual), *whānau* (extended family network), *hinengaro* (the mind), and *tinana* (physical) [20, p. 1141].

In the Australian context, the most used definition of Aboriginal and Torres Strait Islander health is as follows:

> 'Aboriginal health' means not just the physical wellbeing of an individual but refers to the social, emotional and cultural wellbeing of the whole Community in which each individual is able to achieve their full potential as a human being, thereby bringing about the total wellbeing of their Community. It is a whole-of-life view and includes the cyclical concept of life-death-life.... Health to Aboriginal peoples is a matter of determining all aspects of their life, including control over their physical environment, of dignity, of community self-esteem, and of justice. It is not merely a matter of the provision of doctors, hospitals, medicines, or the absence of disease and incapacity. [21, pp. ix–x]

In recent years, several studies have focused on expanding this definition. Garvey and colleagues [22] outlined their *Fabric of Aboriginal and Torres Strait Islander Wellbeing* model based on qualitative research with 359 participants, weaving together eight aspects of well-being: culture; community; family; belonging and connection; holistic health;

purpose and control; dignity and respect; and basic needs. Butler et al. [23] conducted a comprehensive national literature review to identify nine interconnected domains of Aboriginal and Torres Strait Islander well-being, including autonomy, empowerment, and recognition; family and community; culture, spirituality, and identity; Country; basic needs; work, roles, and responsibilities; education; physical health; and mental health. Salmon and her colleagues [19] undertook an international literature review to identify and describe six key cultural domains essential for Aboriginal and Torres Strait Islander well-being: connection to Country; Indigenous beliefs and knowledge; Indigenous language; family, kinship, and community; cultural expression and continuity; and self-determination and leadership. Maintaining and reviving connections to land and culture has been found to be protective of Indigenous health and well-being across a range of studies in Australia and internationally [19, 24].

28.2.3 Indigenous Rights to Data

Indigenous definitions of well-being and its determinants have not been reflected in large-scale epidemiological data collections. For decades, statistics about Aboriginal and Torres Strait Islander communities have been wholly based on the perspective of the White settler-colonial state [25]. Hundreds of Aboriginal and Torres Strait Islander cultural groups were homogenised under the umbrella term 'Indigenous' for comparison to the (equally homogenised) 'non-Indigenous' population. This comparison was based on White settler-colonial definitions of health, social, and economic achievement. Sociologist Maggie Walter (Palawa) argued that the result of this comparison was the production of '5D Data', emphasising the Difference, Disparity, Disadvantage, Dysfunction, and Deprivation experienced within the Aboriginal and Torres Strait Islander population [26]. She writes:

> Current Australian practices in regard to the collection of data on Indigenous people are the cloned descendants of the data imperatives of colonisation. In what I refer to as the deficit data/problematic people (DD/PP) correlation, processes of enumeration have long been used to correlate the highly observable societal Aboriginal and Torres Strait Islander inequality with the concept of racial unfitness. [26]

When data stressing the 'Indigenous problem' present in Australian society are used to inform public health and policy development, the inevitable outcome is a re-colonisation of Aboriginal and Torres Strait Islander communities through programmes and policies designed to correct these perceived deficits. Interventions built on this deficit premise are prone to failure, as has been emphasised time and again by the Australian Government's own monitoring scheme called *Closing the Gap*, established in 2008. The 'Gap' refers to the statistical gaps highlighted by the above-mentioned data, particularly the difference in life expectancy at birth between the Indigenous and non-Indigenous population, which currently sits at 7.8 years for females and 8.6 years for males [27]. According to Government statistics, over half (53 per cent) of the health 'gap' between Aboriginal and Torres Strait Islander Australians and the rest of the Australian population is accounted for by just five social determinants (employment and hours worked, highest non-school qualification, level of schooling completed, housing adequacy, and household income) and six 'health risk factors' (binge drinking, high blood pressure, overweight and obesity status, inadequate fruit and vegetable consumption, insufficient physical exercise, and smoking) [28]. The remaining 47 per cent of the health gap is currently unaccounted for.

Research seeking to measure the health of Indigenous peoples but exclude them from the development of such research is, quite simply, bad science. 'Bad' in this case may be interpreted in two ways. First, in the production of inaccurate, under-powered, and misleading data that, in Australia and Aotearoa at least, have informed decades of largely ineffective public health policy [29, 30]. Indigenous data must have equivalent explanatory power to non-Indigenous data to achieve health equity [31]. Second, it is now widely considered to be unethical to exclude Indigenous peoples from the development of research about their communities. The United Nations Declaration on the Rights of Indigenous Peoples (UNDRIP), which enshrines the right to self-determination for Indigenous peoples [32, Article 3], helped to spur a change in the way Australian human research ethics committees considered applications. Many major research ethics and funding bodies now require applicants to actively partner with Aboriginal and Torres Strait Islander individuals, organisations, or communities involved in the proposed research [33].

To counter the deficit discourse of Indigenous health that has been informed by the 5D data approach, Indigenous Data Sovereignty (IDS) and Indigenous Data Governance (IDG) protocols and principles have been developed for research based on the UNDRIP. For First Nations communities in Canada, this has been solidified through Ownership, Control, Access, and Possession (OCAP®), which became a registered trademark of the First Nations Information Governance Centre (FNIGC) in 2015 [34]. In Aotearoa, the Kaupapa Māori approach has been practised for decades, which upholds Māori self-determination and ways of knowing, doing, and being in research communities. In Australia, possible protocols and principles were discussed at a meeting in 2018 with delegates from the Maiam nayri Wingara Indigenous Data Sovereignty Collective and the Australian Indigenous Governance Institute. They defined Indigenous data as 'information or knowledge, in any format or medium, which is about and may affect Indigenous peoples both collectively and individually' [35]. IDS and IDG were defined as follows:

'*Indigenous Data Sovereignty*' refers to the right of Indigenous people to exercise ownership over Indigenous Data. Ownership of data can be expressed through the creation, collection, access, analysis, interpretation, management, dissemination, and reuse of Indigenous Data.

'*Indigenous Data Governance*' refers to the right of Indigenous peoples to autonomously decide what, how and why Indigenous Data are collected, accessed, and used. It ensures that data on or about Indigenous peoples reflects our priorities, values, cultures, worldviews, and diversity.

In line with these definitions, they determined that Indigenous peoples in Australia have the following rights [35]:

- To exercise control of the data ecosystem including creation, development, stewardship, analysis, dissemination, and infrastructure.
- To have data that are contextual and disaggregated (available and accessible at individual, community, and First Nations levels).
- To have data that are relevant and empower sustainable self-determination and effective self-governance.
- To have data structures that are accountable to Indigenous peoples and First Nations.
- To have data that are protective and respect our individual and collective interests.

Supporting these rights generates 'good data', which is the antithesis of 5D Data. The concept of good data extends existing global conversations around ethical data and data justice and incorporates IDS and IDG principles to describe a resource that Indigenous communities may use to address their self-determined interests and needs [36].

It is only since 2020 that Aboriginal and Torres Strait Islander representative organisations have been meaningfully engaged by Australian governments in the development of the *Closing the Gap* agenda and goals. Part of this engagement involved the recognition that Aboriginal and Torres Strait Islander peoples have the right to define our own needs and priorities in the policy arena. This partnership was formalised through the *National Agreement on Closing the Gap* (the Agreement) that commits to a genuine partnership between all Australian Governments and the Coalition of Aboriginal and Torres Strait Islander Peak Organisations [38]. The goal of this partnership will be to improve the life outcomes of Aboriginal and Torres Strait Islander people, acknowledging that supporting and strengthening Aboriginal and Torres Strait Islander cultures is necessary to achieve this goal [37, p. 4]. Large-scale epidemiological data that reflect Indigenous lifeworlds and reinforce IDS and IDG will be key to driving this national agenda.

28.3 Part 2. Mayi Kuwayu and the Future of the DOHaD

28.3.1 Overview of Mayi Kuwayu

Cohort studies, a type of analytical study, have made a considerable contribution to our understanding of human health and have been at the forefront of identifying the influence of social, environmental, and biological processes on health and well-being outcomes. The goal of analytic studies is to identify and evaluate the causes or risk factors of diseases or health-related events [38]. Cohort studies often involve identifying a 'group' of people to study and plan the research in advance, collecting data over time. Epidemiology, as the study of the patterns and distribution of disease and arguably health, is often the mechanism or method used in telling the story about the presence or absence of disease and what the likely relationships are between social, environmental, and other exposures under study. Due to their long time frames, expense, and difficulties in proving causation, cohort studies are uncommon when compared to other study designs.

Indigenous cohort studies are not common in settler-colonial states such as Australia, Aotearoa, and Turtle Island (referred to collectively as CANZUS) where Indigenous peoples are often incidentally recruited into studies. This limits the ability to conduct robust analytical studies specific to Indigenous groups, and, critically, the variation in Indigenous populations within CANZUS countries presents numerous challenges. The result is a 'tyranny of the majority' and evidence production that is biased towards the majority population while being underpowered for minority groups within those same cohorts. Additionally, these cohorts do not include risk exposures unique to minority groups, nor do they include exposure to unique potentially protective factors.

When the practice of epidemiology is led by Indigenous peoples its potential to contribute towards the achievement of health equity increases exponentially. Mayi Kuwayu is Australia's largest longitudinal cohort study of Aboriginal and Torres Strait Islander well-being. As of January 2024, over 12,000 individuals have participated in the study that surveys Aboriginal and Torres Strait Islander-identified social and cultural determinants of health and well-being [39]. The Mayi Kuwayu baseline questionnaire was developed in consultation with Aboriginal and Torres Strait Islander community members, organisations, and research experts over the course of four years from 2014 to 2018 and is revised every two to three years. It includes a range of metrics that reflect community-identified determinants of health and well-being, such as connection to Country (e.g. 'How much of your life have you lived on your tribe's (mob's) Country or Island?') and cultural knowledge and practice (e.g. 'How much time do you spend learning culture, kinship and respect?'). Mayi Kuwayu data adhere to IDS and IDG principles, and all requests for access to and use of the data must be approved by the Mayi Kuwayu Data Governance Committee, which is a group of Aboriginal and Torres Strait Islander community members and external researchers.

The intent is to conduct world-first analytical work to provide a robust understanding of how settler-colonial risk factors undermine the health and well-being of Aboriginal and Torres Strait Islander peoples, and how culture, a core strength of Aboriginal and Torres Strait Islander communities, can mitigate these adverse effects. This future work aims to understand some of the unexplained 47 per cent health inequity currently experienced by these communities in Australia, while also identifying how the very essence of Indigeneity (cultural maintenance, strengthening, and expression) is fundamental to improving health and well-being and reducing inequities [40, 41]. This work is critical in that settler-colonialism as manifested in historical and contemporary trauma is likely to have a profound impact on adult and intergenerational health.

28.3.2 Mayi Kuwayu Data and Relationship to DOHaD

The Mayi Kuwayu study was developed in response to calls from Aboriginal and Torres Strait Islander peoples to ensure health and well-being concepts were appropriately measured and captured. It is underpinned by a social epidemiological framework, concerned with the influences of social structures, institutions, and relationships on health and well-being [42, 43]. Therefore, the study is designed to enable the examination of health and well-being, taking into account the varied contexts in which Aboriginal and Torres Strait Islander peoples live, including diversity in exposure to settler-colonial factors, and diversity in opportunities to engage in cultural practice and expression. Further, the study is ideally placed to explore and quantify if, and to what extent, culture buffers the impact of settler-colonial risk factors [42].

Since its first release in 2018, analyses of the data collected have shown a positive relationship between connection to Country, culture, and health and well-being outcomes in relation to Aboriginal Ranger work in Central Australia [44]. Being employed as a Ranger, who uses cultural and environmental knowledge to engage in land management activities on Country, was significantly associated with very high life satisfaction and high family well-being [44]. Preliminary analyses of the full Mayi Kuwayu cohort show that key cultural indicators such as spending time on Country, speaking traditional languages, passing on family knowledge and traditions, and feeling in control of one's life are protective against high psychological distress, diagnoses of anxiety, and low life satisfaction [45].

Mayi Kuwayu has also identified a range of settler-colonial exposures experienced by Aboriginal and Torres Strait Islander people and developed measures to capture participants' exposure to these factors from the individual to the systemic level [39, 42]. These exposures have been classified as either Indigenous Historical Trauma (IHT) or Indigenous

Contemporary Trauma (ICT). Indigenous Historical Trauma items included in the study are the following:

1. Tribe/mob forcibly relocated to missions or reserves
2. Being unsure of which tribe/mob you belong to
3. Having a parent who was part of the Stolen Generations
4. Having an aunt or uncle who was part of the Stolen Generations
5. Having a grandparent or great-grandparent who was part of the Stolen Generations

ICT items include the following:

1. Feeling disconnected from culture
2. Being dislocated from Country
3. Worrying about being stolen when they were growing up
4. Growing up in foster care
5. Growing up in a children's home
6. Having children removed in the past 12 months
7. Experiencing interpersonal discrimination
8. Being a part of the Stolen Generations
9. Having a cousin who is part of the Stolen Generations
10. Having child/ren who are part of the Stolen Generations
11. Having grandchild/ren who are part of the Stolen Generations

Over 60 per cent of Mayi Kuwayu participants report at least one exposure to IHT and 85 per cent report at least one exposure to ICT [46]. Exposure to IHT is associated with significant increases in poorer psychological distress and poorer life satisfaction. Stronger links are observed between any experience of ICT and poorer psychological outcomes, poorer general health, and lower life satisfaction. More than half of the Mayi Kuwayu participants have experienced discrimination in some form, and this is significantly associated with a broad range of poor well-being outcomes, ranging from disconnection from culture to high blood pressure and alcohol dependence [47].

These findings strongly support Hoke and McDade's [1] argument that studies on the DOHaD must consider the broader contexts in which we live as well as the intergenerational and transgenerational events that impact our health and well-being. Centring Indigenous lifeworlds in this research has the extraordinary potential to reveal previously 'hidden' factors that either increase the risk for disease or support good health and protect against biosocial harm. With the understanding that such factors and their contribution to health and well-being are heterogeneous across populations, more investment could be made by research institutions and funders in training DOHaD researchers to develop measures for specific salutogenic or risk factors in diverse populations. Intergenerational and transgenerational studies also require secure, long-term funding to provide more robust evidence as it accrues across time.

28.4 Conclusion

The world is currently undergoing a period of disruptive change driven by advances in data science and the convergence of technologies with the potential to enhance and harm Indigenous populations through analytics practice, including cohort studies. This can be addressed by ensuring Indigenous peoples are at the forefront of designing metrics and analytical studies. Data analytics and the translation of resulting insights into practice are key transformations affecting the future of society and its myriad of cultures. These innovations are a double-edged sword for Indigenous peoples, creating potential opportunities to improve well-being through the delivery of healthcare insights through a digital infrastructure that centres Indigenous values and protocols, but also raising concerns about data misuse and collective harm. Further, longitudinal cohort studies are a cornerstone of epidemiology and are central to knowledge production in DOHaD, but few have been developed by and for Indigenous peoples.

This chapter has argued that it is essential that contextual factors, including intergenerational and transgenerational factors, be accounted for by DOHaD research. Centring Indigenous lifeworlds has the extraordinary potential to identify previously 'hidden' factors and lead to the development of lifecourse interventions that could simultaneously reduce risks and increase protective factors. Through the Mayi Kuwayu study, for the first time in Australia and internationally, we have robust, national, longitudinal data on exposure to settler-colonial factors at the individual to systemic level as well as data on cultural practice and expression that may buffer the effects of settler-colonialism. Incorporating IDS and IDG frameworks and applying an Indigenous lens in the DOHaD research space has the potential to produce better science, better data, and better outcomes for our communities. Mayi Kuwayu is just one example of how Indigenous lifeworlds can be centred to produce a good data story about the origins of health and disease.

References

1. Hoke MK, McDade T. Biosocial inheritance: A framework for the study of the intergenerational transmission of health disparities. Annals of Anthropological Practice. 2014;**38**(2):187–213. doi: 10.1111/napa.12052

2. Paradies Y. Colonisation, racism and indigenous health. Journal of Population Research. 2016;**33**(1):83–96. doi: 10.1007/s12546-016-9159-y

3. Mitchell TA, Arseneau C, Thomas D. Colonial trauma: Complex, continuous, collective, cumulative and compounding effects on the health of Indigenous peoples in Canada and beyond. International Journal of Indigenous Health. 2019;**14**(2):74–94. doi: 10.32799/ijih.v14i2.32251

4. Williams AN. A new population curve for prehistoric Australia. Proceedings of the Royal Society B: Biological Sciences. 2013;**280**(1761):20130486. doi: 10.1098/rspb.2013.0486

5. Australian Bureau of Statistics. Table 9. Indigenous census counts and estimates of the population, states and territories, 1836 onwards. Australian Historical Population Statistics. Cat. No. 3105065001. Canberra, ABS. 2006.

6. Australian Institute of Health and Welfare. Aboriginal and Torres Strait Islander Stolen Generations and descendants: Numbers, demographic characteristics and selected outcomes. Cat. No. IHW 195. Canberra, AIHW. 2018.

7. Warin M, Kowal E, Meloni M. Indigenous knowledge in a postgenomic landscape: The politics of epigenetic hope and reparation in Australia. Science, Technology, & Human Values. 2019;**45**(1):87–111. doi: 10.1177/0162243919831077

8. King M, Smith A, Gracey M. Indigenous health part 2: The underlying causes of the health gap. Lancet. 2009;**374**(9683):76–85. doi: 10.1016/S0140-6736(09)60827-8

9. Sherwood J. Colonisation – It's bad for your health: The context of Aboriginal health. Contemporary Nurse. 2013;**46**(1):28–40. doi: 10.5172/conu.2013.46.1.28

10. Czyzewski K. Colonialism as a broader social determinant of health. International Indigenous Policy Journal. 2011;2(1) :Article 5. doi: 10.18584/iipj.2011.2.1.5

11. Priest NC, Paradies YC, Gunthorpe W, et al. Racism as a determinant of social and emotional wellbeing for Aboriginal Australian youth. The Medical Journal of Australia. 2011;194(10):546–50. doi: 10.5694/j.1326-5377.2011.tb03099.x

12. Priest N, Paradies Y, Stewart P, et al. Racism and health among urban Aboriginal young people. BMC Public Health. 2011;11(1):1–9. doi: 10.1186/1471-2458-11-568

13. Paradies Y. Race, racism, stress and Indigenous health. PhD thesis. Melbourne, University of Melbourne. 2006.

14. Paradies Y, Harris R, Anderson I. The Impact of Racism on Indigenous Health in Australia and Aotearoa: Towards a Research Agenda. Darwin, Cooperative Research Centre for Aboriginal Health. 2008.

15. Thurber KA, Colonna E, Jones R, et al. Prevalence of everyday discrimination and relation with wellbeing among Aboriginal and Torres Strait Islander adults in Australia. International Journal of Environmental Research and Public Health. 2021;18(12):6577. doi: 10.3390/ijerph18126577

16. Australian Institute of Health and Welfare. Aboriginal and Torres Strait Islander Stolen Generations and descendants: Numbers, Demographic Characteristics and Selected Outcomes. Canberra, AIHW. 2018.

17. Tuck E, Yang KW. Decolonization is not a metaphor. Decolonization: Indigeneity, Education & Society. 2012;1(1):1–40. doi: 10.25058/20112742.n38.04

18. Dudgeon P, Bray A. Cathedrals of the spirit: Indigenous relational cultural identity and social and emotional well-being. In: Adams BG, van de Vijver FJR, eds. Non-Western Identity: Research and Perspectives. Cham, Springer International Publishing. 2021; 199-214.

19. Salmon M, Doery K, Dance P, et al. Defining the indefinable: Descriptors of Aboriginal and Torres Strait Islander peoples' cultures and their links to health and wellbeing. Canberra, Research School of Population Health, The Australian National University. 2019.

20. Durie M. Understanding health and illness: Research at the interface between science and Indigenous knowledge. International Journal of Epidemiology. 2004;33(5):1138–43. doi: 10.1093/ije/dyh250

21. National Aboriginal Health Strategy Working Party. A National Aboriginal Health Strategy. Canberra, National Aboriginal Health Strategy Working Party. 1989.

22. Garvey G, Anderson K, Gall A, et al. The fabric of Aboriginal and Torres Strait Islander wellbeing: A conceptual model. International Journal of Environmental Research and Public Health. 2021;18(15):7745. doi: 10.3390/ijerph18157745

23. Butler TL, Anderson K, Garvey G, et al. Aboriginal and Torres Strait Islander people's domains of wellbeing: A comprehensive literature review. Social Science and Medicine. 2019;233:138–57. doi: 10.1016/j.socscimed.2019.06.004

24. Bourke S, Wright A, Guthrie J, et al. Evidence review of Indigenous culture for health and wellbeing. The International Journal of Health, Wellness, and Society. 2018;8(4):11–27. doi: 10.18848/2156-8960/CGP/v08i04/11-27

25. Lovett R, Prehn J, Williamson B, et al. Knowledge and power: The tale of Aboriginal and Torres Strait Islander data. Australian Aboriginal Studies. 2020;2:3–7.

26. Walter M. Data politics and Indigenous representation in Australian statistics. In: Kukutai T, Taylor J, eds. Indigenous Data Sovereignty: Toward an Agenda. Canberra, ANU Press. 2016; 79–98.

27. Australian Institute of Health and Welfare. Deaths in Australia. Cat. no. PHE 229. Canberra, AIHW. 2019.

28. Australian Institute of Health and Welfare. Social Determinants and Indigenous Health. Canberra, AIHW. 2020. www.aihw.gov.au/reports/australias-health/social-determinants-and-indigenous-health (Accessed 6 June 2022.)

29. Kukutai T, Walter M. Recognition and indigenizing official statistics: Reflections from Aotearoa New Zealand and Australia. Statistical Journal of the IAOS. 2015;31(2):317–26. doi: 10.3233/sji-150896

30. Walter M. The voice of Indigenous data: Beyond the markers of disadvantage. Griffith Review. 2018:60:256–263. www.griffithreview.com/articles/voice-indigenous-data-beyond-disadvantage/ (Accessed 27 January 2022.)

31. Reid P, Paine S-J, Curtis E, et al. Achieving health equity in Aotearoa: Strengthening responsiveness to Māori in health research. The New Zealand Medical Journal. 2017;130(1465):96–103.

32. United Nations. United Nations Declaration on the Rights of Indigenous Peoples 2007. A/RES/61/295. Geneva, UN. 2007. www.un.org/development/desa/indigenouspeoples/declaration-on-the-rights-of-indigenous-peoples.html (Accessed 6 June 2022.)

33. Australian Institute of Aboriginal and Torres Strait Islander Studies. Code of ethics. Canberra, AIATSIS. 2020. https://aiatsis.gov.au/research/ethical-research/code-ethics (Accessed 27 January 2022.)

34. First Nations Information and Governance Centre. The First Nations Principles of OCAP®. Akwesasne, FNIGC. 2022. https://fnigc.ca/ocap-training/ (Accessed 22 June 2022.)

35. Maiam nayri Wingara. Key principles. 2019. www.maiamnayriwingara.org/key-principles (Accessed 22 June 2022.)

36. Lovett R, Lee V, Kukutai T, et al. Good data practices for Indigenous data sovereignty and governance. In: Daly A, Devitt K, Mann M, eds. Good Data. Amsterdam, Institute of Network Cultures. 2019; 26–36.

37. Department of the Prime Minister and Cabinet. National Agreement on Closing the Gap. Canberra, Commonwealth of Australia. 2020. www.closingthegap.gov.au/national-agreement/national-agreement-closing-the-gap (Accessed 25 January 2022.)

38. Song JW, Chung KC. Observational studies: Cohort and case-control studies. Plastic and Reconstructive Surgery. 2010;126(6):2234–42. doi: 10.1097/PRS.0b013e3181f44abc

39. Lovett R, Brinckley M-M, Phillips B, et al. Marrathalpu mayingku ngiya kiyi. Minyawaa ngiyani yata punmalaka; wangaaypu kirrampili kara [Ngiyampaa title]; In the beginning it was our people's law. What makes us well; to never be sick. Cohort profile of Mayi Kuwayu: The National Study of Aboriginal and Torres Strait Islander Wellbeing [English title]. Australian Aboriginal Studies. 2020;2:8–30.

40. Dudgeon P, Milroy H, Walker R. Working together: Aboriginal and Torres Strait Islander Mental Health and Wellbeing Principles and Practice. Canberra, Australian Government Department of the Prime Minister and Cabinet. 2014. www.telethonkids.org.au/globalassets/media/documents/aboriginal-health/working-together-second-edition/working-together-aboriginal-and-wellbeing-2014.pdf (Accessed 25 January 2022.)

41. Australian Institute of Health and Welfare. National Aboriginal and Torres Strait Islander Health Plan 2021–2031. Canberra, AIHW. 2021. www.health.gov.au/resources/publications/national-aboriginal-and-torres-strait-islander-health-plan-2021-2031 (Accessed 22 June 2022.)

42. Jones R, Thurber KA, Chapman J, et al. Study protocol: Our cultures count, the Mayi Kuwayu Study, a national longitudinal study of Aboriginal and Torres Strait Islander wellbeing. BMJ Open. 2018;8(6):e023861. doi: 10.1136/bmjopen-2018-023861

43. Krieger N. Epidemiology and the People's Health: Theory and Context. Oxford, Oxford University Press. 2011.

44. Wright A, Yap M, Jones R, et al. Examining the associations between Indigenous Rangers, culture and wellbeing in Australia, 2018–2020. International Journal of Environmental Research and Public Health. 2021;**18**(6):3053. doi: 10.3390/ijerph18063053

45. Lovett R. Culture as a salutogenic factor for indigenous health in Australia. Unpublished.

46. Lovett R, Brinckley M-M, Colonna E, et al. Quantifying exposure to settler-colonial risks and links to Aboriginal and Torres Strait Islander people's wellbeing outcomes in Australia: Evidence from the Mayi Kuwayu Study. Unpublished.

47. Thurber KA, Colonna E, Jones R, et al. Prevalence of everyday discrimination and relation with wellbeing among Aboriginal and Torres Strait Islander adults in Australia. International Journal of Environmental Research and Public Health. 2021;**18**(12):6577. doi: 10.3390/ijerph18126577

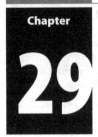

Chapter

29

DOHaD in the Anthropocene
Taking Responsibility for Anthropogenic
Biologies

Jörg Niewöhner

29.1 Entering the Anthropocene

As this volume has shown, the 'developmental origins of health and disease' framework
(DOHaD) inquires into health and disease in adult human life as a function of environmental factors acting upon the human organism prior to conception, ante-/perinatally,
in early life, and increasingly also throughout the lifecourse, respectively [1]. In its
current form, which has been developed over the last three decades, it has not only
helped to address the temporal and environmental dimensions of human disease aetiologies. This predominantly biomedical – in the broad sense of the term – framework has
also proved useful to the social sciences and humanities to think through questions of
human–environment relations, embodiment, and the role of the material environment
in understanding 'development'. The preceding sections in this volume attest to this
generative role. They demonstrate how the framework acts as a boundary object, that is
how it mediates between distinct disciplinary cultures. It also, however, carefully sensitises scholars to significant theoretical commitments, implicit assumptions, and practical
consequences of current research on DOHaD conducted in these different disciplinary
traditions. Many of these commitments are neither universally nor uncritically shared
across academic disciplines. Attending to these differences is an important process in the
development of DOHaD research.

In this final contribution to the volume, I want to look ahead and provide some tentative
ideas about how the DOHaD framework might be translated into the Anthropocene.
I understand the Anthropocene as the geological epoch following the Holocene and
characterised by the acknowledgement that human action has developed into a formidable
force shaping the planet in its entirety. More specifically, human action has been structured
by the world's dominant political economies into patterns of living and working that put
immense pressure on the planet. So-called 'planetary boundaries' have been calculated that
help to make visible how the planet responds [2]. These boundaries, such as climate, land
use, biodiversity, ocean acidification, or the abundance of novel entities, have reached a
point where the earth system might shift into radically different states that are likely to be
far less amenable to human and social life than provided by the Holocene. Systems-speak
aside, what this means is that deeply Western modern assumptions about progress, growth,
and the stability of social expectations cease to exist as the unquestioned bedrock underpin-
ning development and social welfare.

Today, tomorrow is less likely to be like yesterday. Instead, we are entering a phase of
new extremes, new volatilities, and new non-linear dynamics and tipping points [3]. The
Anthropocene challenges social and natural scientists to always also think in planetary

terms. The key distinction between local and global, which has shaped academia and politics for decades, needs rethinking. The 'terrestrial' has instead been suggested as a way of conceptualising all social-ecological action in planetary terms [4]. Whichever way one frames the issue, one key question remains: how can societies worldwide establish and sustain this planet such that humans and other species can continue to inhabit it? Or as anthropologists today phrase it: how can more-than-human liveability on this planet be achieved? [5] The notion of 'liveability' indicates that this is not only a question of biological survival for human societies and beyond. It is a question of what a decent life can be. Hence, it is fundamentally a political and ethical question that is today reposed under conditions of rapid planetary environmental change and resultant social-ecological struggle and suffering.

Addressing the challenges of more-than-human liveability is a vast field. I want to focus here on one aspect only, namely the need to understand biology as anthropogenic [6]. By that I mean that both human bodies and the environments they inhabit are deeply shaped by human actions and the political economies within which these actions are organised. The steep rise of non-communicable, often chronic, as well as infectious diseases and mental health concerns correlates in astonishing ways with Western industrialisation and the global rise of capitalist means of organising human co-existence [7]. Natural resource exploitation, expanding industrial production, and the creation and mass production of novel biological and chemical entities at an unprecedented rate characterise this period of unchecked progress and development [8]. The result is landscapes, bodies, and metabolisms that are shaped by the dominant patterns of economic exchange and their violent histories of colonial extraction. These are landscapes, bodies, and metabolisms that can be meaningfully understood only as human-made: anthropogenic biology.

How then can the DOHaD framework address anthropogenic biology? How can it contribute to more-than-human liveability on this planet and to emerging thinking and research on planetary health? I offer my tentative line of argument in three steps: first, I want to make more graspable the challenges of more-than-human liveability to the DOHaD framework. To do so, I briefly discuss developments in environmental epigenetics, microbiome research, and the emergence of planetary boundaries. All three developments demand cooperation between natural and social sciences. I believe that the DOHaD framework currently does not offer a unifying solution as to how to organise this cooperation. Hence in a second step, I outline three different modes of interdisciplinarity between natural and social science following the excellent work of Andrew Barry and Georgina Born [9]: service, integration, and agonism. In a final third step, I set out what I consider important research questions and perspectives in each of these three modes that address more-than-human liveability while retaining the key concerns of the DOHaD framework. I conclude that the DOHaD framework must take responsibility for the emerging politics of habitability.

29.2 Rethinking Origins and Development in DOHaD in the Anthropocene

In this section, I reflect on recent research on epigenetics, the human microbiome, and planetary boundaries to draw out the implications for the notions of 'origins' and 'development' in the DOHaD framework.

29.2.1 Environmental Epigenetics

Environmental epigenetics denotes the study of changes in gene expression that occur without changes in DNA sequence [10]. Such changes may occur in response to environmental challenges to an organism, including both material (e.g. nutrients and toxicants) and social factors (e.g. discrimination and adversity). They operate through a number of mechanisms. The three most important currently known are methylation, histone- and RNA- modifications. Some of these changes have shown to be mitotically and meiotically heritable, that is they may propagate across generations. Many of the specifics of this field and its implications for DOHaD have been discussed elsewhere in this volume. I therefore keep this point brief.

Epigenetic research challenges the developmental origins of Western biomedical thinking in Mendelian genetics, Weissmann's germ plasm theory, and – more broadly – the autonomous subject of Western modernity. If indeed heritable changes in germline functionality occur without DNA sequence change, individual human organisms are far more open to their past and present environments than so far appreciated. The DOHaD framework has begun to embrace these findings as they suggest mechanisms for phenomena that have so far only been shown through correlations [1]. The 'tracking' of physiological parameters over time from early life into adulthood might in fact be encoded at least to some degree in epigenetic processes. The details and some implications of this have been debated intensely over the last two decades. I want to focus on three lessons that follow from an epigenetics-inflected DOHaD understanding and that have received somewhat less attention.

First, 'environments' are diverse, dynamic, and never innocent. From my own fieldwork in a molecular biology lab working on environmental epigenetics, I have learned that epigenetic response mechanisms are far more subtle than the dominant digital logic of knock-out genetic thinking gives credit for [11]. Oftentimes, the handling of rodents in experimental settings appears to produce stronger epigenetic changes than the actual substance whose epigenetic effects were under investigation. This demonstrates that it might well be very difficult to isolate individual 'factors' or 'causes' from a complex environment. Instead, material and social factors readily interact in manifold ways with an organismic epigenome (if that term even makes sense), which is in itself a highly dynamic system. Mental models of human–environment relations derived from carcinogenicity and acute toxicity assume a unidirectional and non-reversible dose–response relationship between the environment and human organism (see Rossmann and Samaras in this volume). Epigenetics on the other hand suggests a reversible (e.g. *de novo* de/methylation) and perhaps bidirectional relationship where dose–response is likely to occur in a non-linear fashion; if indeed it is the right model at all. Lastly, environments are never politically and ethically innocent. The proof of principle experiments around the Dutch Winter Hunger cohort [12], the studies of licking and grooming behaviour under conditions of reduced nesting material and displacement [13], or the forensic psychiatric reconstruction of life histories in child abuse and suicide completers [14], all demonstrate that 'environmental factors' occur in politically, ethically, and socially charged settings that need to be appreciated in their economic, racial, and gendered complexity (see also the contributions by Meloni et al., Valdez and Lappé, and Cohen in this volume).

Second, while the notion of 'origins' in DOHaD was developed against genetic determinisms, it nevertheless still carries unwanted implicit remnants of Mendelian and Weissmannian biological temporality. Origins suggests a starting point that is defined if not genetically then still by some kind of non-human nature. This might not be a blank slate, but it is a starting point that is often reified through methodological designs that rarely reflect the constructed and contingent nature of study subjects – be they ready-to-study mice or Romanian orphans. The dynamic environmental conditions that have evolved historically and cross-generationally – from nutritional environments to political regimes – are seldom explored in social-ecological detail. Epigenetics makes us attentive to these conditions and thus to the historical and social contingency of any starting point. 'All the way down' [15] in the body, we do not encounter some kind of pure biological matter. Rather the body is as much ecosocially entangled at the molecular level as it is at the organismic level. For 'environments', the scientific construction work and the ecosocial entanglements are even more obvious. Finding a plausible starting point for one's research design is a question of cutting the network and making the cut accountable to the field [16], one's own discipline, and scientific practice at large. Epigenetics thus helps to challenge the idea of 'origins' as a largely unreflected, somehow natural starting point of a developmental process.

Third, for all the attention to environmental factors, the notion of development centres the framework on the human organism. That is perfectly acceptable as it is a framework in human medicine. Epigenetics, however, shows the human organism to be remarkably open to its manifold environments. And *vice versa*: the human organism contributes to making its own livelihoods and niches. Most ecologists today subscribe to the idea that organisms do not find or adapt to existing niches but that organisms and environments interact in co-producing niches [17]. In social scientific terms, 'niching' as a material and social everyday practice might be the more apt analytic for these forms of world-making [18]. Perhaps, then, one ought to refer to 'genealogies' instead of 'origins' and 'development'. This would help to address the multiple histories that run through any origin as well as the necessary contingency of multiple struggles of power/knowledge that mark any genealogy. Genealogies of Health and Disease: GoHaD?

Appreciating the multi-directionality of human–environment relations casts doubt on the developmental thinking in environmental factors, mechanisms, and linear causality for all but the most pervasive and drastic isolated health effects. Most human–environment interaction research, however, remains rooted in a thinking premised on distinct entities. It is either enviro-centric suggesting that the environment as an independent variable causes certain responses in the body or it is organism-centric and thus focused on how human action shapes the environment [19] or how humans may act as niche modifiers [20]. These are all entity-based ways of thinking about human–environment interactions. They start from entities with certain characteristics (organisms and niches) that enter into interaction. One might also, however, start from the action and investigate how action produces entities. This results in a process-based approach [21]. Drawing on the French philosophers Gilles Deleuze and Félix Guattari, British anthropologist Tim Ingold proposes to think of humans in environments not in terms of interacting entities but as 'lines of flight'[22]: 'The line of flight, write Deleuze and Guattari, "is not defined by the points it connects, or by the points that compose it; on the contrary, it passes between points, it comes up the middle"'. What Ingold is essentially challenging his readers to do is think that humans and environments 'should not be understood as interacting entities, . . . but as trajectories of movement, responding to each other in counterpoint, alternately as melody and refrain'. The result is a process- or practice-based biology in which organisms and environments are constantly in becoming and in which development occurs rhizomatically rather than along a linear path. The notion of development in DOHaD does not usually take this into account. It rests on the understanding of an entity that is exposed to an environment as a set of factors. I am not suggesting that lines of flight readily translate into biomedical research designs. Yet they present an important conceptual challenge that sensitises researchers to the fact that evolutionary, structural, and systemic thinking never quite captures the situational specificities of human practice and its effects. These require process-based approaches.

29.2.2 Microbiome Research

The human microbiome denotes the aggregate of all microorganisms living on or in human tissue or fluids. Research efforts to better understand the components and dynamics of the human microbiome have rapidly increased over the last decade. The human microbiome comprises around 10–100 trillion symbiotic microbial cells per human individual [23]. They match if not outnumber human somatic cells, and their genetic material by far exceeds that of the 'human proper'. Cells belong to around 500–1000 different species at any given moment within a human [24]. The genetic diversity and hence flexibility of this crowd by far exceed that of human genetic material. Over the last ten years, the field of microbiome research has begun to transition from the description of components to mechanisms and to the tentative development of clinical interventions. It has also invited a rich scene of lay 'bio hackers' to self-experiment alongside the emerging science with everything from probiotic foodstuffs to faecal transfer. A scientific understanding of how the microbiome impacts human somatic and mental health and disease onset and progression directly, as well as through complex interactions with the immune, endocrine, and nervous system, is only just emerging. Yet already today it is becoming clear that microbiome research will be another insult to human narcissism and anthropocentrism. After Copernicus, Darwin, and Freud, microbiome research demonstrates that 'man' is not even somatically speaking the master in his own house. While the skin as 'philosophy's last line of defense' [25] remains intact if porous, inside that skin shell emerges a multiplicity of inhabitants and agencies in complex and finely balanced interaction and oftentimes symbiosis.

In the preceding section, I used epigenetics to question whether we should move from origins to genealogies and from development to lines of flight. Microbiome research extends this questioning. Anthropologist Myra Hird discusses how human subjectivity and social form need to be understood as also shaped by bacteria [26]. She demonstrates how deeply biological and economic notions of the self are enshrined in Western modern thought. Westerners think of themselves as individual cognitive agents that act autonomously, often in competition with each other to increase fitness. Society is often understood as synchronised individuals. The vast majority of biological and medical research designs presume the existence of human individuals who act autonomously and are structurally closed to their environments. The subsequent distinction between self and other (along the skin) is foundational to Western self-understanding. Taking bacteria and their actions seriously challenges this understanding. Hird focuses on the understandings of symbiogenesis and a very corporeal interdependence of human and microbial life. The human 'I' becomes a multitude or collective. Similar to Ingold, she thus arrives at a world in becoming that is made up of encounters: encounters, for example, between humans and microorganisms that then develop ways of co-existing. Continuous encountering is what makes us what we are. Hence 'we' are not only epigenetically open to 'outside' environments, but 'we' are also open to 'inside' environments in the form of microorganismic collectives and their respective habitats.

It is this continuity of encounters that DOHaD also needs to address. Whether framed as contagion, as multi-species thinking, or as making kin, health and disease can rarely be sensibly understood as states of a single organism isolated in interaction from its environment. Dose–response simply does not capture the fact that exposure occurs in dynamic patterns of encounters. Even in the simplest scenario of an isolated single toxicant having an impact on a human organism, it is not only human cells and organs reacting. It is a symbiogenetically evolved social organism that responds. And while this social organism exhibits a distinct meta-stability that most people readily accept as human subjectivity, responses to substances are multiple and differentiated. Substances that occur at levels in the environment that are commonly considered well below toxicity thresholds not only interact to complicate exposure. They interact in differential ways with the human microbiome such that effects may occur that might well then surface as a human health issue. Hence environments are never really environments for only one organism as Uexküll suggested. The 'environment multiple' is a direct result of understanding the human body as a multiplicity of encounters.

29.2.3 Planetary Boundaries and Planetarity

So far, I have addressed molecular, cellular, and organismic dynamics. Let me now briefly turn to planetary dynamics and how they might challenge DOHaD. Earth system science is understanding with increasing certainty that the planet's capacity to sustain life as we know it has boundaries that we are already transgressing through human action [2]. Environmental factors are thus ceasing to be local phenomena and instead need to be contextualised within planetary environmental change and its manifold repercussions for social-ecological systems across the globe. Philosopher Bruno Latour rightly challenges us to develop across all forms of scholarly activity a consciousness for the fragile and restricted conditions of habitability of the earth and life on it [4].

This planetary dimension challenges the DOHaD framework to understand 'the environment' and its health-relevant factors as part of earthly subsystems and its associated complexities and non-linear dynamics [20]. Major efforts have been underway for some years now to better understand and quantify both the global burden of disease [27] and the bio-geo-physical and increasingly social dynamics of earth's subsystems as well as their stable state boundaries [2]. Suggestions are being made to integrate earth system science and global health through international consortia and (big) data approaches [28]. Such approaches are commonly shaped by systems thinking and various forms of computational modelling that foster data-driven integration. The rise of earth system modelling from the late 1980s onwards has undoubtedly been an amazing process of knowledge production culminating in the 6th Assessment Report of the IPCC on the 'physical science basis' of global climate change. Never has a comparable global evidence machine been built of such scale and with such rigour. This evidence machine runs on a positivist epistemology that addresses 'the planet' through data aggregation and integration as part of system dynamics modelling. Its dominant if not its only mode of speaking about large phenomena (aka 'the planet') is through scaling up by means of data aggregation and integration. Everything else is anecdotal or an opinion, that is not considered evidence. This approach aligns well with the data-driven calculations of global burdens of disease and exposomes.

Yet feminist literary theorist Gayatri Spivak [29] and others use the notion of 'planetarity' [30] to point to the data-driven construction of the planet asking where this leaves significant differences in ways of thinking and being on this planet – differences to which the social sciences and humanities attend. An altogether different perspective on this new planetary dimension is thus possible and important. The social sciences and humanities have long developed conceptual and empirical alternatives to address large-scale phenomena such as globalisation. Thinking in scapes and flows [31], global assemblages [32], global entanglement [33], and post- and decolonial critique [34] approaches 'the global' very differently. These approaches start from significant social differences and ask how they spread, reach, infect, travel, transform, and resonate. These approaches either focus on the forces that make phenomena graspable as 'global' or they move around inside the phenomena understood as global, showing their heterogeneity and multiplicity. Globality is about differences and what these differences (can) mean for respective others. Planetarity, in contrast, is often about trying to produce the one true representation of a whole. Of course, globality has been concerned with primarily social dynamics, while planetarity is rooted in biogeophysical phenomena. In the Anthropocene, however, this neat division of labour is being challenged as social inquiry becomes interested in material dynamics and ontological questions, while modellers of physical systems are incorporating not only economic exchanges into their models but increasingly also social dynamics.

Latour's 'Terrestrial' [4] might be a useful point of contact between these very different ways of addressing phenomena that span the world in various ways. It is these reconfigurations of socio-material relations and the ensuing debate of how to address them that form the context within which the DOHaD framework can make an important contribution. How do we conceptualise 'environmental factors' when they cease to be local phenomena; when we try to understand them within a terrestrial context? One response would be to scale 'environmental factors' up, for example, to produce global estimates of 'novel entities', that is 'new substances, new forms of existing substances and modified forms of life' [8], and assess their impact on earth's subsystems. Microplastics, lead, or persistent organic pollutants serve as examples. This might be related to the global burdens of disease in a data-driven integrative approach. In a very different approach, one might contextualise 'environmental factors' in highly political patterns of exposure related to colonial and racialised histories of exploitation and production, imperial debris, and the ruins of capitalism [35].

The Anthropocene and its demand to think in planetary terms, then, challenge biomedically and epidemiologically established notions of environment, environmental factors, exposure, dose–response, temporality, and scale. These notions are also embedded within the DOHaD framework. However, the framework does not inherently offer a singular and straight path to address these challenges. It is not a foregone conclusion that these challenges will be solved with data collected and analysed in the empirico-analytical frameworks of twentieth-century biomedicine. Rather, the DOHaD framework might afford a reflexive moment, a moment of producing 'theory out of science' [36], which might enable a diverse set of approaches to address anthropogenic challenges and to address more-than-human liveability on a fragile planet. The DOHaD framework might offer a space within which data-driven approaches might complement other approaches that open up environments to a politics of exposure and habitability and that understand the human body as historically shaped, socialised, and habituated in patterns of practice [37]. Realising this potential and situating DOHaD in this sense, however, requires a diversity of approaches.

29.3 Modes of Interdisciplinarity: Ecosocial Co-laboration

29.3.1 Three Modes of Interdisciplinarity

Moving DOHaD into the Anthropocene cannot be achieved with a single logic or methodological approach. It would be a futile task to try to develop an overarching framework that can fully integrate the existing conceptual and methodological diversity, the desire to reduce and explain with the need to contextualise and interpret, and the strengths of rigorous data-based analysis with the strengths of critical inquiry. The present volume features this diversity, and it is clear that this does not cohere in an overarching heuristic or integrative framework – nor should it. Instead, it might be useful to distinguish between different forms of interdisciplinary engagement and forms of collaboration to give orientation and take away some of the pressure towards integration.

Andrew Barry and Georgina Born [9], drawing on their investigation of using ethnography within various other epistemic cultures, usefully outline three modes of interdisciplinarity: subordination–service, integration–synthesis, and agonistic–antagonistic. In the subordination–service mode, the research question and design come from one lead discipline, while the other discipline delivers additional data to extend or deepen the analysis. This is a fundamentally asymmetrical approach shaped by one discipline. In the integration–synthesis mode, two different disciplines readily find ways of addressing problems that are of interest to both. Biochemistry is the typical example within the natural sciences. It is a little less obvious across the natural/social science divide. This approach is symmetrical with both disciplines staying within their comfort zone but addressing a new topic in a shared way [3]. The agonistic–antagonistic mode is perhaps the most demanding. It arises when two disciplines differ in their understanding of the research object. Often, this disagreement is ontological in nature. For example, human differences might be considered a material and bodily phenomenon by biologists while social scientists would insist on it being primarily a social phenomenon constructed through the social interaction of subjects positioned in social space. In an agonistic–antagonistic mode, these differences between disciplinary perspectives are not levelled. Instead, they need to be worked with to turn them into something generative from which both disciplines can learn without necessarily agreeing to the respective other perspective. This approach is symmetrical but not as comfortable as in the integration mode. It is about letting oneself be irritated by other ways of thinking and designing research and by sustaining significant differences to learn and develop one's own perspective.

In opening up DOHaD further to social science thinking, this form of agonistic interdisciplinarity will play a key role. It is important to note that co-laboration [38] is possible: co-laboration is temporary joint knowledge production between two disciplines without necessarily having a shared goal. Two scholars from different disciplines might work together without necessarily getting a shared result. Rather they might take different results and insights away from the co-laboration and integrate those into their respective disciplines. To make this rather abstract typology of possible interdisciplinary research more tangible, I want to briefly sketch examples of research questions and designs for each of these three modes of interdisciplinarity that might help the current DOHaD framework embrace the challenges of the Anthropocene.

29.3.2 Subordination–Service

Environmental epigenetics offers an obvious entry point for subordination–service interdisciplinarity. Currently, research within the DOHaD framework tends to operationalise environmental factors as independent variables, for example social disadvantage, zip code, and nutritional status (cf. Liz Roberts in this volume). For many social situations and structural inequalities [39], such operationalisations are not only too crude. They also miss the entire dimension of subjective and collective experience that social science would consider fundamental to the emergence of 'the social' and thus to pathways from 'objective' disadvantage to actually 'living inferiority' [39] and associated individual bodily health and disease. Hence social science could contribute its understanding of social dynamics to research on social drivers within the DOHaD framework. At a time where many countries – and in particular the major metropoles – are undergoing fundamental transformations trying to meet climate targets, this kind of social science service work could also contribute to making sure that ambitious climate targets are not reached at the expense of increasing inequality and thus worsening individual and public health outcomes.

Subordination–service approaches might also work the other way around. The long-term social inquiry into living with chronic respiratory diseases, for example, might benefit from global to local climate projections, air quality modelling, and associated health data. The Anthropocene foregrounds the dynamics of nature–culture relations, making such social inquiries into 'natural' phenomena such as disease aetiologies even more relevant [40]. Planetary health is currently conceptualised largely in biomedical and public health terms with the social sciences adding knowledge about social dynamics. This could be – perhaps ought to be – turned around placing well-being and environmental justice at the centre and putting the medical disciplines in the service role.

29.3.3 Integration–Synthesis

Recent work at the interface of sociology and biogeochemistry presents an outstanding example of biosocial interdisciplinarity in the integration–synthesis mode [6]. Hannah Landecker, a sociologist and historian of science, and Cajetan Neubauer, a biochemist, in rather serendipitous fashion, began to work on the planetary availability and bodily effects of methionine together. Methionine is an essential amino acid, that is it cannot be synthesised by the human body and needs to be taken up through food. Working together on the methionine metabolism both globally and within the body, the two perspectives together were able to 'establish the scale and historical trajectory of the methionine industry and provide a preliminary model for tracing this amino acid through the food supply into the human body' [6]. The study shows how planetary-scale anthropogenic activity changes 'environments' and consequently also human metabolisms with so far largely unknown consequences. Human biology and ecology, that is both environment and body, are understood as anthropogenic. The DOHaD framework thus requires biosocial, or rather ecosocial, collaboration as it is the social science perspective that can reveal how environmental factors come to be what they are through anthropogenic activity, specifically through analyses of dominant political economies and ecologies.

Hannah Landecker reflects on the back of the methionine study: 'I have always felt that my contribution has been to enable the asking of experimental questions, the parameterisation of models, and the forming of hypotheses that would not otherwise have been possible ... What Harry Collins termed "interactional expertise" has also been important in helping teams of different kinds of knowledge practitioners recognise ways in which they don't understand one another, or facilitating the synthesis of different modes of proof or reasoning. . . .' [41] Landecker reports her interdisciplinary research as an example of integration–synthesis cooperation, that is both disciplines, biochemistry and history, contribute from within their comfort zone to arrive at a new question and analysis. This is cleverly done, and it is this approach that enables Landecker to conduct a historical and social study of chemicals of metabolic significance – as a social scientist, albeit one with deep knowledge of natural science and the dynamics of the particular field in question.

29.3.4 Agonism–Antagonism

Oftentimes, however, social science perspectives do not readily complement or integrate with existing natural science or medical knowledge. Take approaches to social dynamics as an example. Biomedical or public health operationalisations of social dynamics often do not resonate with state-of-the-art social scientific knowledge and critique. The reason for such dissonance often lies in profound differences in the understanding of the research object. Much medical expertise works with a concept of 'the social' that is based on individuals interacting within a value system or culture. The notion of the individual tends to be under-socialised, that is based on ideas of individual decision-making that might be found in behavioural economics. Whereas the notion of the 'value system' tends to be over-socialised, that is assuming a firm grip of an abstract but homogeneous set of values on the framing of individual behaviour. Social dynamics from most social science perspectives sit in between these two perspectives and often work with notions of agency, subjectivity, and practice that combine structural ('value system') and individual ('decision-making') elements in highly dynamic and reflexive ways.

The agonistic–antagonistic approach starts from such dissonances and tries to make them generative. Agonism here refers to the work of political scientist Chantal Mouffe, who argued for agonism as a democratic form that does not solely rely on consensus but rather is able to work with differences as a potentially positive democratic force. Agonism within interdisciplinary research then means working with and through differences rather than searching for an integrative framework. This takes some work between the right partners. Working with differences requires explicating methodological, epistemological, and ontological assumptions. Differences need to come out to enable research that searches for common ground while critically reflecting on one's own disciplinary perspective.

In this regard, the DOHaD framework needs to address the question of how much it can allow environments and bodies to be 'situated' in a social science sense [42]. As it stands, DOHaD often rests on a universal body that responds to environmental factors.

While this rests on a perfectly plausible set of assumptions, it does appear to underestimate what anthropogenic biology means. If all-pervasive anthropogenic activity has begun to change environments and bodies in significant ways, the 'universal' body is perhaps not the most prudent assumption anymore. Of course, at some general level, most bodies share some basic structures and processes. Yet these structures and processes are shaped by widely different trajectories through individual life histories and start to differentiate in significant ways. Most study designs assume a universal body and investigate the response to exposure. Yet 'exposure' to chemicals, social disadvantage, infrastructural violence, and to colonial legacies is systematically patterned and has been so for many centuries. The 'inward laboratory' of the body adjusts and contributes to these patterns and to living in, with, and through these patterns in significant ways. Rather than starting from the universal body at a national or even global scale, is it not high time that we should also try to scale approaches a little differently? Sure, trying to assess the global burden of disease, the global presence of chemicals and novel entities, and planetary boundaries remains important. Systems thinking and data-based integration remain important, and attempts at measuring the exposome and conducting exposome-wide association studies will certainly be productive in many ways even if they are bound to never reach their objective [43]. Yet other exposure patterns also matter. We might start with landscapes and how they have been shaped by political histories and economies, social dynamics and forms of dwelling, as well as biogeophysical contexts of climate, topography, and ecology. Urban and rural landscapes [5] can be investigated in great ecosocial detail to better understand how they afford particular exposure patterns and how these contribute to shaping deeply situated bodies [44]. Inside such landscapes, situated bodies are thoroughly historicised, socialised, and politicised and constantly in becoming. They are not simply local as they relate to many transnational exchanges and flows of people, goods, and information as well as planetary environmental change. Such ecosocial analyses of the situated genealogies of health and disease require the agonistic and antagonistic struggle between critical social science perspectives and rather more solution-oriented medical perspectives.

29.4 The Future of DOHaD: Taking Responsibility for Anthropogenic Biologies

Translating the DOHaD framework into the Anthropocene requires an opening up of its underlying biomedical and epidemiological thought style. It needs to be opened up, because the human body and the complex social-ecological environments within which it dwells can only be understood as anthropogenic. They have ceased to be 'natural' in any meaningful sense. In an epoch where human action and its political economy are thoroughly transforming life at a planetary scale, the material agencies of more-than-human liveability cease to be universal and innocent – if they ever were. Situating bodies and environments is one response. Situating means understanding how 'environmental factors' are embedded within landscapes that are shaped thoroughly by land use practices and metabolisms reflecting dominant natural, social, and moral orders. And it means appreciating the habituated nature of the human body-in-practice that fends for its livelihood in such landscapes.

The DOHaD framework offers sufficient openness to pursue health and disease in emerging and dynamic patterns of everyday practice. The key to such an approach is the constant careful calibration of a balance between on the one hand appreciating the singularity of life as such [45] and its multi-species encounters and on the other recognising structural continuities in life itself [46] shaped by hegemonic patterns of bio- and geopolitics regulating bodies and landscapes. Methodologically, this has to be a programme that starts from an in-depth understanding of the regularities and patterns that shape health and disease over time in situated cases. Long-term social-ecological field sites that can understand exposure as practice rather than correlation seem promising. Ethnographic, micro-sociological, and micro-historical approaches need to be brought into conversation with, on the one hand, biomedical and epidemiological methods and, on the other, with methods that can assess drivers of landscape change, for example earth observation, land use science, and climate impact modelling. Such multi-method approaches need not be fully integrated into a single framework. They can explore the tension between the singularities and regularities of more-than-human liveability by exploring both statistical and analytical generalisation; by situating numerical models of social-ecological dynamics; and by deconstructing knowledge claims but also by reconstructing alternatives.

Starting from situated cases and possibly community-based research into more-than-human liveability also offers the chance to embrace the necessarily political nature of this work. Long-term multi-method field sites offer the opportunity to align knowledge production with the co-production of interventions rooted in a thoroughly situated understanding of the developmental origins of multi-species health and disease. In such an approach, the DOHaD framework begins to take responsibility for how bodies and environments are known and problematised. It begins to take responsibility for the worlds people live in and for possible futures.

References

1. Rosenfeld CS, editor. The epigenome and developmental origins of health and disease: Amsterdam: Academic Press; 2016.

2. Steffen W, Richardson K, Rockström J, Cornell SE, Fetzer I, Bennett EM, et al. Planetary boundaries: Guiding human development on a changing planet. Science. 2015; 347(6223).

3. Otto IM, Donges JF, Cremades R, Bhowmik A, Hewitt RJ, Lucht W, et al. Social tipping dynamics for stabilizing Earth's climate by 2050. Proceedings of the National Academy of Sciences. 2020;117(5):2354–65.

4. Latour B. Down to Earth: Politics in the new climatic regime: Cambridge: John Wiley & Sons; 2018.

5. Tsing AL, Mathews AS, Bubandt N. Patchy anthropocene: Landscape structure, multispecies history, and the retooling of anthropology: An introduction to Supplement 20. Current Anthropology. 2019;60(S20):S186–S97.

6. Neubauer C, Landecker H. A planetary health perspective on synthetic methionine. The Lancet Planetary Health. 2021;5(8):e560–e9.

7. Khan A, Plana-Ripoll O, Antonsen S, Brandt J, Geels C, Landecker H, et al. Environmental pollution is associated with increased risk of psychiatric disorders in the US and Denmark. Plos Biology. 2019;17(8):e3000353.

8. Persson L, Carney Almroth BM, Collins CD, Cornell S, de Wit CA, Diamond ML, et al. Outside the safe operating space of the planetary boundary for novel entities. Environ Science Technology. 2022;56 (3):1510–21.

9. Barry A, Born G. Interdisciplinarity: Reconfigurations of the social and natural sciences: London: Routledge; 2013.

10. Bollati V, Baccarelli A. Environmental epigenetics. Heredity. 2010;105 (1):105–12.

11. Niewöhner J. Epigenetics: Embedded bodies and the molecularisation of biography and milieu. Biosocieties. 2011;6(3):279–98.

12. de Rooij SR, Painter RC, Phillips DIW, Osmond C, Michels RPJ, Bossuyt PMM, et al. Hypothalamic-pituitary-adrenal axis activity in adults who were prenatally exposed to the Dutch famine. European Journal of Endocrinology. 2006;155 (1):153–60.

13. Weaver I, Meaney M, Szyf M. Maternal care effects on the hippocampal transcriptome and anxiety-mediated behaviors in the offspring that are reversible in adulthood. Proceedings of the National Academy Science USA. 2006;103:3480.

14. McGowan PO, Sasaki A, Huang TCT, Unterberger A, Suderman M, Ernst C, et al. Promoter-wide hypermethylation of the ribosomal RNA gene promoter in the suicide brain. PLoS ONE. 2008;3(5): e2085.

15. Haraway DJ. Staying with the trouble: Making kin in the Chthulucene: Durham: Duke University Press; 2016.

16. Strathern M. Cutting the network. Journal of the Royal Anthropological Institute. 1996;2:517–35.

17. Odling-Smee FJ, Laland KN, Feldman MW. Niche construction: The neglected process in evolution. Princeton: Princeton University Press; 2003. xii, 472 p.

18. Bister MD, Klausner M, Niewöhner J. The cosmopolitics of 'niching': Rendering the city habitable along infrastructures of mental health care. Urban Cosmopolitics: Agencements, Assemblies, Atmospheres 2016. pp. 187–205.

19. Williams M, Zalasiewicz J, Waters CN, Edgeworth M, Bennett C, Barnosky AD, et al. The Anthropocene: A conspicuous stratigraphical signal of anthropogenic changes in production and consumption across the biosphere. Earth's Future. 2016;4(3):34–53.

20. Gluckman PD, Low FM, Hanson MA. Anthropocene-related disease: The inevitable outcome of progressive niche modification? Evolution, Medicine, and Public Health. 2020;2020(1):304–10.

21. Bapteste E, Dupré J. Towards a processual microbial ontology. Biology Philosophy. 2013;28(2):379–404.

22. Ingold T. The textility of making. Cambridge Journal of Economics. 2010;34(1):91–102.

23. Ursell LK, Metcalf JL, Parfrey LW, Knight R. Defining the human microbiome. Nutrition Reviews. 2012;70(suppl_1): S38–S44.

24. Gilbert JA, Blaser MJ, Caporaso JG, Jansson JK, Lynch SV, Knight R. Current understanding of the human microbiome. Nature Medicine. 2018;24(4):392–400.

25. Bentley AF. The human skin: Philosophy's last line of defense. Philosophy of Science. 1941;8:1–19.

26. Hird M. The origins of sociable life: Evolution after science studies: New York: Palgrave Macmillan; , 2009.

27. Murray CJ, Abbafati C, Abbas KM, Abbasi M, Abbasi-Kangevari M, Abd-Allah F, et al. Five insights from the global burden of disease study 2019. The Lancet. 2020;396(10258):1135–59.

28. Whitmee S, Haines A, Beyrer C, Boltz F, Capon AG, de Souza Dias BF, et al. Safeguarding human health in the Anthropocene epoch: Report of The Rockefeller Foundation–Lancet Commission on planetary health. The lancet. 2015;386(10007):1973–2028.

29. Spivak G. Imperatives to re-imagine the planet. Vienna: Passagen Forum; 2013.

30. Spivak GC. Planetarity. Paragraph. 2015;38(2):290–92.

31. Appadurai A. Modernity at large. Cultural dimensions of globalization. Minneapolis: University of Minnesota Press; 1991.

32. Ong A, Collier SJ. Global assemblages: Technology, politics, and ethics as anthropological problems. Malden, MA: Blackwell Publishing; 2005. xiii, 494 p.

33. Conrad S, Randeria S. Geteilte Geschichten–Europa in einer postkolonialen Welt. In: Conrad S, Randeria S, Römhild, R. Jenseits des Eurozentrismus. Postkoloniale Perspektiven in den Geschichts-und Kulturwissenschaften. Frankfurt am Main: Campus; 2002:9–49.

34. Escobar A, Mignolo W. Globalization and the decolonial option. London & New York: Routledge. 2010.

35. Nading AM. Living in a toxic world. Annual Review of Anthropology. 2020; 49:209–24.

36. Roosth S, Schrader A, Jentsch LJ. Feminist theory out of science differences. Duke University Press. Durham.2012;23(3).

37. Roepstorff A, Niewöhner J, Beck S. Enculturing brains through patterned practices. Neural Networks. 2010;23 (8–9):1051–59.

38. Niewöhner J. Co-laborative anthropology: Crafting reflexivities experimentally. In: Jouhki J, Steel T, editors. Etnologinen tulkinta ja analyysi Kohti avoimempaa tutkimusprosessia. Helsinki: Ethnos; 2016. pp. 81–124.

39. Charlesworth SJ, Gilfillan P, Wilkonson R. Living inferiority. British Medical Bulletin. 2004;69:49–60.

40. Timmermans S, Haas S. Towards a sociology of disease. Sociology of Health & Illness. 2008;30(5):659–76.

41. Landecker H. From Archives to Isotopes: Studying the Transit of Petroleum-Derived Nutrients through Social and Biological Worlds. 4S; Toronto: unpublished; 2021.

42. Niewöhner J, Lock M. Situating local biologies: Anthropological perspectives on environment/human entanglements. BioSocieties. 2018;13(4):681–97.

43. Vermeulen R, Schymanski EL, Barabási A-L, Miller GW. The exposome and health: Where chemistry meets biology. Science. 2020;367(6476):392–96.

44. Pentecost M, Cousins T. Strata of the political: Epigenetic and microbial imaginaries in post-apartheid Cape Town. Antipode. 2017;49(5):1368–84.

45. Fassin D. Another politics of life is possible. Theory, Culture & Society. 2009;26(5):44–60.

46. Rose N. The politics of life itself. Theory, Culture & Society. 2001;18(6):1–30.

Index

Printed in the United States
by Baker & Taylor Publisher Services